The Total
Food
Allergy
Health and Diet Guide

The Total Food Allergy

Health and Diet Guide

Includes 150 recipes
for managing food allergies and intolerances
by eliminating common allergens and gluten

Alexandra Anca, MHSc, RD
with Dr. Gordon L. Sussman, MD, FRCPC, FACP, FAAAAI

Robert
ROSE

For complete cataloguing information, see page 342.

Disclaimer
This book is a general guide only and should never be a substitute for the skill, knowledge, and
experience of a qualified medical professional dealing with the facts, circumstances, and symptoms
of a particular case.

The nutritional, medical, and health information presented in this book is based on the research,
training, and professional experience of the author, and is true and complete to the best of her
knowledge. However, this book is intended only as an informative guide for those wishing to
know more about health, nutrition, and medicine; it is not intended to replace or countermand the
advice given by the reader's personal physician. Because each person and situation is unique, the
author and the publisher urge the reader to check with a qualified health-care professional before
using any procedure where there is a question as to its appropriateness. A physician should be
consulted before beginning any exercise program. The author and the publisher are not responsible
for any adverse effects or consequences resulting from the use of the information in this book. It
is the responsibility of the reader to consult a physician or other qualified health-care professional
regarding his or her personal care.

This book contains references to products that may not be available everywhere. The intent
of the information provided is to be helpful; however, there is no guarantee of results associated
with the information provided. Use of brand names is for educational purposes only and does
not imply endorsement.

The recipes in this book have been carefully tested by our kitchen and our tasters. To the best of
our knowledge, they are safe and nutritious for ordinary use and users. For those people with food
or other allergies, or who have special food requirements or health issues, please read the suggested
contents of each recipe carefully and determine whether or not they may create a problem for you.
All recipes are used at the risk of the consumer. We cannot be responsible for any hazards, loss,
or damage that may occur as a result of any recipe use. For those with special needs, allergies,
requirements, or health problems, in the event of any doubt, please contact your medical adviser
prior to the use of any recipe.

Design and production: Kevin Cockburn/PageWave Graphics Inc.
Editors: Bob Hilderley, Senior Editor, Health; and Sue Sumeraj, Recipes
Copy editor: Sheila Wawanash
Proofreader: Kelly Jones
Indexer: Gillian Watts
Illustrations: Kveta/threeinabox.com

We acknowledge the financial support of the Government of Canada through the Book Publishing
Industry Development Program (BPIDP) for our publishing activities.

Published by Robert Rose Inc.
120 Eglinton Avenue East, Suite 800, Toronto, Ontario, Canada M4P 1E2
Tel: (416) 322-6552 Fax: (416) 322-6936
www.robertrose.ca

Printed and bound in Canada.

1 2 3 4 5 6 7 8 9 FP 20 19 18 17 16 15 14 13 12

Contents

Top 10 Food Allergies and Intolerances

- **①** Peanut allergy
- **②** Tree nut allergy
- **③** Fish, shellfish, and crustacean allergy
- **④** Milk allergy and lactose intolerance
- **⑤** Egg allergy
- **⑥** Soy allergy
- **⑦** Wheat allergy
- **⑧** Sesame seed allergy
- **⑨** Sulfite sensitivity
- **⑩** Mustard allergy

Other Allergies and Intolerances

Corn allergy

Fruits and vegetables allergies

MSG sensitivity

Introduction

We probably all know someone who has a food allergy or intolerance, and the closer to home, the more troubling this may be. Food allergies can range from simple rashes and runny noses to life-threatening anaphylactic episodes and even death. And allergies can affect children and seniors, the physically fit and the overweight. They do not discriminate.

After several decades of scientific trials, we now know that any one of more than 270 foods can trigger an allergic reaction. The majority of allergies, however, are triggered by 10 common allergens:

- Peanuts
- Tree nuts
- Seafood (fish, shellfish, and crustaceans)
- Milk
- Eggs
- Soy
- Wheat
- Sesame seeds
- Sulfites
- Mustard

Sulfites produce allergic-like reactions but are not, in and of themselves, allergens. While they may be listed as allergens under different labeling laws, they do not trigger true IgE-mediated allergic reactions.

Treating Food Intolerances and Allergies

Common sense suggests that the best way to treat these food allergies and intolerances is to avoid the foods that trigger them, but that is not as easy as it sounds. For one thing, we have ingrained eating habits that are difficult to change. Even if I have an allergy to milk, how can I give up my ice cream? And many allergens are hidden in our food supply as a component in processed foods. How do we find these hidden foods? Read food labels and call the manufacturer or supplier for a list of ingredients.

Seems simple enough, but when we look for a diet program that achieves the dual goals of being allergen-free and nutritionally balanced, we encounter a number of options, none wholly satisfactory and some potentially dangerous. Especially problematic are the popular elimination and exclusion diets.

Q What is the difference between a food allergy and a food intolerance?

A Food allergies differ from food hypersensitivities or intolerances in many ways, yet they are often confused with one another, leading to misunderstandings about the way each is diagnosed and treated. Here are several terms for describing reactions to food:

- A food hypersensitivity is an adverse reaction to a food that other people can safely eat and includes food intolerances and food allergies.
- A food intolerance is a food sensitivity that does not involve the individual's immune system. Unlike food allergies or chemical sensitivities, where a small amount of food can cause a reaction, it generally takes a more normal-sized portion to produce symptoms of food intolerance. While the symptoms of food intolerance vary and can be mistaken for those of a food allergy, food intolerances are more likely to originate in the gastrointestinal system and are usually caused by an inability to digest or absorb certain foods, or components of those foods. Lactose intolerance is a well-known example of a food intolerance.
- A food allergy is an unexpectedly strong response of the body's immune system to food proteins that are usually harmless to most people. Food allergies are the focus of this book.
- A chemical sensitivity occurs when a person has an adverse reaction to chemicals that occur naturally in or are added to foods. Examples of chemical sensitivities include reactions to caffeine in coffee, to tyramine in aged cheese, and to the flavor enhancer monosodium glutamate.

Elimination Diets for Diagnosis of Food Intolerances

How do we know what food is causing the intolerance? Although there is no standard test to confirm or rule out a food intolerance, the elimination diet has become a popular option. To diagnose whether you have an intolerance to soy, for example, you can eliminate soy foods from your diet for several weeks and then reintroduce them. If your symptoms return, it may be because of the soy products you are now eating (this is sometimes referred to as an oral challenge). If you now know that soy causes these symptoms, you should avoid eating soy products for a period of time. You may then try reintroducing them at a later time to monitor whether you continue to develop symptoms of intolerance. However, if you are diagnosed with IgE-mediated allergy to soy, you will need to completely avoid it.

Step-by-Step Elimination Diet Instructions

Johns Hopkins University provides this set of instructions for conducting a simple diagnostic elimination and challenge for various foods:

1. Completely eliminate the food from your diet for 2 weeks. While you are doing this, eat simple foods that you prepare yourself, to avoid the possibility of cross-contamination. For example, if you are eliminating soy, eat fresh fruits, veggies, and meats rather than anything that comes in a package or is prepared in a restaurant, unless it has been made in a certified soy-free facility.

2. Keep track of your symptoms to see if they improve. If they don't improve, then the food you eliminated was most likely not the problem.

3. If they do improve, reintroduce the food in its most basic form to see if you have a reaction. This is called a "challenge." In the case of soy, a good challenge would be a soybean, rather than soy sauce or a food with multiple ingredients.

4. If your symptoms get worse after eating the food, try the process of elimination and challenge again to confirm the results. It is possible that the first time was a coincidence. For example, perhaps the food you used for your challenge is greasy and upset your stomach, but you can tolerate the food in another form.

 What is the difference between an elimination and an exclusion diet?

 In the case of food intolerances, an elimination diet may be used as a diagnostic tool. Once you find out your specific food intolerances, an exclusion diet that eliminates those foods becomes a long-term treatment plan.

Limitations of an Elimination Diet

This elimination process can help link symptoms to specific foods, but it is not foolproof and can be dangerous.

Reintroduction Risks

Because there is no universally accepted protocol for the order, amounts, and specific forms in which foods should be introduced back into the diet, the elimination diet is more an art than a science. For example, reintroducing too small a quantity of the test food may not be sufficient to provoke symptoms. You need to have clear guidance from your health-care providers on the forms of food to be reintroduced. Simple forms of food should be introduced before packaged foods or other meals containing multiple ingredients. The reintroduction process is also a very slow one — it may take several months while you slowly reintroduce different foods and monitor symptoms. You will need to be highly committed to the process, and you will need plenty of support from your health-care providers and family.

Self-Diagnosis Danger

Often, adult patients or parents of children experiencing symptoms initiate elimination diets on their own without medical guidance and appropriate dietetic follow-up. For children, this is very problematic because nutritional needs corresponding to the stage of development have to be balanced with eliminating allergenic proteins that are typically high in nutritional value. For adults who may be dealing with food intolerances, initiating elimination diets may lead to further confusion and unnecessary long-term avoidances that affect their quality of life and give rise to nutritional deficiencies.

Nutrient Deficiencies and Malnutrition

Poorly planned elimination diets can increase the risk of nutrient deficiencies and malnutrition. In extreme elimination practices, most foods associated with sensitivities, intolerances, and allergies are removed from the diet, including corn and soy products and all food sources of gluten, casein, simple carbohydrates, and yeasts along with fried food, junk food, added sugars, and artificial colors and preservatives. To restore nutritional balance to the diet, large doses of vitamins A, C, E, B, along with probiotics, omega-3 fatty acids, digestive enzymes, and antifungal medication, are added. This type of diet may lead to restricted eating preferences and a fear of trying new foods. In the case of children, elimination procedures may affect nutritional status and growth in the long term.

Stress

Some patients find that implementing elimination diets becomes disruptive and upsetting, mostly when resistance to change and difficulty transitioning to new experiences is a barrier.

Children

Elimination diets, such as the specific carbohydrate diet (SCD), should not be administered to children because it puts them at risk of a poorly balanced and nutritionally deficient diet during a critical period of growth and development.

Monitoring

Before embarking on an elimination diet for the diagnosis of food intolerances and allergies, consult your family doctor, who will likely refer you to an allergy specialist and registered dietitian to plan a safe course of action for:

- Selecting suspect foods to eliminate.
- Discovering all the possible sources of allergens, including hidden food ingredients.
- Ensuring the elimination diet will be nutritionally sound.
- Identifying foods to replace the nutrients you may be missing while on the diet.
- Reintroducing foods in a specific order, amount, and form.
- Monitoring symptoms while you are carrying out the reintroduction phase.
- Handling practical issues that may arise during the elimination and reintroduction stage, such as how to deal with social outings and meals eaten outside the home.

All these details need to be clearly outlined for you, because failing to address these issues will make the process of identifying food intolerances confusing and may ultimately prevent you from reaching your goal.

Food Exclusion Diets for Treatment

To follow up on a diagnosis of a food intolerance, a number of food exclusion diets have been proposed, but there is not enough evidence to show that the benefits of carrying out these diets outweigh the difficulties in implementing and maintaining them, as well as the risk for developing nutritional deficiencies in the long run. These exclusion diets should be considered, at best, short-term trials and should only be pursued in the long term if medical or behavioral benefits are clearly seen in the individual. These "experiments" should be made under the guidance of a knowledgeable health-care professional.

Gluten-Free, Casein-Free Diet (GFCF)

This variation on the multiple food exclusion diet focuses on eliminating two allergens. It is based on the theory that gluten (wheat protein) and casein (cow's milk protein) are poorly digested in the gut and poorly absorbed into the bloodstream through a leaky gut. It is speculated that gluten and casein interfere with behavior by affecting neurological processes in the brain. No part of the GFCF diet has been proven, and a thorough, systematic review of the studies that do exist has found insufficient evidence to recommend GFCF diets.

Yeast-Free Diet

This diet is based on the premise that an overgrowth of yeast triggers a leaky gut, making individuals more prone to food allergies and intolerances. This diet will typically exclude yeasts — found in bread, vinegar, cheese, soy sauce, and processed foods — and the simple sugars believed to feed the growth of those yeasts. However, there is no evidence that eating less sugar and dietary yeasts helps prevent food allergies or intolerances. This diet is unscientific and has not been clinically proven and validated. It is not recommended.

Feingold Diet

This once popular diet aims to eliminate food additives — artificial colorings, flavorings, and preservatives, such as sodium benzoate. It also advocates the exclusion of salicylates and aspartame. There is no proven benefit for implementing the Feingold diet, and it has not been proven useful in the treatment of attention deficit disorders.

Combined Allergen-Free and Balanced Diet

The challenge for managing food allergies, intolerances, and sensitivities is to identify offending foods and exclude them from your diet without jeopardizing balanced nutrition. To achieve this goal, your allergist and dietitian will work with you to:

1. Assess your current nutritional status and measure dietary intake for calories, carbohydrates, fats, proteins, fiber, and micronutrients.
2. Avoid hidden sources of foods being excluded and find appropriate foods that can replace or substitute for those being excluded.
3. Ensure appropriate supplementation when nutrients are lost by exclusion. In the case of a casein-free diet, for example, to avoid compromising growth and health status, your dietitian needs to ensure adequate intake of calcium, vitamin D, magnesium, and alternative sources of protein from food sources or nutritional supplements.

Recipes for Success

It is possible to create recipes that avoid one or more of the top 10 allergens yet constitute the balanced diet our national food guides recommend to ensure normal growth among children and adolescents and long-term good health among adults and the elderly. In this book, we use the term "combination diet" to describe a diet that excludes the allergens that affect your health adversely yet provides adequate nutrients to maintain good health. Understanding in greater depth what causes food allergies and how they develop will enable you to avoid threats to your wellbeing and achieve good health, despite your food allergies and intolerances.

Part I

Understanding Food Allergies, Intolerances, and Sensitivities

CHAPTER 1
The Immune System

Case Study

Fear and Loathing

Michael is a 36-year-old, relatively healthy man who maintains a fairly active lifestyle. Two years ago, he went abroad on vacation and suffered a stomach infection and a bad bout of diarrhea. Although he recovered from this, his bowels never really returned to normal: he was plagued by recurrent diarrhea and, sometimes, constipation, severe bloating, and gas. Eating makes him uncomfortable.

When the situation continued to worsen, Michael consulted with his physician for a diagnosis. After taking a count of his symptoms, and knowing Michael's medical history, the doctor referred Michael to a gastroenterologist for further testing. Screening colonoscopy revealed no significant abnormalities; likewise, routine endoscopy and biopsies for celiac disease were negative. Michael was also referred to an allergy specialist and no outstanding allergies were detected. Following this battery of tests, Michael was diagnosed with irritable bowel syndrome (IBS). He was then referred to a dietitian for dietary counseling. Lifestyle-modification strategies were also recommended.

When Michael came to see me, his symptoms were extremely bothersome. He reported being fearful of social situations because he could never predict when symptoms of diarrhea would set in. It seemed like eating the same foods would cause no symptoms one day and full-on pain and unpredictable trips to the bathroom the next!

I asked Michael to keep a thorough food and symptom diary for a full week. It became very clear that most of his bouts of diarrhea occurred after consuming rich meals, often in restaurants. He also reported symptoms of bloating and gas after his mid-morning and mid-afternoon snack, which usually consisted of 1 serving of fruit. Knowing that fructose and sorbitol (a natural sugar in fruits such as plums, prunes, apples, cherries, and nectarines) are not fully digested, we agreed on a plan to cut back on the amount of fat consumed at mealtimes and switch to low-fructose and low-sorbitol fruits at snack time. After 2 weeks of making leaner meal choices and eating smaller meals for lunch and dinner, he reported that his symptoms of diarrhea had subsided. He also found that avoiding fruits high in fructose and sorbitol and pairing them with a lean source of protein helped diminish the bloating and gas.

Food allergy is a serious health problem affecting both children and adults worldwide. A growing number of people have adverse reactions, ranging from temporary skin rashes and indigestion to life-threatening anaphylactic shock, to eating specific foods. Oddly enough, foods consumed without adverse reactions by most people can provoke allergic reactions and intolerances in some people. What causes these reactions and how to avoid them has become the subject of considerable medical research in the past few decades as the incidence of allergic disease has increased. These studies have focused on the complex functions of the immune system in defending us against infections.

Prevalence of Food Allergies and Intolerances

According to the World Allergy Organization, the prevalence of food allergies is increasing in both developed and developing countries. Globally, 250 to 520 million people suffer from food allergies. While children are the largest population affected by food allergies, adults are a growing population. It has been reported that 3% of adults may suffer from one or more food allergies. Childhood allergies to milk, eggs, soy, and wheat are eventually outgrown and, according to the American Academy of Asthma, Allergy and Immunology, about 20% of children with peanut allergy and about 9% of children with tree nut allergy will outgrow it.

The key distinction between a food allergy and a food intolerance is that an allergy affects the immune system, while an intolerance does not.

Food Allergy

Food allergies trigger a strong reaction of the immune system to a specific food. When the reaction is severe and occurs every time you are exposed to the allergen, identifying the cause of the reaction is straightforward. If you develop hives every time you consume shrimp, for example, and you eliminate shrimp from the diet and then notice that the skin symptoms do not return until you consume shrimp again, you know that shrimp is the culprit for the symptoms. Diagnosis for food allergies should always be confirmed by an allergy specialist through blood tests and skin prick tests. You will need to carry an epinephrine auto-injector with you to treat possible future recurrences of allergic reaction to the food in question.

Did You Know?

Food Allergy Statistics
According to a study released by the Centers for Disease Control and Prevention, there was an 18% rise in food allergies in the United States between 1997 and 2007 in children under the age of 18. In Canada, recent research shows that 1.3 million people are affected by food allergies. While the exact prevalence is unknown, current estimates show that food allergies affect as many as 5% to 6% of young children and 3% to 4% of adults in Western countries.

Estimated Prevalence of Adult Allergies to Various Foods Worldwide

Specific Allergy	Canada	United States	Other Countries
Peanuts	0.71%	0.6% (all ages) 1.3% (peanut, tree nut or both)	France, Germany, Israel, Sweden, UK: 0.06%–5.9%
Tree nuts	1.00%	0.4%–0.5% (all ages) 1.3% (peanut, tree nut or both)	France, Germany, Israel, Sweden, UK: 0.03%–8.5%
Fish	0.56%	0.5%	Europe: 0.2%–0.3% (all ages)
Crustaceans	1.69%	2.3% (all ages)	Europe: 0.53%
Cow's milk	Data not available	2.5%	Denmark: 2.2% Other European countries: 0.6%–0.9% (all ages)
Egg	Data not available	1.5%–3.2%	Norway: 1.6% Other European countries: 0.3%–0.9% (all ages)
Sesame	0.05%	Data not available	Data not available
Mustard	Data not available	Data not available	Data not available

Food Intolerance

Food intolerance does not affect the immune system, manifesting itself in more subtle ways. The symptoms tend to be milder but may get progressively worse with time. They develop slowly in response to intake of regular amounts of a food as opposed to the very small amounts needed to trigger an allergic reaction. In some cases, the intolerance disappears in response to changes in diet, stress, and lifestyle, only to reappear again some time later. What makes the picture of food intolerance more complicated is the lack of reliable quantitative tests to diagnose it. The only way to diagnose non-allergic food sensitivity is an elimination diet followed by reintroduction of the food, otherwise known as a food challenge.

Key Terms

Besides the distinction between food allergies and food intolerances, there are other special terms involved in describing the immune system.

Allergens: Antigens that trigger an allergic response.

Antibodies: Specific blood proteins that arise in response to foreign antigens in the body. Each antigen induces the production of an antibody, which is meant to act against that specific antigen only. The role of the antibody is to destroy or neutralize the antigen.

Antigens: Food proteins and other chemicals or pathogens that have the ability to induce the production of antibodies by the body's immune system. Some antigens trigger the production of protective antibodies, responsible for destroying pathogens and preventing infections in the future.

Autoimmunity: The body's immune system response against its own cells and tissues as a result of failing to recognize those components as "self." For reasons not fully understood, the immune system will turn against itself, destroying its own body cells, in an autoimmune response.

Autoimmune conditions include celiac disease, thyroid disease, type 1 diabetes, and rheumatoid arthritis.

Celiac disease: An autoimmune disease triggered by the consumption of gluten. The main sources of gluten in the diet are cereal grains. The only treatment for this disease is a strict gluten-free diet for life.

Haptens: Molecules too small to induce an immune response by themselves but that, when coupled with body proteins in tissues and blood, induce an allergic response. Drug molecules, such as penicillin, are an example of haptens.

Pathogens: Infectious microbes, such as viruses and bacteria, capable of causing disease.

Immune Function

At the center of food allergies, intolerances, and sensitivities is the immune system, which defends our bodies from infections. These infections are caused by the millions of microorganisms in our environment, including viruses, bacteria, fungi, algae, and protozoa. Collectively, these microorganisms are call pathogens.

The various components of our immune system prevent infectious diseases and rid the body of the infecting agent when we do succumb to disease — most of the time. But when any component of the immune system is lacking, whether from an inherited defect or an acquired deficit, the body is unable to resist the proliferation of disease-causing microorganisms and is susceptible to infections it would normally suppress.

Pathogen Defence

The body is physically and chemically equipped to fend off infections. The skin, for example, provides a physical barrier, and hydrochloric acid in the stomach offers a line of chemical defense against pathogens. When we refer to the immune system, however, we are primarily talking about immunity at the cellular level, specifically the functions of the white blood cells (leukocytes) in defending against pathogens.

Q What is the role of inflammation in the immune response?

A Inflammation is the first sign and, most often, the only visible evidence of the complex series of events that constitute the immune response — the mobilization of cells that interact in a regulated manner to defeat the threats from outside the body. You may experience this firsthand when a cut or skin abrasion becomes infected. The area becomes red, swollen, and painful. The redness is due to increased blood flow to the area; the swelling is caused by expansion of the blood vessels (known as dilation), often resulting in leakage of fluid-containing plasma proteins; and the pain is due to the pressure of the swollen tissues on the nerve endings and by other irritating chemicals. The inflammatory response occurs whenever pathogens come in contact with body tissues, such as the digestive tract, the lungs, and skin.

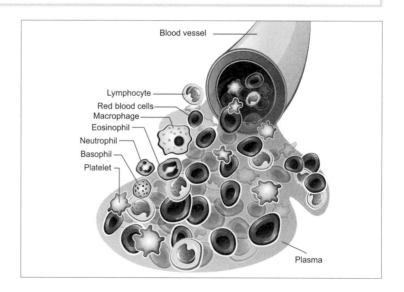

Specialized Blood Cells

All immune system cells are blood cells derived from a common stem cell produced in the bone marrow. The bone marrow stem cell is an immature cell that will differentiate into one of three major categories of specialized blood cells:

- Erythrocytes (red blood cells) carry oxygen and other nutrients throughout the body.
- Platelets are involved in blood clotting but also in the immune response.
- Leukocytes (white blood cells) protect the body from pathogens and allergens and other harmful chemicals. Some leukocytes, called phagocytes, devour invading cells, while others attack with "chemical weapons" stored in granules within the cells.

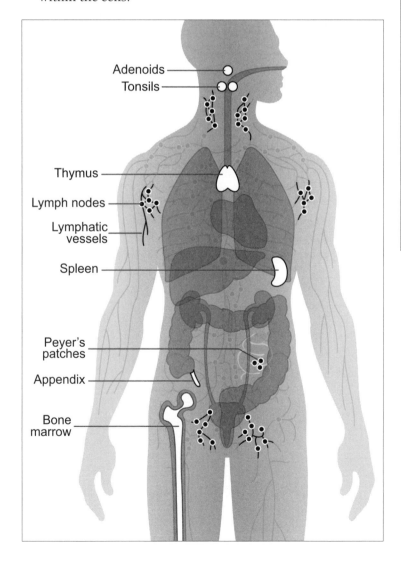

Adenoids
Tonsils
Thymus
Lymph nodes
Lymphatic vessels
Spleen
Peyer's patches
Appendix
Bone marrow

White Blood Cells

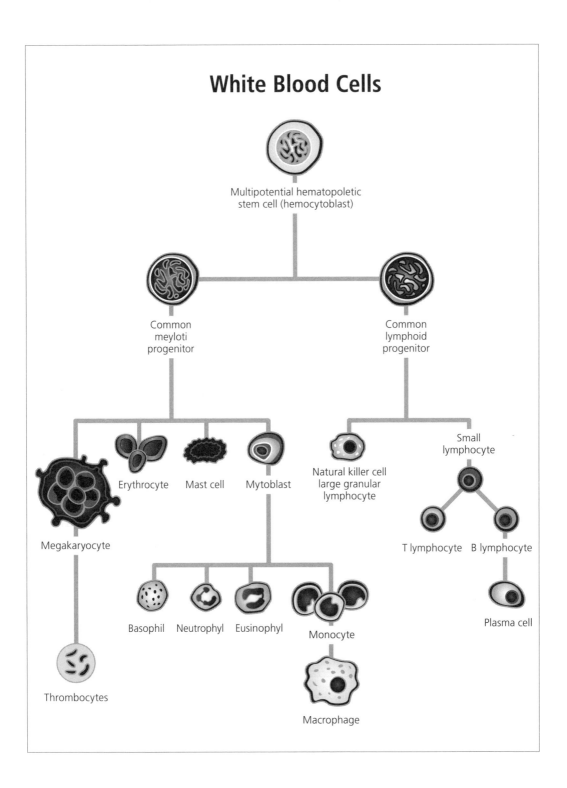

Kinds of Leukocytes

Granulocytes
- Basophils
- Neutrophils
- Eosinophils

Agranulocytes
- Monocytes
- Lymphocytes

Leukocytes

The five types of leukocytes — basophils, neutrophils, eosinophils, monocytes, and lymphocytes — are divided into two groups: those that are filled with microscopic granules (granulocytes) and those that have no distinct granules in their cytoplasm (agranulocytes).

Basophils

These granulocytes release powerful chemicals, capable of destroying invaders, from their granules into the surrounding tissues and bloodstream, a process known as degranulation. The most important of these released chemicals are:

- *Heparin*: A powerful anticoagulant that prevents the blood from coagulating.
- *Histamine*: A chemical that causes contraction of smooth muscle, for example, in the lungs. Digestive tract dilation of the blood vessels allows more blood cells to the area, which is experienced as swelling. An increase in the blood vessel permeability allows fluid to easily pass from the bloodstream to tissues, allowing more white blood cells and chemicals to flood the infected area.
- *Enzymes*: Biological molecules that break down components of the allergen, bacteria or virus.

Neutrophils

Neutrophils are the first to respond to the presence of infection. When they pass from the bloodstream into the tissues at the site of inflammation, they engulf and destroy the foreign substance at its point of entry into the body.

Eosinophils

Eosinophils are found in small numbers in a healthy individual, but they multiply enormously in response to infections by parasites and allergic and inflammatory

Did You Know?

Mast Cells
Mast cells also play an important role in allergic response. They are fixed in many body tissues, but are most numerous in the lungs and uterus, in connective tissue and around blood vessels. Their role is very similar to that of basophils, but they are more powerful and can release up to 20 times more histamine than basophils. In addition to histamine, mast cells release other chemicals that contribute to the inflammatory response.

conditions. Like the other granulocytes, they release toxic chemicals from their granules to attack invading cells. In addition, when encountering an allergen, they can transform into phagocytes, or "eating cells," to devour the allergen.

Monocytes

These small phagocytes circulate freely in the blood, attacking infected cells. When they migrate from the blood vessels into other tissues, such as the spleen, lymph nodes, liver, or lungs, they transform into large eating cells called macrophages, which stay fixed in the tissue.

Lymphocytes

The primary cells of the immune system, lymphocytes are responsible for activating and regulating the functions of the other leukocytes. Lymphocytes make up 20% to 40% of white blood cells and are present in large number in the lymph nodes (from which their name is derived), spleen, and thymus. Many lymphocytes mature into T-cells and B-cells, which have various special functions.

Q What is a cell-mediated immune response?

A This is a protective immune response that does not involve antibodies. Instead, cell-mediated immune responses activate macrophages, natural killer cells, and cytotoxic T lymphocytes in response to an antigen and go on to isolate and neutralize it.

T-Cells

Named for the thymus lymph gland, where they mature, T-cells mediate the entire immune response and are the cornerstone of cell-mediated immunity. They control the immune response by initiating, directing, and terminating the process. T-cells also play a central role in Type IV hypersensitivity response.

T-Cells in Concert

T-cells work together to coordinate the immune response. T-helper cells are key to initiating the immune response. These white blood cells warn the immune system about being attacked by harmful pathogens or antigens. When first exposed to food proteins that are not actually harmful, such as peanut or seafood proteins, T-cells respond by stimulating the production of other white blood cells and specific antibodies, such as immunoglobulin E (or IgE), responsible for the majority of allergic reactions. In addition to mounting a specific immune response, T-cytotoxic cells also have the ability to kill foreign cells within the body. Finally, T-suppressor cells help finalize the immune response after the antigen has been destroyed, and T-memory cells remain behind to be rapidly activated when the same antigen enters the body at a later time.

Kinds of T-Cells

There are four main types of T-cells, each of which has very specific functions in the immune response.

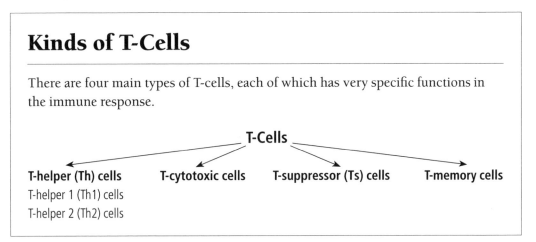

T-helper (Th) cells
T-helper 1 (Th1) cells
T-helper 2 (Th2) cells

T-cytotoxic cells

T-suppressor (Ts) cells

T-memory cells

1. T-helper (Th) Cells

These cells mediate the immune response by directing other cells to perform the tasks of phagocytosis (the process of "eating" cells), killing infected cells, and clearing pathogens. They can recognize the foreign antigen presented by an antigen-presenting cell (APC) and decide, through the intermediacy of messenger molecules called cytokines, which type of immune response to initiate. The types of responses may include activation of B lymphocytes to produce specific antibodies or activation of T-cytotoxic cells to induce cell-mediated (protective) immune responses. There are two important subgroups of T-helper cells:

- *T-helper 1 (Th1) cells:* These cells trigger the release of macrophages and participate in the generation of T-cytotoxic cells, which are essentially part of a protective cell-mediated immune response. Th1 cells also activate B-cells to produce neutralizing antibodies — otherwise known as IgG-type antibodies.
- *T-helper 2 (Th2) cells:* These cells trigger B lymphocytes to produce IgE-type antibodies, mast cells, basophils, and

eosinophils, all of which are responsible for the allergic response and typically lead to Type I hypersensitivity reactions.

2. T-cytotoxic Cells
These T-cells are able to attack organisms directly and kill infected cells even in the absence of antibodies.

3. T-supressor (Ts) Cells
These T-cells limit and suppress the immune system, and thus may function to control abnormal immune responses to self-antigens and the development of autoimmune disease.

4. T-memory Cells
These are the few T-cells that remain once the infection has been cleared. They become more easily activated upon subsequent interaction with a foreign antigen, mounting a faster and more effective immune response.

B-Cells
Named for the organ in birds, the bursa of Fabricius, where original research showed they matured from precursor cells, B-cells are responsible for producing antibodies. When they encounter an antigen, or when they are activated by Th2 cells, B-cells differentiate into plasma cells, which manufacture and release antibodies, such as IgE antibodies, specific to the antigen that triggered their production. B-cells oversee humoral immunity (acquired immunity in which the role of circulating antibodies is predominant).

Null Cells
Null cells are neither B-cells nor T-cells but rather large granular lymphocytes that secrete toxic proteins able to kill tumor cells and virus-infected cells. One subgroup of null cells are natural killer (NK) cells, which are very important in antiviral and antitumor immunity.

Five Common Foods and Four Ways They Can Make You Sick

Food	Allergy	Sensitivity or Intolerance	Contamination or Innate Poison	Other
Wheat	Wheat protein	Gluten sensitivity (causes gastric distress and flu-like symptoms)	Bacillus cereus contamination	Celiac disease (autoimmune reaction to gluten that damages the small intestine)
Milk	Milk protein	Lactose intolerance	Gastroenteritis from raw or unrefrigerated milk	
Eggs	Egg protein		Gastroenteritis from raw or unrefrigerated eggs	
Fish	Fish protein		Poisoning from puffer fish, which contains a neurotoxin	Scromboid poisoning (allergy-like reaction from histamine released by spoiled fish)
Peanuts	Peanut protein		Gastroenteritis from contaminated peanut butter	

Excerpted with permission from "Food Allergy, Intolerance, and Sensitivities." March 2012, Harvard University. For more information, visit health.harvard.edu.

Innate and Adaptive Immune Systems

The immune system has two major divisions: the innate (non-specific) and the adaptive (specific). The innate immune system is our first line of defense against invading organisms, while the adaptive immune system functions as the second line of defense and allows the body to protect itself against the same pathogen if it encounters it again. Although the two systems have distinct functions, they interact and complement each other.

Functions of the Innate and Adaptive Immune Systems

Innate Immune System	Adaptive Immune System
Mobilizes cells and defense mechanisms immediately to protect against infection	Takes time to build the arsenal of immunological components to react to an invading organism
Reacts equally to all invading organisms	Reacts only against the specific microorganism that provoked the reaction
Does not have a "memory" for specific invaders	Has the ability to "remember" invaders

Innate Immune System

The first line of defense in our bodies consists of physical and chemical barriers:

- The skin blocks pathogens and allergens unless there is an opening, such as a scratch, cut, or bruise.
- Coughing and sneezing abruptly expel all living and non-living microorganisms from the respiratory tract.
- Tears, saliva, and sticky mucus force pathogens from the body.
- Stomach acid and powerful protein-digesting enzymes help destroy many pathogens.
- Fever and inflammatory response contribute to this non-specific line of defense.
- Monocytes, macrophages, polymorphonuclear granulocytes, natural killer cells, basophils, eosinophils, mast cells, and platelets are generated and distributed in response to infectious diseases.

Adaptive Immune System

There are two fundamental mechanisms that help the immune system to better track the invading antigen: cell-mediated immunity and humoral immunity.

Cell-Mediated Immunity

T-cells mount an inflammatory response against a foreign antigen. Cell-mediated immunity protects against:

- Microbes inside our cells
- Fungal infection
- Protozoan parasites
- Cancer cells

Humoral-Mediated Immunity

In this type of immune response, another kind of white blood cell, known as B-cell lymphocytes, produces antibodies that bind to and neutralize specific antigens. Humoral-mediated immunity works best in targeting pathogens that enter our bodies through:

- Viruses
- Allergens
- Bacteria
- Other foreign molecules

Cellular Components of the Immune System

Type of Immune System	Specific Cellular Components
Innate (non-specific) immune system	Monocytes, macrophages, polymorphonuclear granulocytes, basophils, eosinophils, mast cells, platelets
Adaptive (specific) immune system	T-cells, B-cell lymphocytes

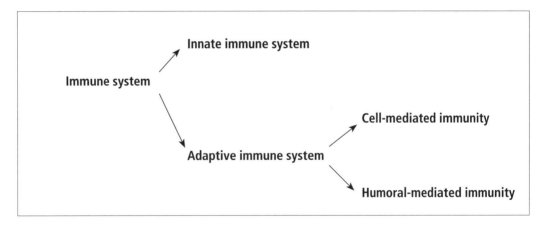

Lymph System

The immune system is closely linked to the lymph system, a network of organs, nodes, ducts, and vessels that produces and transports lymph from tissues to the bloodstream. The lymph system is a major component of the body's immune system. Lymph is a clear or white fluid that contains proteins and fats and is made of lymphocytes and fluid from the intestines called chyle.

Q What is the function of the lymph system in immunity?

A The main role of the lymphatic system is to collect and transport fluids from all the tissues of the body back to the veins in the blood system. Its function as part of the immune system is to transport new lymphocytes produced in the lymph nodes in the event of an immune response against a pathogen or antigen.

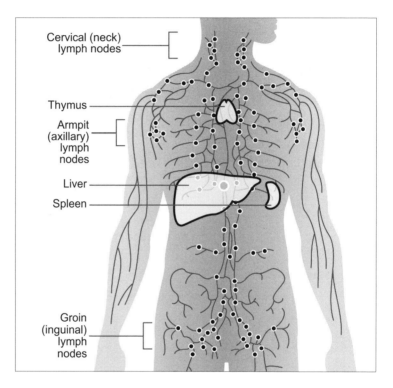

Antigens and Allergens

Antigens stimulate the immune system into producing antibodies to destroy them. For example, when a virus enters the body, it promotes the production of protective antibodies that aid in the destruction of the virus and help prevent reinfection with the same virus again in the future.

Other antigens, however, do not lead to the usual production of protective antibodies but to an allergic response — these antigens are then called allergens. Allergens are substances that vary widely in origin, from plants (ragweed pollen, trees, grasses) and wasp and bee venom to foods (eggs, grains, nuts, and milk), inhaled chemicals, and medications. They enter the body through the respiratory and digestive tracts, from direct contact with the skin or mucous membranes, or from insertion into the bloodstream by injection or insect bites.

Some allergens enter the body as molecules too small to induce immune response by themselves but then couple with body proteins in tissues or with blood cells to induce the allergic response. The antibiotic penicillin is one such example.

Kinds of Food Allergens

Class 1: These large, water-soluble glycoproteins (proteins with sugar chains) are stable in the presence of heat, acid, and enzymes. They can remain intact even after processing, storage, cooking, and digestion.

Class 1 Food Allergens
- Caseins (milk)
- Vicilins (legumes and nuts)
- Ovomucoids (eggs)
- Non-specific lipid transfer proteins (present in many different plant foods)

Class 2: These highly soluble substances are easily destroyed by heat, acid, and enzymes. Because of their unstable nature, they usually do not cause sensitization through ingestion but rather through skin contact or absorption through the oral mucosa.

Class 2 Food Allergens
- Pollens (e.g., birch, grass)
- Fruit and vegetable allergens (e.g., apples, carrots, peaches)

Antibodies (Immunoglobulins)

Antibodies are special kinds of blood proteins produced by B-cell lymphocytes in response to encountering foreign antigens in the body. Antibodies are also known as immunoglobulins, for convenience designated as Ig. Each antigen leads to the production of an antibody active specifically against that antigen alone. When an antigen meets its corresponding antibody, the antigen and antibody link together in a complex, rather like a lock and key, and the antigen is neutralized. The complex stimulates a further response of the immune system, which will finally destroy the antigen.

Kinds of Antibodies

- *IgG antibodies:* These are the most predominant kind of antibody, making up 75% of immunoglobulin in the body. This kind of antibody is important in neutralizing bacterial toxins; it binds to other macrophages and monocytes and allows them to better internalize the antigen and make its destruction (phagocytosis) more efficient. IgG antibodies are the only kind to cross the placenta, providing passive immunity to the newborn.

- *IgA antibodies:* The second most common immunoglobulin in the body is found in secretions — saliva, tears, colostrums, and mucus. Because it is found primarily in secretions, it is most important in local (secretory) immunity. One such example is celiac disease, where the lining of the intestine is damaged in response to the presence of gluten. The antibodies useful in detecting the presence of celiac disease are of the type IgA.

- *IgM antibodies:* This is the first antibody produced when a new antigen enters the body. It is especially important in neutralizing bacteria and other toxins in the blood and is the third most common antibody.

- *IgE antibodies:* These make up only 0.002% of all immunoglobulins, but they bind very tightly to basophils and mast cells even before interacting with an antigen and become highly associated with allergic reactions. Binding of the allergen to the IgE antibody on the cells leads to the release of various chemicals that result in allergic symptoms.

- *IgD antibodies:* These are found in very low quantities in plasma and their role is uncertain. They may act as an antigen receptor on B-cell lymphocytes or they may be involved in recognition of "self" and "foreign" antigens.

Hypersensitivity Reactions

In 1963, Patrick Gell and Robin Coombs developed a comprehensive classification of hypersensitivity reactions based on the underlying immune mechanisms. Since then, as knowledge of cellular and molecular immune systems has evolved, there have been various attempts to reinterpret or revise this classification. To this day, however, it remains the most valid and useful framework for understanding food hypersensitivities. The Gell-Coombs system identifies four distinct types of food hypersensitivity reactions, though there is very little evidence that Types II and III play a role in food-related reactions.

- *Type I hypersensitivity:* Also known as immediate hypersensitivity, this is the IgE-mediated, classic allergic response and induces symptoms of urticaria (hives); angioedema (swelling, often in the face); stuffy nose; itchy, watery eyes; asthma; digestive tract upset; and, the most severe response, anaphylaxis. The reaction usually takes 15 to 30 minutes from the time of exposure to the antigen, although rarely it may have a delayed onset, generally for up to a few hours.
- *Type II hypersensitivity:* Unlike Type I reactions, Type II hypersensitivity is caused by direct antibody-mediated cell damage and may affect a variety of organs. These types of hypersensitivities involve antibodies of the IgG or IgM class, which trigger the onset of a unique sequence of immunologic reactions leading to the final destruction of the invader through a process of "splitting" (known as lysis) of the foreign cell. Examples of Type II hypersensitivity reaction include autoimmune anemia and allergic reaction to penicillin, which can result in distinct symptoms, including a rash, painful joints, and hives. Type II hypersensitivity reaction is very rare and can take anywhere from 2 to 24 hours to develop.
- *Type III hypersensitivity:* Also known as immune complex hypersensitivity, this type involves antibodies of both the IgG and the IgM class. The reaction may be general (e.g., serum, or blood, sickness) or may involve individual organs, including the skin (e.g., systemic lupus erythematosus), kidneys, lungs, blood vessels, joints (e.g., rheumatoid arthritis), or other organs. The reaction may take hours, days, or even weeks to develop and it is usually treated with anti-inflammatory and corticosteroid drugs.
- *Type IV hypersensitivity:* This hypersensitivity is a delayed response caused by T-cells. This type of hypersensitivity can manifest as a variety of symptoms, such as enterocolitis and eczema, and is the major mechanism involved in the defense against certain parasites and fungi. It also plays a major role in transplant rejection and tumor immunity. Contact dermatitis caused by poison ivy is an example of a Type IV hypersensitivity reaction.

Development of Food Allergies

Given the different components of the immune system and classifications of immune responses to allergens, how do food allergies develop?

IgE-Mediated Food Allergy

Food proteins are broken down by digestive enzymes into small fragments called peptides and amino acids. In normal circumstances, these small particles are prevented from entering the tissues by physical and chemical barriers in the gut. Sometimes, however, small amounts of intact food proteins may be absorbed through the gastrointestinal tract or lungs.

Take, for example, an individual consuming nuts. During a classic IgE-mediated allergic response, intact nut protein fragments get trapped by antigen-presenting cells (APC) and are presented to T-helper (Th) cells. In individuals with a genetic predisposition to developing allergies — also known as atopic individuals — the process stimulates the production of T-helper 2 (Th2) cells, which, in turn, stimulates B-cells to produce IgE food-specific antibodies to the amino acid sequence found in that protein. These IgE antibodies then bind to mast cells in tissues or basophils circulating in the blood.

Sensitization

Although IgE antibodies in plasma have a very short life, once bound to mast cells in tissues, they can remain there for months, waiting to come into contact with the allergen. This is called sensitization. Once the individual is sensitized to an allergen, the body reacts more strongly and rapidly. The specific IgE antibodies recognize certain areas of the food protein, called epitopes, and allow the protein and antibody to couple in the typical key-and-lock type of complex, leading to degradation of these cells and the release of histamine and other chemicals, such as prostaglandins, leukotrienes, platelet activation factors, and bradykinin. These white blood cells cause dilation of the blood vessels and increased permeability, which attracts more cells into tissues, leading to inflammation.

Anaphylaxis

The most severe allergic reaction is called anaphylaxis. Unless treated promptly, anaphylaxis may lead to death. Sensitization can be present without necessarily triggering a clinical reaction — this means that IgE antibodies to nuts are present, but no reaction occurs with exposure. Only a small percentage of those exposed to a protein allergen will become sensitized. Research suggests that this depends on population genetics, the individual's unique immune response, and possible environmental factors.

Late-Phase Reaction

A subsequent, more pronounced reaction, known as late-phase reaction, occurs a few hours after the initial reaction. This is mainly caused by the presence of eosinophils, but mononuclear cells, other lymphocytes, and neutrophils are also involved.

Food Hypersensitivity Stages

Stage 1 — Foreign antigen (allergen) is introduced.
Stage 2 — Macrophage cell ingests the allergen.
Stage 3 — T-helper (Th) cell lymphocyte is activated.
Stage 4 — Antigen binds to Th.
Stage 5 — Formation of antigen-MHC II complex (antigen presentation to B-cells).
Stage 6 — Production of antigen-specific antibodies by B-cells — in the case of food allergies, IgE antibodies.

Non-IgE-Mediated Food Allergies

Although food-induced reactions are not always well understood, the absence of IgE antibody production during an adverse reaction to food has been clearly demonstrated. Unfortunately, this type of allergy is poorly defined both clinically and scientifically. Non-IgE-mediated food allergies are typically delayed in onset and occur 4 to 28 hours after ingestion of the offending food(s). They also tend to primarily affect the GI tract. Better diagnostic tools and evidence through well-designed scientific studies are needed to clarify this type of food allergy and the best way to diagnose it.

One emerging alternative diagnostic tool has focused on measuring IgG antibodies as indicators of food hypersensitivity reactions that do not involve IgE antibodies. It is thought, however, that IgG-level responses to a particular food indicate the level of food consumption rather than reaction to a particular food. This is one of the many reasons why IgG testing is not recommended for diagnosing this type of allergy. Further research with well-designed, robust studies is needed to determine whether this method of testing is at all useful.

Non-Allergic Food Hypersensitivity

Also known as food sensitivity or food intolerance, this type of reaction is most often characterized by a delayed reaction, occurring hours or even days after eating certain foods. It can be described as an adverse reaction to food other than a non-IgE-mediated food allergy or a true food allergy in which the involvement of the immune system is uncertain because reliable tests for allergy are negative. It is difficult at this point to ascertain whether the immune system is involved in all food intolerance reactions. What we do know is that the immune system may play a role, but it is only part of the story — other factors are involved in the development of intolerance to foods.

Food Hypersensitivity Terms

The European Academy of Allergy and Clinical Immunology task force recommends these terms for differentiating food hypersensitivities:

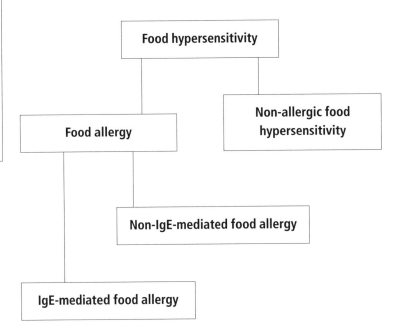

Severe, generalized allergic reactions to food are classified as anaphylaxis.

Q How do you know whether you have a food allergy and not a food intolerance?

A Food allergies involve the immune system, and the symptoms are acute, affecting the skin, the gut, and the respiratory and cardiac systems. They are fairly straightforward for an allergy specialist to diagnose. Food intolerances, on the other hand, are mainly felt in the gastrointestinal tract and may manifest with bloating, gas, cramping, and, sometimes, diarrhea. Because intolerances share some similarities with food allergies, the two are often confused. Unfortunately, there are currently no adequate, reliable tests for diagnosing a food intolerance — with the exception of a couple that have been well documented: lactose intolerance and fructose intolerance. "Gluten sensitivity" is a new term for individuals who cannot tolerate gluten in wheat, barley, rye, spelt, Kamut, triticale, or commercial oats and test negative for celiac disease, an autoimmune condition that damages the lining of the small intestine in response to gluten.

Cross-Reactivity

A phenomenon called cross-reactivity may occur when an antibody reacts not only with the original allergen but also with a similar allergen. In food allergies, cross-reactivity occurs when a food allergen shares structural or sequence similarity with another food allergen or an airborne allergen, which may then trigger an adverse reaction similar to that triggered by the original food allergen. Cross-reactivity is common, for example, among different shellfish and tree nuts. Cross-reactivity is also responsible for symptoms of oral allergy syndrome (OAS), which is a cross-reaction between various pollens and fresh fruits and vegetables.

Oral Allergy Syndrome

Also known as pollen–food allergy syndrome, this condition occurs when the immune system, which is already sensitized to environmental allergens, such as pollen, grass, or ragweed, responds in a similar fashion to proteins in fruits and vegetables. This happens because certain fruits and vegetables have allergens that are very similar to those found in pollen, grass, and ragweed.

The symptoms of oral allergy syndrome are typically limited to the lips, mouth, and pharynx and are characterized by a tingling and burning sensation. Fortunately, symptoms may be avoided by choosing cooked or canned fruits and vegetables, because the allergens are denatured during heating

Did You Know?

Latex Cross-Reactivity

Latex cross-reactivity is another example of possible food cross-reactivity. Individuals who are allergic to latex may also develop allergies to banana, avocado, kiwi, chestnut, papaya, passion fruit, mango, tomato, pepper, potato and celery. Some of these reactions may be anaphylactic.

Cross-Reactions Between Proteins in Pollen and Fresh Fruits and Vegetables

Pollen	Fruit/Vegetable
Birch pollen	Almond, apple, apricot, Brazil nut, carrot, celery, cherry, coconut, fennel, hazelnut, kiwi, nectarine, peach, peanut, pear, plum, potato, rutabaga (turnip), tomato, walnut
Ragweed	Banana, cantaloupe, cucumber, honeydew, watermelon, zucchini
Grass	Cherry, kiwi, orange, melon, peach, peanut, potato, tomato, Swiss chard, watermelon
Birch/mugwort	Carrot, celery, sunflower seeds, honey
Plane (Platanus genus, *Platanaceae* family)	Apple, chickpea, corn, hazelnut, green beans, kiwi, lettuce, melon, peach, peanut

Did You Know?

Fish and Shellfish Allergy

Fish and shellfish are the most common trigger of adult-onset allergies. According to the Food Asthma and Anaphylaxis Network, nearly 40% of those with fish allergy first experienced the allergic reaction as an adult. Very little is known about the cause of this allergy, and theories are speculative at this point.

or digestion. Examples of cooked and canned fruits and vegetables include jams, preserves, pies, cobblers, soups, and stews — all of which may be well tolerated.

Allergy skin tests with fresh extract from the fruit or vegetable itself are generally positive. In a small proportion of oral allergy syndrome, there may be progression to systemic symptoms.

Food-Dependent Exercise-Induced Anaphylaxis (FDEIA)

This is a rare disorder that develops when an individual is physically active within a few hours of consuming food. Neither food nor physical activity alone produces anaphylaxis. Any food may be implicated in FDEIA. Likewise the same type of exercise does not necessarily induce allergic episodes consistently in everyone. The advice to individuals who suffer from this type of allergic reaction is to avoid the trigger foods and wait for several hours before starting any type of physical activity. In addition, they should carry additional doses of epinephrine and work out with a partner who recognizes the symptoms of anaphylaxis and is trained to handle epinephrine injections.

Adult-Onset Allergies

While most allergies develop during childhood and only a subset of individuals have persistent allergies to peanuts, tree nuts, fish, and shellfish, there are cases in which people who do not suffer from allergies or have a family history of allergies develop hypersensitivity to foods they have enjoyed all their lives. The reaction is sudden and unexpected, and can range from a tingling sensation around the mouth to hives to full-blown anaphylactic reactions.

What Causes Food Allergies?

Not surprisingly, there is a genetic and an environmental factor involved in the development of food allergies.

Genetics

Food allergies develop when there is a genetic predisposition, or atopy. However, the recent rise in the prevalence of allergies cannot be explained by genetics alone. While the causes are multiple and still not fully understood, a few hypotheses have been postulated.

Hygiene

This theory suggests that children exposed to a variety of microbes are protected from developing allergies because this exposure strengthens their immune system, while children not exposed to a variety of pathogens are prone to develop allergies. There is scientific evidence to show that children who are in close contact with other children and experience a wide range of infections are less likely to develop allergies later in life than children not in close contact with other children.

Scientists also believe that, particularly in the Western world, modern, improved living standards and more rigorous cleanliness, including the rise of a large variety of potent household cleaning products, such as disinfectant cleaners, have exposed children to fewer microbes, which, in turn, has had a weakening effect on their immune system. These conditions have undeniably cut the risk of infectious diseases and morbidity, but the rate of allergies is increasing worldwide, and the trend in Western developed countries is higher than that in the developing world. However, many factors other than a clean environment contribute to the development of allergies.

Did You Know?

Filaggrin Gene
There may be an association between the filaggrin gene and peanut allergy. A defect in this gene has been previously linked to eczema, but research has shown that the same defect was also found in individuals who suffered from peanut allergy. Research on the filaggrin gene is still experimental at this time.

Antibiotic Overexposure

The extensive use of antibiotics has lessened the burden on the immune system to fight common bacterial infections. With the proliferation of antibacterial soaps, gels, and cleaning wipes, children today are more sheltered from infection than they were in the past and fail to build immune system tolerance as adults.

Evidence also exists showing that exposure to microbes and infections trains the immune system not only to recognize pathogens but also to suppress reaction when it encounters proteins in foods and other environmental allergens. However, this hypothesis fails to explain the increased incidence of allergies and asthma in poor inner-city neighborhoods.

Delayed Introduction of Solid Foods

Delaying introduction of some foods, such as peanuts, until 1 year of age may be associated with higher risk of developing an allergy. In parts of the world where peanuts are introduced very early on in a child's diet, the incidence of peanut allergy is very low. Current guidelines from American-based pediatric allergists recommend delaying solids until 4 to 6 months. Beyond this age, there are no further recommendations to delay introduction of "at risk" foods for allergic reasons, but there are still restrictions about food for developmental or infectious reasons. Studies are ongoing to come to a consensus on this issue.

CHAPTER 2
Associated Health Conditions

Case Study

Gluten-Free

Murray is a 38-year-old man with a successful career in the information technology industry who came to our office with symptoms of gluten sensitivity. He had been diagnosed with ADHD at the age of 6 and had learned to manage symptoms mostly through behavior modification and drug treatments. Murray told the story of successfully managing hyperactivity with sessions of intense exercise, mountain biking, and long-distance running, along with dietary strategies, such as reducing the amount of sugars and simple carbohydrates he consumed. He also described having eczema since the age of 16, with symptoms getting worse during the winter.

He had recently read about the gluten-free, casein-free diet and decided to eliminate gluten from his diet to see if symptoms of ADHD would improve. Although a gluten-free diet did not help improve his focus in reading and writing, his eczema went away.

Back at the doctor's office, blood work for celiac disease came up negative and the doctor concluded that the gluten-free diet had prevented him from obtaining accurate results. Murray was advised to reintroduce gluten into his diet. After 6 months, he had a referral to a gastroenterologist for a small bowel biopsy, which resulted in a negative diagnosis for celiac disease. He also had blood testing that did not reveal an IgE-mediated allergy to wheat.

While on the gluten-free diet, Michael had experienced constipation, which was due to a lower fiber intake from gluten-free starches, such as rice, potatoes, and corn. We helped Murray implement a gluten-free diet corresponding to his degree of tolerance and taking into consideration total daily amount of fiber, fluid, probiotics, and fruits, which help relieve constipation. Overall, Murray found a gluten-free, dairy-free, and soy-free diet best for his digestive system and overall health. But it was extremely important to take into account his calorie, fiber, protein, and micronutrient needs in order to avoid any nutrient deficiencies that could develop as a result of his long-term avoidance.

Food allergies and sensitivities can affect many body systems and produce a multitude of symptoms. Symptoms of IgE-mediated or non-IgE-mediated food hypersensitivity reactions are experienced as a result of ingesting a specific food and may develop within minutes to hours or days of ingestion. While food sensitivities (non-allergic) may be similar to those of food allergy, they tend to develop more slowly and require larger amounts of food to be ingested before symptoms appear. The amount of food that leads up to the development of symptoms varies from person to person. And anaphylactic reactions are not seen in non-allergic food sensitivities.

Skin Disorders

Skin reactions can be caused by IgE-mediated, non-IgE-mediated, or mixed IgE- and non-IgE-mediated immune responses to food allergens. Toxic substances, irritants, or other non-specific properties of foods may also trigger skin reactions, but they would not involve the immune system. The most common reactions include urticaria (hives), angioedema (swelling), pruritus (itching), and atopic eczema.

Skin reactions are common in IgE-mediated food allergies, with acute onset urticaria (with or without angioedema) being very common. Symptoms can develop shortly after ingesting the offending food, but in many cases, even skin contact with food (contact urticaria) can trigger severe allergic reactions. However, skin reactions can also commonly occur without identifiable food allergies.

Skin Disorder Symptoms

Disorder	Symptoms
Urticaria	Otherwise known as hives, urticaria manifests as itchy red areas with white raised central circles that resemble mosquito bites. Acute urticaria usually shows up a few minutes after contact with the allergen and can last for a few hours to several weeks. Chronic urticaria lasting longer than 6 weeks and physical urticaria (for example, exercise-induced) are not caused by allergies.
Angioedema	Angioedema is similar to hives, but the swelling occurs in the deeper layers of the skin or mucous membrane. The swelling can occur around the mouth (lips, tongue), in the throat, in the abdomen, and in areas of loose connective tissue, such as the face and eyelids. In severe cases, such as anaphylaxis, the swelling of the throat can be fatal.
Pruritus	Prutitus is characterized by an intense itching sensation.
Eczema	Also known as atopic dermatitis, eczema is a chronic, relapsing, itchy, and inflammatory skin disease. Scratching the skin makes it worse.

Skin Hypersensitivity Reactions

Mechanism	Disorder	Onset	Possible Food Triggers
IgE-mediated	Urticaria	Immediate	Eggs, milk, wheat, soy, fish, peanuts, tree nuts
	Contact urticaria	Immediate	Raw or processed foods: fruit (especially citrus, pineapple, berry fruits, and tomato), vegetables, meat, fish, chicken, spices, oatmeal, milk, eggs
	Angioedema	Immediate; often occurs with urticaria	Eggs, milk, wheat, soy, fish, peanuts, tree nuts
	Pruritus	Immediate	Eggs, milk, wheat, soy, peanuts, tree nuts
	Flushing	Immediate	Eggs, milk, wheat, soy, peanuts, tree nuts, alcohol, histamine-containing foods (e.g., Parmesan cheese)
Non-IgE mediated	Contact dermatitis	Delayed	Various fresh fruits, vegetables, spices
	Dermatitis herpetiformis (celiac disease)	Delayed	Gluten-containing grains (wheat, barley, rye, spelt, Kamut, triticale)
Mixed IgE- and non-IgE-mediated	Eczema (atopic dermatitis)	Immediate or delayed Usually chronic and recurrent	Eggs, milk, wheat, soy, peanuts, tree nuts, foods that cross-react with pollen (e.g., apples, carrots, hazelnuts, sesame seeds)

Respiratory Disorders

Respiratory symptoms are not common manifestations of food hypersensitivity but may include laryngeal edema (acute inflammation of the larynx that can lead to obstruction of airflow and shortness of breath), rhinorrhea (runny nose), and bronchospasm (constriction of the bronchioles in the lungs that may lead to difficulty in breathing).

Asthma

According to the American Academy of Allergy, Asthma and Immunology, food allergy fatalities are associated with severe asthma, particularly in the case of peanut allergy. Respiratory symptoms may often be observed in fatal or near-fatal food anaphylaxis. Increased respiratory symptoms are also reportedly linked to egg allergy. There may be a relationship between asthma, allergic rhinitis (hay fever), and food allergy in school-aged children.

Hay Fever

According to one report of food allergy in adults, allergy is frequently associated with hay fever (allergic rhinitis, or irritation of the nose). Specifically, the study reported that nearly 73% of those affected with a reported food allergy were also affected by hay fever. It is important to stress, however, that the study did not suggest symptoms of hay fever to be the result of the food allergy; rather, they are concomitant allergic conditions. In spring and fall, hay fever is generally reported in patients suffering from the oral allergy syndrome due to primary allergens in birch and ragweed pollen.

Respiratory Hypersensitivity Reactions

Mechanism	Symptoms and Conditions
IgE-Mediated (immediate reactions)	• Asthma • Allergic rhinitis • Laryngeal edema (swelling of the larynx) • Rhinorrhea (runny nose) • Bronchospasm • Nasal congestion • Cough • Chest tightness • Wheezing
Non-IgE-Mediated (delayed or chronic conditions)	• Heiner syndrome

Q I've been told that if I drink cow's milk, my mucus production will increase and rhinitis, blockage, and wheezing will follow. Is that true?

A Several well-designed studies using double-blind, placebo-controlled challenges have found nothing to back up claims that milk increases nasal secretions, coughing, or congestion. When milk was tested on asthmatic patients, no effects were observed on the severity of symptoms. It is believed that milk may thicken saliva and coat the throat, which gives the perception of increased mucus production.

Gastrointestinal Disorders

Food sensitivities tend to bring milder but chronic symptoms usually associated with irritable bowel syndrome. Gastrointestinal (GI) symptoms of food allergy include nausea, vomiting, abdominal pain, and diarrhea.

Gastrointestinal Symptoms of Food-Induced Allergic Reactions

Anatomy	IgE-Mediated (immediate reactions)	Non-IgE-Mediated (delayed reactions)
Upper GI	• Swelling of the lips, tongue, or palate • Oral pruritus (itchy mouth)	
Lower GI	• Nausea • Colicky abdominal pain • Reflux • Vomiting • Diarrhea	• Nausea • Abdominal pain • Reflux • Vomiting • Diarrhea • Irritability and refusal to eat in young children

Gastrointestinal Disorders Associated with IgE- and non-IgE-Mediated Hypersensitivities

Disorder	Symptoms
Gastrointestinal anaphylaxis	An IgE-mediated reaction characterized by quick onset of nausea/vomiting and abdominal pain/cramps with or without diarrhea. Skin or respiratory disorders are often present.
Allergic eosinophilic esophagitis ("asthma of the esophagus," or EoE)	Mixed IgE- and non-IgE-mediated reaction to food and environmental allergens. Characterized by gastroesophageal reflux, nausea, vomiting, dysphagia (pain on swallowing), pain, irritability, sleep disturbance. EoE does not respond to conventional reflux treatment. Typical onset is seen in childhood, but disease can be found in all age groups, with varying degrees of symptoms. Treatment includes empirical elimination diet and corticosteroid treatment.
Allergic eosinophilic gastroenteritis	A non-IgE-mediated reaction characterized by inflammation of stomach and intestines. Milk, soy, egg, wheat, and fish allergies are the most common causes. Symptoms resolve within 6 weeks on elimination of the foods. May present in any age group, including infants.
Food protein–induced enterocolitis	A non-IgE-mediated reaction that affects infants and young children, characterized by vomiting, bloody diarrhea, weight loss and failure to thrive.

Gastrointestinal Disorders Associated with IgE- and non-IgE-Mediated Hypersensitivities (continued)

Disorder	Symptoms
Food protein–induced proctocolitis	A non-IgE-mediated reaction to cow's milk protein or soy protein appearing in the first 2 months of life. Symptoms include bloody stool and occasional anemia, but otherwise infants are thriving and look well. Eosinophil infiltrations, swelling, and tissue erosions are observed in the rectum and sigmoid portion of the large intestine. Symptoms disappear within 72 to 96 hours of elimination of the protein.
Food protein–induced enteropathy	A non-IgE-mediated reaction characterized by diarrhea, fatty stool, and weight loss. Gut shows villous atrophy (degeneration of villi) and presence of eosinophils and mononuclear cells.
Celiac disease	Celiac disease leads to more extensive damage to the intestinal villi caused by the presence of the gluten protein in wheat, barley, rye, spelt, Kamut, and triticale, along with highly contaminated oats. This is an autoimmune disease and not an allergy. Symptoms vary but may include nausea, vomiting, weight loss, failure to thrive (in children), diarrhea, and IBS-like symptoms.

Irritable Bowel Syndrome

Irritable bowel syndrome (IBS) is a chronic condition characterized by a variety of symptoms, including bloating, abdominal pain, and inconsistent bowel behavior that may include diarrhea or constipation or a combination of both. IBS is considered a functional gastrointestinal disorder; in other words, the gastrointestinal system does not function correctly. IBS may affect up to 20% of the population, with twice as many women affected as men. IBS is usually classified into three groups: constipation-predominant (IBS-C), diarrhea-predominant (IBS-D), and alternating, or mixed, diarrhea and constipation IBS (IBS-A).

Whether food hypersensitivity in IBS is due to food allergy or food sensitivities is the subject of much debate. Currently, there is no evidence to indicate that IgE-mediated immune responses to specific food allergens are the cause of IBS. A large number of studies have shown that in patients suffering from IBS, there is an increased presence of mast cells in the small intestine. Mast cells found on the lining of the small intestine, known as mucosal mast cells, contain numerous granules rich in histamine and tryptase. These substances are important for wound healing and defense against pathogens and are also responsible for allergic-type symptoms. Unfortunately, these results have been too inconsistent, due to limitations in diagnostic tools in clinical practice, to suggest that they are due to local hypersensitivity or to food antigens. Other studies have linked IgG-mediated food reactions with IBS, although no correlation between symptom severity and elevated levels of IgG antibodies to specific food antigens has been shown.

Cardiovascular Conditions

IgE-mediated food allergic reactions may lead to symptoms of low blood pressure, such as dizziness, fainting, and loss of consciousness. According to the American Academy of Asthma, Allergy and Immunology, tachycardia (abnormally rapid heartbeat), low blood pressure (hypotension), dizziness, fainting, and loss of consciousness are all immediate symptoms that may develop during an anaphylactic reaction.

Behavioral Conditions

The impact of food hypersensitivity and intolerance on behavior, particularly in children with hyperactive disorders, has been a long-standing topic of debate.

Attention Deficit Hyperactivity Disorder

The main symptoms of attention deficit disorder (ADD) and hyperactivity (ADHD) are reduced attentiveness and concentration, and excessive levels of activity, distractibility, and impulsiveness. Many children learn to manage symptoms or simply outgrow them. Sometimes, however, symptoms may persist through adulthood, making it more difficult for individuals to pursue career opportunities and achieve satisfying social interactions.

The hypothesis that food dyes, along with artificial flavors, preservatives, and naturally occurring salicylates (compounds found in a variety of foods, such as berries, apricots, eggplant, tomatoes, and many others), could trigger symptoms of hyperactivity in children was spearheaded in the 1970s by Dr. Benjamin Feingold, Chief Emeritus of the Department of Allergy at the Kaiser Permanente Medical Center, the joint administrative division for Kaiser Foundation Hospitals and the Permanente Medical Group, in California. Children most likely to respond to elimination of food dyes and additives, such as sodium benzoate, are those with a history of allergic conditions or a family history of atopy or food sensitivity.

Feingold Diet

This diet advocates the elimination of artificial colorings, flavorings, and preservatives, such as sodium benzoate. It also advocates exclusion of salicylates and aspartame. Ironically, some of the foods allowed in the diet actually contain salicylates thanks to outdated information on the amount of salicylates in foods. For example, while bananas used to be considered salicylate-free, they have been found to contain 0.4 mg/kg of salicylic acid.

While anecdotal reports have claimed dramatic improvements in some hyperactive children, evidence from controlled trials showed a "limited positive association" between defined Feingold diets and decreased hyperactivity, and a review of 23 studies that focused on the Feingold diet did not find that dietary modification had any significant effect on behavior.

More recently, a U.S. Food and Drug Administration (FDA) panel concluded that there was no clear indication that food colorings cause hyperactivity among children in the general population and that the evidence was not strong enough to warrant public health warnings about food dyes. The panel did acknowledge, however, that the chemicals can cause problems for some children, including those who already have hyperactivity disorders. Previously, the National Institutes of Health had similarly concluded that food additives do, indeed, affect a small number of children with hyperactive disorders. The general consensus was that more studies are needed to evaluate the safety of color additives.

However, a recent British study of 300 children without ADHD, aged 3, 8, and 9, found significantly more hyperactive behavior after consumption of fruit drinks to which food dyes and sodium benzoate had been added. The researchers concluded that artificial color or a sodium benzoate

Q Do kids with ADHD become more hyperactive if they consume sugar?

A None of the studies conducted to date support the belief that sugar or artificial sweeteners such as aspartame worsen symptoms of hyperactivity. However, foods high in sugar, such as fruit juices, pop, candy, and frozen desserts such as Popsicles and freezies, are also the ones that contain food dyes and preservatives, which have been linked to hyperactivity.

preservative (or both) in the diet resulted in increased hyperactivity in 3-, 8- and 9-year-old children in the general population. Of note is that the amount of artificial color administered daily was quite high — for the group of 3-year-olds, the amount of artificial coloring was roughly equivalent to that found in two 2-ounce (56 g) bags of candy and for the 8- and 9-year-olds the amount equivalent to that found in four bags of candies a day. Also, there was a wide variation in the effects of these additives on the children's behavior.

Autism and Autistic Spectrum Behaviors

"Autism spectrum disorders" (ASD) is a term used to describe a group of developmental disorders, including autism; Asperger syndrome; pervasive developmental disorders; Rett syndrome; and childhood disintegrative disorder.

ASD affects many aspects of emotional and social development. It is common for a child or adult with ASD to have repetitive behavior patterns, resistance to change in routine, and under- or oversensitivity to sensory stimuli. Autistic disorders are commonly managed by behavioral and education techniques. Medical treatment is also available to help manage the hyperactivity, motor coordination problems, anxiety, and epilepsy.

Elimination Diets for ASD and ADHD

Although interest in dietary and biochemical interventions for the treatment of ASD and hyperactivity disorders dates back to the late 19th century, no specific diet is routinely recommended by medical or dietetic professionals as treatment for ASD and ADD/ADHD. Despite evidence to the contrary, however, many parents of children with behavioral disorders, as well as adults with behavioral disorders, continue to undertake dietary approaches, often soon after diagnosis and with very little professional supervision. While there is insufficient evidence to recommend the use of any particular type of diet, the role of a dietitian or other health-care professional, preferably one who specializes in counseling children and adults with hyperactive disorders, is to provide evidence-based information and support when individuals or parents of a child express the desire to try dietary changes.

CHAPTER 3

How Is Food Allergy Diagnosed?

Case Study

Validity

Carol is a 55-year-old teacher. She describes herself as "always having had stomach and digestive issues." She believes that she suffers from food intolerances and, at the advice of a friend, had decided to undergo an IgG ELISA test for food intolerances. The blood test listed 34 foods to which her blood serum had been found to react, including cheese, cow's milk, goat's milk, baker's and brewer's yeast, herbs (such as sage, thyme, and parsley), along with vanilla, paprika, and various fruits and vegetables. She was confused and depressed about how she was going to incorporate these results into her day-to-day living. She asked us to help her interpret these results and affirm their validity. We emphasized that IgG testing was not useful in explaining her symptoms and was unnecessary, but explained that it was valuable to explore her symptoms and take the results in the context of her medical history, along with an analysis of a week-long food and symptom diary.

First, we needed to ensure that there were no outstanding medical issues. We asked her to follow up with her gastroenterologist for a battery of tests, including colonoscopy, endoscopy with small bowel biopsy — to confirm presence or absence of celiac disease — and additional pertinent blood tests. The colonoscopy and endoscopy results revealed no abnormalities and no presence of celiac disease, but blood test results confirmed lactose intolerance. She also reported experiencing symptoms of bloating when consuming wheat-based products.

Based on this information, we proceeded with planning a nutritionally balanced lactose- and wheat-free diet. After 2 weeks on the diet, she reported almost full resolution of symptoms. Follow-up at 6 months revealed that she was managing the lactose-free diet very well and could also occasionally tolerate a slice of bread without ill effects.

Recent analysis evaluating the prevalence of food allergies has shown that up to 35% of individuals who report a reaction to food believe that they are experiencing an allergic reaction. Studies that confirmed food allergies by means of appropriate diagnostic tests suggest a much lower percentage of the population — 3.5% — suffers from true food allergies. In many cases, reactions to foods are not allergic in nature. For example, lactose intolerance causing bloating, diarrhea, and abdominal pain may be confused with an allergy to dairy when, in fact, it is a metabolic disorder; that is, an insufficient amount of the enzyme lactase is available to break down lactose in milk and milk products.

Diagnostic Procedures

- Medical history
- Physical examination
- Nutrition status and habits
- Food and symptom diary
- Elimination diets
- Skin prick test
- Allergen-specific serum IgE test
- Oral food challenges

Medical History and Physical Examination

If you present to your doctor with possible symptoms of food allergy or intolerance, the initial evaluation typically begins with a thorough history and physical examination. This evaluation takes into account what is known as differential diagnosis — that is, consideration of other health conditions, diseases, or disorders that could lead to similar symptoms as those triggered by food allergies. Examples include metabolic disorders (e.g., lactose intolerance), anatomic abnormalities, malignancy, pancreatic insufficiency, and non-immune system reactions to foods and other substances. For example, foods rich in tyramine, such as aged cheese, may be the cause of migraines and allergy-like symptoms in some individuals.

During the physical examination, the physician will be looking for symptoms to support evidence of atopic disease — for example, atopic dermatitis (eczema), allergic rhinitis, and asthma.

Nutrition Status and Habits

To narrow down the source of the allergic response, your doctors will inquire about common suspect foods. These are some of the questions the physician may ask:

- What quantity of food was ingested when symptoms occurred?
- How long after exposure did the symptoms appear?
- Was the reaction immediate (occurring within minutes to a few hours, known as IgE-mediated reactions) or delayed (occurring within several hours to a few days, thought to involve cellular mechanisms)?
- What was the duration of the symptoms?
- What was the severity of symptoms? Various scales from mild to severe may be used to answer this question.
- Can the food ever be eaten without these symptoms occurring?
- How was the food prepared (cooked or raw)?
- What other ingredients were used in food preparation, such as spices, sauces, and seasonings?
- Were other factors present, such as exercise, alcohol consumption, or use of aspirin or nonsteroidal anti-inflammatory drugs (NSAIDs)?

Food and Symptom Diary

At this stage, keeping a food and symptom diary for 1 to 2 weeks may be recommended. The food and symptom diary helps document symptoms and uncovers any trends or relationship between symptoms and food intake that may not be apparent from recall. This record also serves as a baseline for future intervention.

Use this scale to rank the severity of symptoms, from 0 to 5:
0 — None
1 — Mild
2 — Mild to moderate
3 — Moderate
4 — Moderate to severe
5 — Severe

For each meal, record the foods you eat and make notes in your diary before leaving the table so you don't forget the details later on. If symptoms do arise later, be sure to note this.

Meal	What did I eat?	How much?	Describe your symptoms and severity on a scale of 0 to 5
Breakfast	Milk	½ cup (125 mL)	Stomach cramps: 3
Snack			
Lunch			
Snack			
Dinner			
Snack			

Elimination Diets for Identifying Food Intolerances

For those individuals with food intolerances, diagnosis can only be made by means of a combination of clinical history, a food and symptom diary, and diagnostic elimination diets followed by the reintroduction of foods. There are several kinds of elimination diets for food sensitivities or intolerances.

Single-Food Elimination Diet

This type of diet excludes only one allergen (e.g., soy protein) as identified from the individual's food and symptom diary. All food sources containing the chosen allergen and all sources of cross-contamination, including those that may occur during food preparation, must be avoided. The diet may be followed for up to 30 days, followed by reintroduction of the allergen in its simplest form. When testing tolerance for soy protein, for example, you may reintroduce cooked tofu as the first step in the challenge.

Multiple-Food Exclusion Diet

This type of diet involves the exclusion of two or three foods at the same time. The decision regarding which foods to eliminate should be made based on your food and symptom diary along with a list of suspicious foods. This elimination diet may also last for 30 days and should be monitored for nutritional adequacy by an experienced health-care professional, such as a dietitian specializing in the treatment of food allergies and sensitivities.

Few Foods Elimination Diet

This type of diet includes only foods that are known to be hypoallergenic. Only about 10 foods are allowed on this diet (that is, two meats, two grain products, two fruits, two vegetables, and water). Because this diet is considered a semi-starvation diet, it should be followed for a limited time only. Here again, recommendations differ about the length of this exclusion diet and range from 7 to 21 days. If it does not lead to any improvement in symptoms, it should be discontinued immediately.

Laboratory Tests

While effective for detecting food intolerances, elimination diets are not sufficiently rigorous to detect food allergies and cannot be used as the only means of diagnosis. For diagnosing food allergies, the World Allergy Organization states in a position paper that "the final say in terms of diagnosis of all IgE-mediated allergies should rest with the hospital-based allergist." Diagnostic tests for food allergies should be performed by an allergy specialist in a laboratory or clinic equipped to run skin prick tests, allergen-specific serum IgE tests, and oral food challenges.

Laboratory Tests

* Skin prick test (SPT)
* Allergen-specific serum IgE test
* Oral food challenges

Skin Prick Test

A skin prick test (SPT) is one of the most commonly used types of test for diagnosis of allergy. During the test, a drop of extract of each potential allergen is placed on corresponding marks on the skin. Two additional drops are then added to the skin's surface: a negative control, or the fluid used to dilute the allergen extract, and a positive control, usually histamine, used to test the skin's reactivity to histamine. A pricking needle is then used to scratch the surface of the skin — the epidermis — in the middle of the allergen extract. A test will be considered positive when the diameter of the wheal is $1/8$ inch (3 mm) or greater than the negative control. It is the size of the wheals, or flares on the skin, that help the allergist determine the degree and type of allergy.

Because of the difficulty in measuring the size of the wheals, the SPT only indicates the presence of allergen-specific IgE antibodies; it does not necessarily suggest that you are allergic to a particular food. It is important to work with an allergy specialist who can interpret the results in the context of your medical history, physical examination, and food and symptom diary. If you were to conclude that you had a food allergy based on a skin prick test alone, you might end up unnecessarily avoiding that food for life.

Allergen-Specific Serum IgE Test

As the name implies, an allergen-specific serum IgE test is used to measure the amount of IgE antibodies to specific allergens (such as milk, egg, peanut, fish, wheat, or soy) in a blood sample extracted from a patient. Serum IgE levels used to be measured using the radio allergo sorbent test, also known as RAST, but this has now been replaced by the enzyme-linked immunosorbent assay (ELISA), which is much more sensitive and specific. In general, the higher the level of specific IgE antibody, the more likely the individual is to be allergic, but there is no clear cutoff point between being allergic and not.

As with the skin prick test, the allergen-specific IgE test does not predict the severity of the reaction. This test also comes with limitations:

• With food allergies, circulating IgE antibodies may remain undetected, leading to a false negative result. This may be due to the way allergens in the food for which the patient was tested may have been altered by cooking methods, industrial processing, or digestion. The American Academy of Asthma, Allergy and Immunology recommends that in cases where the clinical history is highly suggestive of food allergy, additional investigations, such as a physician-led oral food challenge, is necessary before making the final diagnosis.
• A false positive test may result from cross-reactivity with similar allergens and not the specific allergen tested.

For both tests, the detection of IgE in the skin or blood only indicates that the individual is sensitized to an allergen, not that allergy clinically exists. For this reason, neither of these tests is an absolute indicator of food allergy and neither should be used on its own as a means for diagnosis.

Other skin and blood tests, such as intra-dermal tests and measurement of total serum IgE, are not recommended for the diagnosis of food allergy because insufficient data exist to warrant their use.

Oral Food Challenges

Oral food challenges are used to identify, confirm, or rule out a suspected allergy to foods. The double-blind, placebo-controlled oral food challenge is considered the gold standard for diagnosing food allergy and includes a properly conducted elimination diet followed by oral food challenge with foods suspected of causing allergic reaction (based on the medical history and skin or blood testing results). Food challenges should only be administered under the medical supervision of an allergy specialist in a setting equipped to handle the outcomes of an anaphylactic reaction.

During an oral food challenge, the suspect food is consumed in carefully measured amounts, which are gradually increased. With double-blind, placebo-controlled food challenges, neither the physician nor the patient knows which sample contains the allergen that is being trialed and which contains the placebo (a harmless, non-allergic substance). This is done to ensure the most objective results from both patient and physician — that is, to ensure that whatever reaction the patient is experiencing is the result of ingesting the allergen-containing food and not because of other factors, such as anxiety about coming into contact with the allergen.

During an oral food challenge, the allergy specialist is not trying to trigger a severe allergic reaction. On the contrary, the test is designed to minimize the chance of severe reactions. The patient receives the test food containing the allergen in gradually increasing amounts, starting with a dose that is unlikely to trigger symptoms. If any signs of a reaction appear, the testing stops. In this way, most reactions experienced, such as flushing or hives, are mild, and medication such as antihistamines are available for symptomatic relief. In the rare event that an anaphylactic reaction may occur, epinephrine is available to provide resolution of symptoms.

While very useful and accurate, double-blind, placebo-controlled oral food challenges are time consuming and expensive and, like any other form of oral food challenge, subject the patient to potentially severe allergic reactions. As a result, single-blind or open food challenges are often used instead to screen patients for food allergies.

Food Challenge Procedure

With the single-blind food challenge, the suspect food is disguised so the patient is unaware of the challenge food's contents. This type of challenge helps minimize patient bias during the procedure. With the open food challenge, both the specialist and the patient know the content of the test food being tested. If the results are negative, food allergy may be ruled out. If the results are positive, they may be used to diagnose food allergies in patients with a supportive medical history and laboratory data. These tests should never be performed at home, even if the chance of developing severe symptoms is remote.

Oral Food Challenge Considerations

- When specific IgE test results are positive, eliminating these foods from the diet can result in a resolution of symptoms. In this case, an oral challenge for each food eliminated would be recommended to help increase variety in the diet.

- When elimination of the food in question has not resolved allergic symptoms but the specific food remains highly suspicious, the oral food challenge can help settle the issue.
- When considering reintroduction of a food known to cause acute anaphylaxis, an oral challenge can help determine whether the individual has lost clinical reactivity to the food.
- In the cases of non-IgE-mediated reactions, the oral food challenge may be the only means of diagnosis.

Alternative Tests

If you do not get clear results from blood or skin prick tests, the search for answers to explain your food intolerances can be frustrating. Unfortunately, there are no validated tests to diagnose food intolerances. This remains a gray area of practice in dealing with food hypersensitivity.

Although unproven diagnostic tests are available on the market, their use is viewed with much skepticism because they are costly and divert attention from actual allergies and true food intolerances, thus delaying treatments that offer relief. Often, clients are provided with a long list of foods labeled "highly reactive," "moderately reactive," or "tolerable." Some people have to avoid up to 30 to 40 foods at one time and follow general rotational diets, which lack detail on implementation and are nutritionally incomplete. Food-intolerant individuals are, unfortunately, left without much guidance and knowledge about how to deal with or manage the new "prescribed diet."

Besides the inconvenience and impact on lifestyle and social interactions, people who embark on such elimination diets run the risk of inadequate nourishment. This is why it is so important to consult with your doctor for appropriate monitoring and referral to a qualified dietitian.

Non-Validated Alternative Tests

None of the tests listed below has been proven to be effective at diagnosing food allergies.

- *Cytotoxic testing:* A suspect food allergen is added to a blood sample. The mix is examined under a microscope to check for any white blood activation.
- *Immune complex assay:* A suspect food allergen is added to a blood sample. The mix is examined under a microscope

to check whether antibodies bind to the allergen. This test is invalid because antibodies bind to a variety of food molecules during digestion.

- *Vega testing (electro-dermal screening):* An electrical circuit is created between a machine, the test technician, and the person being tested. The patient holds a negative electrode in one hand and a positive electrode is applied to acupuncture points over fingers or toes. Small amounts of food or environmental allergens are added to the circuit and the machine registers any dips in electrical current as a sign of sensitivity to that substance.
- *Applied kinesiology (muscle testing):* This test relies on energy fields in the body to diagnose allergy and intolerance. The patient is asked to hold a vial containing the food allergen mix and a counterforce is applied to the client's arm or shoulder muscle. If the muscle appears weak, it indicates a sensitivity to the particular food being tested.
- *Hair analysis:* A hair sample is analyzed for vitamin and mineral deficiencies, allergies, or heavy metal toxicity. There is currently no scientific evidence to support this testing method.
- *IgG testing:* This test measures the levels of IgG antibodies in blood. There are tests measuring IgG- and IgG4-type antibodies, which typically develop in all individuals after exposure to food. Their detection in the bloodstream indicates a normal, non-specific response of the immune system to exposure to food and not sensitization. According to the American Academy of Asthma, Allergy and Immunology, IgG and IgG subclass antibody tests for food allergy do not have clinical relevance, are not validated, lack sufficient quality control, and should not be performed.

Prognosis

In general, most infants and young children outgrow or become tolerant of their food hypersensitivities. By following a proper allergen avoidance diet, most allergy symptoms in adults and children eventually resolve. Studies show that approximately one-third of all adults and children lose their clinical reactivity to specific food allergens after 1 to 2 years of proper food allergen avoidance diets. However, patients with peanut, tree nut, or fish and shellfish allergies rarely lose their reactivity.

Part 2

Managing Food Allergies, Intolerances, and Sensitivities

CHAPTER 4
Managing Anaphylaxis

> ## Case Study
>
> ### Crab Attack
>
> *Vanessa was a healthy teenager who had been following a mainly vegetarian diet since the age of 12. On her 18th birthday, her family and friends organized a party at a restaurant and ordered one of her favorite treats: crab cakes. Within minutes of taking her first bite, Vanessa's mouth and tongue began to swell. Her face was flushed and swollen. She complained of itchiness and began to have trouble breathing. One of the restaurant staff responded quickly and called 911 right away. Once the paramedics arrived, they were able to give Vanessa the life-saving medication she needed. As epinephrine was administered by intramuscular injection, Vanessa quickly recovered and was immediately taken to the hospital. After being referred to an allergy specialist, she was diagnosed with anaphylactic reaction to shellfish. Although the experience was traumatic, she is now very conscientious about avoiding all shellfish in her diet, and she always carries two doses of epinephrine that can be administered by auto-injector to treat such attacks in case of emergency.*

The only available treatment for food allergies is to avoid the offending allergen. That sounds relatively simple, but not so. First, you will need to consult with an allergy specialist, who will make the diagnosis. Then you will need to consult with a knowledgeable dietitian to learn how to avoid offending allergens and how to plan a nutritious, balanced diet that makes up for any nutrient losses or imbalances.

Guidelines for Avoiding Allergens

1. Outline *all* the possible sources of the allergen, including foods, hidden food ingredients, and sources of contamination.
2. Become adept at reading labels and identifying obvious and hidden sources of the allergen, including sources of cross-contamination.
3. Choose alternative foods and ingredients that are appropriate while taking into consideration your tolerance for those foods, along with food likes and dislikes.

4. Ensure nutritional adequacy of the diet after offending foods are excluded, to prevent the development of long-term nutritional deficiencies.
5. Learn how to manage food allergies at home, at restaurants, and in other social situations.
6. Find additional ongoing support, including reliable sources of information on the Internet and in print, and consider joining a peer support group.
7. Be prepared for emergency situations brought on by anaphylactic reactions.

Anaphylaxis

If you have a food allergy, you need to have a plan for handling situations if you accidentally ingest a food you are allergic to. Unfortunately, many cases of anaphylactic reactions occur when individuals are caught off guard and are not prepared to handle a severe reaction. Between 40% and 100% of food-induced anaphylactic reactions involve ingestion of catered foods or foods prepared outside the home.

Symptoms of Anaphylaxis

Anaphylaxis is a severe allergic reaction that can involve several body systems and potentially lead to death if untreated. Trace amounts of specific food allergens can trigger very serious anaphylactic reactions, as can allergens combined with exercise. Anaphylactic symptoms include:

- Hives, rashes, swelling
- Itching
- Changes in skin color
- Cold, clammy skin
- Tingling in the mouth
- Fear, panic, sense of doom
- Nausea and/or vomiting
- Diarrhea and/or cramps

- Coughing, wheezing, choking, changes in voice
- Difficulty breathing and/or swallowing
- Dizziness and/or light-headedness
- Loss of consciousness, coma, even death

Emergency Treatment for Anaphylaxis

Symptoms of acute anaphylaxis can include gastrointestinal, skin, respiratory, and cardiovascular reactions, as listed above. These symptoms may be similar to those you have experienced during a previous allergic reaction, or they may be more severe than you have experienced before. Either way, if you believe you are experiencing anaphylaxis, react immediately. Early recognition and treatment with an epinephrine auto-injector (EpiPen or Twinject) can be lifesaving, and using it when it is not really needed will do no harm.

Carry two doses of epinephrine administered by auto-injector with you at all times. As soon as you recognize that you are having a severe allergic reaction, use your auto-injector to give yourself a dose of epinephrine (or ask someone to do this for you). Then call 911.

Always wear a medical alert bracelet or necklace so you can easily communicate with any available person who might know first-aid procedures for anaphylactic allergy. If you are allergic to any medications, your bracelet should also specify this.

Quick Steps for Managing Anaphylactic Reactions
1. Seek medical help immediately.
2. Administer epinephrine using your auto-injector (EpiPen or Twinject) at the first signs of an allergic reaction.
3. Call 911 or your local emergency medical services and tell them that you are having an anaphylactic reaction (or ask someone to do this for you).
4. Give yourself a second dose of epinephrine in 5 to 15 minutes if the reaction continues or gets worse.
5. Go to the nearest hospital right away, ideally by ambulance, even if symptoms are mild or have stopped. The reaction could get worse or come back after using epinephrine. You should stay in the hospital to be observed, generally for about 4 hours.
6. Call your emergency contact person — parent, guardian, spouse.

Epinephrine Facts

Epinephrine is the drug used to treat anaphylaxis. Epinephrine should be administered even if there is uncertainty about the diagnosis. There is no danger in giving epinephrine by intramuscular injection in the recommended dosage. You will feel shaky, and your heart will pound, but this will pass quickly. There are currently two epinephrine auto-injectors available in North America: EpiPen and Twinject. Both products come in two dosages, 0.15 mg and 0.30 mg, and are prescribed according to weight. They should be stored away from extreme temperatures and replaced before the expiration date.

Q If I think I have a food allergy or intolerance to a certain food, should I exclude that food and all others related to it from my diet?

A A number of reactions may occur shortly after consuming a food, and these may be caused by conditions other than a food allergy. Excluding entire food groups without medical advice could lead to serious nutritional deficiencies. Consult with your doctor as soon as possible so that you may be referred to an allergy specialist for appropriate testing and diagnosis.

New Therapies

Although managing food allergies involves avoiding all traces of allergens, some novel therapies suggest promise for increasing tolerance in atopic individuals.

Oral Immunotherapy

In these clinical tests, increasingly higher doses of food allergens are administered during multiple food challenges, over the course of several months, until a maintenance dose is reached. The tests must be carried out in research facilities with all emergency equipment available and proper ethics board approval. This is a promising future treatment for patients with food allergies, but it is still in its experimental stages and is not ready for use in clinical practice.

Targeted Treatments

Although the treatment is fairly recent, clinical trials on the effectiveness of antibodies to IgE are very promising. A recent study reported positive results in a group of children with milk allergies who were treated with a combination of immunotherapy and omalizumab (Xolair), a drug approved for asthma. Nine of 11 children were able to tolerate 1 cup (250 mL) of milk per day after 16 weeks of treatment. Similar results had previously been reported for treatment with an anti-IgE drug in adolescents and adults who were allergic to peanuts. However, some patients have had serious allergic reactions to this treatment, and for this reason, it is only carried out in research facilities properly equipped to deal with emergency reactions that may arise.

CHAPTER 5

The 10 Most Common Allergens

Peanut Allergy

Did You Know?

Legume Tolerance
Peanuts and tree nuts are not botanically related. The peanut belongs to the legume family (peas, beans, and lentils). The majority of individuals with peanut allergy can tolerate other legumes but may develop allergies to other foods.

Peanut allergy accounts for the majority of severe allergic reactions to foods. Many studies have shown that the incidence of peanut allergy has doubled in the past 10 years, and it is now estimated to affect 1.3% to 1.5% of the North American population. Allergic reactions to peanuts frequently occur on the first exposure to the food. It takes as little as $\frac{1}{7000}$ to $\frac{1}{70000}$ of a peanut to trigger a reaction in some individuals. Although once considered a lifelong allergy, recent studies have shown that 20% of children outgrow it by the age of 5.

Association with Tree Nut Allergy

The makeup of a peanut is 26% protein, which contains nine known allergens, Ara h 1 to Ara h 9. Ara h 1 is responsible for the most severe reactions, but everyone with peanut allergy will be sensitized to Ara h 2, which has been found to share common IgE-binding epitopes with almond and Brazil nut allergens, even though they are from different botanical

Q If I have a peanut allergy, should I exclude other legumes from my diet?

A Peanut-allergic individuals are often faced with the question of whether to avoid other legumes, such as soy, lentils, peas, and other members of the Fabaceae family. Laboratory experiments frequently confirm cross-reactivity between peanut and soy, most likely due to similarities in their respective epitopes, those coupling sites that are recognized by IgE antibodies and lead to the onset of allergic reactions.

However, this link does not translate in practice — in fact, a number of studies have failed to confirm that peanut-allergic individuals also react to soy and it has been shown that up to 90% of peanut-allergic individuals can tolerate soy. Avoiding legumes, such as soy, lentils, beans, and peas, is only necessary when allergy to the individual foods has been identified. The only exception is the risk of cross-reaction between peanut and lupine.

Legume Family

Peanuts are a member of the legume family, but not all legumes are allergens.

- Acacia/acacia gum
- Adzuki beans
- Alfalfa
- Black-eyed pea
- Broad bean
- Black turtle bean
- Black-eyed bean
- Carob bean
- Cassia
- Chickpea (garbanzo bean)
- Cowpea
- Fava bean
- Field pea
- Great Northern bean
- Green bean
- Guar gum
- Gum arabic
- Gum talha (derived from *Acacia seyal*)
- Karaya gum
- Kidney bean
- Lentil
- Licorice
- Lima bean
- Locust bean gum
- Lupine bean
- Mung bean
- Navy bean
- Pinto bean
- Soy bean
- Snap bean
- Split pea
- String bean
- Tamarind
- Tragacanth gum
- Urd flour
- Wax bean

Sources of Peanut Allergen

- Peanut kernels
- Peanut protein
- Hydrolyzed peanut protein
- Peanut oil
- Cold-pressed peanut oil
- Peanut butter
- Peanut flour
- Beer nuts
- Arachis oil
- Goober nuts
- Goober peas
- Groundnuts
- Mandelonas
- Monkey nuts
- Nu-Nuts
- Nut meats
- Valencias
- Hydrolyzed vegetable protein

families. This explains why people with peanut allergy are at greater risk — at a rate of 1 in 5 — of also having a tree nut allergy. Having a peanut allergy is clearly associated with developing a tree nut allergy.

Smell

Despite some speculation otherwise, there is no evidence that the smell of a food, such as peanut butter, causes allergic reaction, simply because there is no protein in scent. Peanut-allergic individuals will generally feel uncomfortable or even unwell when smelling peanut butter, but this is due to a strong aversion rather than allergy. Inhalation of airborne peanut

Q Are seeds safe to eat when I have peanut allergy?

A Yes. You should be safe consuming seeds, such as pumpkin, sunflower, sesame, mustard, safflower, and canola, unless you are allergic to them. However, there is a great risk of cross-contamination with peanuts or tree nuts, so any seed product whose ingredient list warns it "may contain" or "may contain traces of" peanuts must be strictly avoided.

particles, however, *can* cause allergic reaction. Particle dust may occur when peanuts are being shelled in large quantities or if many bags are opened at once. Proteins could also be released during cooking, boiling, or processing.

Peanut-Free Diet

The list on pages 68–73 is set up to mimic the organization of a grocery store, with fresh foods arranged around the outside walls and processed foods in the inner aisles. The list is not exhaustive. **Please read the food label every time.**

Foods to Enjoy, Question, and Exclude if You Have a Peanut Allergy

Aisle by Aisle	Foods to Enjoy	Foods to Question	Foods to Exclude
Produce section	• All fresh fruits and vegetables • All pure fruits and fruit juice • Freshly cut ready-to-eat fruits • Freshly cut ready-to-eat vegetables • Packaged salads • Fresh, frozen, and canned fruit juices • Salad dressings and dips made without peanut-derived ingredients, in peanut-free facility	• Dried fruit — ensure no cross-contamination with peanuts • Fruit pie toppings • Salad toppings	• Fruit or vegetable salads with toppings including peanut ingredients • Fruit or vegetable dishes prepared with peanut or undisclosed source of oil • Date rolls • Dried fruit and nut trail mixes

Aisle by Aisle	Foods to Enjoy	Foods to Question	Foods to Exclude
Bakery and crackers	• Homemade breads and baked goods (e.g., doughnuts, muffins, pancakes) prepared without peanut ingredients • Commercial breads (French, Italian, rice, oatmeal, rye, Kamut, whole wheat) made without peanut-derived ingredients, in a peanut-free facility	• Soda crackers • Angel or sponge cake • Pita • Rye crackers and rye crisps • Seasoned croutons • Party wafers • Sesame sticks	• Fruit and nut cakes • Danishes topped with peanuts • Buns topped with peanuts • Muffins containing peanut ingredients (e.g., multiseed and nut muffins) • Baklava (contains a mixture of peanuts and tree nuts) • Doughnuts (even when tree nuts are listed, peanut-based fillers may be added) • Meringues • Breads, biscuits, muffins, pancakes, cakes, and pies made with peanut-derived ingredients • Lavash • Croissants • Cinnamon rolls • Tarts
Dairy/dairy alternatives and eggs section	• All fresh milk, cheese, yogurt, cottage cheese, aged cheese • Coconut milk • Soy beverages • Rice milk • Hemp milk • Oat milk • Potato-based milk • Non-dairy creamers • Vegan margarine • Fresh eggs (boiled, fried, poached)	• Flavored yogurts • Flavored cheese spreads • Flavored coffee whiteners	• Yogurts with muesli topping • Cheese balls covered with peanuts • Dairy foods made with peanut-based ingredients • Egg rolls

Aisle by Aisle	Foods to Enjoy	Foods to Question	Foods to Exclude
Deli section	• All processed deli meats made without peanut-derived ingredients (e.g., chicken breast, turkey breast, ham, salami, prosciutto)	• Sausages • Weiners • Vegetarian deli meats — check for peanut flour/peanut oil • Marinated olives	• All deli products made with undeclared hydrolyzed vegetable protein, oils, or peanuts • Mortadella with nuts
Meat, poultry, and fish section	• All fresh or frozen meat, poultry, fish/seafood • Fish or meat canned in broth, water, or non-peanut oils	• Vegetarian meat substitutes (meatless burgers)	• Meat, poultry, or fish prepared with hydrolyzed vegetable protein — check source • Nut roasts • Foods made with extruded, cold-pressed peanut oil • Fish canned in peanut oil or undisclosed oils
Aisle 1 Breakfast cereals, hot cereal, jam, peanut butter, canned fruit, syrup	• All plain boxed cereal made without peanuts in a peanut-free facility • All plain cooked or ready-to-eat cereal made without peanuts in a peanut-free facility • Plain cream of wheat • Plain oatmeal • All jams, jellies, preserves • All plain canned fruit • Honey • Maple syrup • Pancake syrup • Granola bars made without peanuts in a peanut-free facility	• Cereal bars • Pancake or waffle mixes • Hot chocolate • Mixed hot cereal • Nut and seed butter — ensure no cross-contamination with peanuts • Soy butter — ensure no cross-contamination with peanuts	• Fruit and nut cereal • Honey nut cereal • Granola • Granola bars • Muesli • Protein bars • Nut-flavored oatmeal (banana nut) • Peanut butter–flavored cereal • Peanut butter

Aisle by Aisle	Foods to Enjoy	Foods to Question	Foods to Exclude
Aisle 2 Cookies, confectionery, crackers, potato chips, snacks, popcorn, nuts and seeds, desserts	• Plain popcorn • Plain corn tortilla chips • Rice cakes • Plain candies clearly labeled peanut-free • Plain potato chips • Hard candy • Caramel candy • Plain or flavored gelatins • Homemade cookies, cakes, and pies made without peanut ingredients	• Candy • Pudding • Seasoned potato or corn chips • Roasted seeds — check for risk of cross-contamination • Seasoned rice crackers • Seasoned tortilla chips	• All dry-roasted and oil-roasted peanuts (plain or seasoned) • Trail mix • Peanut butter cookies • Chocolate bars • Brownies • Cookies containing peanuts • Brownies with peanuts • Chocolate-covered peanuts • Trail mix • Turkish delight • Crushed or ground peanut toppings for cakes • Marzipan • Nougat • Nut substitutes • Fudge
Aisle 3 Spices, flour, baking supplies, sugar and other sweeteners	• All pure spices and herbs • All single plain grain flours • Sugar • Molasses • Artificial sweeteners • Fruit glazes	• Herb mixtures • Seasoning mixes • Icing • Baking mixes — ensure no cross-contamination with peanuts	• Seasoning mixes with undisclosed ingredients • Baking mixes containing peanut ingredients

Aisle by Aisle	Foods to Enjoy	Foods to Question	Foods to Exclude
Aisle 4 Oils, vinegars, sauces, salad dressings, condiments	• All vegetable oils except peanut oil • All animal fats • All vinegar products • Mustard, ketchup, soy sauce, relish, pickles • Pickled vegetables (e.g., sauerkraut) • Oil-based salad dressings without peanut oil • Homemade gravy without peanut oil or peanut-derived ingredients • Mayonnaise	• Hot sauce • Gravy • Mole sauce • Salad dressings — check for undeclared or unrefined peanut oil • Dried salad dressings • Seasoning packets with undisclosed ingredients • Vegetables packed in oils — check for undisclosed oil	• Peanut oil • Pesto sauce • Peanut sauce • Satay sauce
Aisle 5 Soup, canned vegetables, pasta, pasta sauce, Mexican rice and other side dishes	• Homemade, prepared, canned, or refrigerated soups made without peanut-derived ingredients • Pasta sauce made without peanut-derived ingredients • Bruschetta • Salsa • Plain macaroni and other pasta • Plain rice or mixed rice • Guacamole • All plain dried canned beans, peas, and lentils (as tolerated) • Plain whole grains (e.g., quinoa, barley, millet)	• Spaghetti sauce • Chili sauce • Seasoned rice pilaf	• Dried soups • Canned chili • Vietnamese meals (often with crushed peanut topping) • Spring rolls • Satay • Thai meals (e.g., curries) • Chinese meals (especially Schezuan) • Mexican meals (e.g., enchiladas) • Indonesian meals • Malaysian meals • Indian meals (e.g., curry with peanut protein) • Nutted seasoned couscous

Aisle by Aisle	Foods to Enjoy	Foods to Question	Foods to Exclude
Aisle 6 Water, soft drinks, sport drinks, fruit juices, alcoholic beverages	• Coffee, tea, decaffeinated coffee • Carbonated beverages • All milks • Cocoa • Water, flavored water • Fresh fruit juices • Shelf-stable juices • Soft drinks • Alcoholic beverages		• Peanut punch
Aisle 7 Frozen fruits and vegetables, frozen meals and desserts	• Plain frozen fruits and vegetables • Sorbet or sherbet manufactured in a peanut-free facility • Frozen yogurt made without peanuts in a peanut-free facility	• Ice creams from parlors — cross-contact occurs with shared scoops • Frozen waffles • Frozen pancakes • Frozen french fries • Frozen scalloped potatoes • Frozen entrées • Frozen muffins	• Ice creams flavored with peanuts • Frozen yogurts flavored with peanuts • Frozen meals made with peanut sauce or peanut-derived ingredients
Other		• Cosmetics • Sunscreen • Craft materials • Medications • Pet food • Vitamins • Mushroom growing medium • Stuffing in toys	• Ant baits • Bird feed • Mouse traps

What's in a Kiss?

Kissing someone who has just consumed peanuts or peanut products may give enough exposure to trigger an allergic reaction. While it may be uncomfortable to address these issues in the early stages of a relationship, it is extremely important to discuss your allergy with your partner to avoid the threat of anaphylaxis.

Tree Nut Allergy

Tree nut allergies affect about 1.8 million Americans. In Canada, a recent survey indicated the prevalence of perceived tree nut allergy at 1.2%. Tree nut allergies vary along geographical lines: walnut, almond, and pecan allergy are commonly seen in North America, whereas Brazil nut, almond, and pecan allergy seem to be more common in the United Kingdom. In Australia, cashew nut allergy is most commonly seen in infants, followed by hazelnut and walnut allergy.

Association with Oral Allergy Syndrome

Tree nut allergies, especially to hazelnuts, are also often seen in patients suffering from oral allergy syndrome. Hazelnuts, when eaten along with peaches, apples, melons, and kiwi, cross-react with pollen from the plane tree. It is extremely important that the diagnosis of true allergy be confirmed, as it can be easily confounded with symptoms of oral allergy syndrome.

Cross-Reactivity Among Tree Nuts
- Cashews and pistachios are highly cross-reactive
- Walnuts and pecans are highly cross-reactive

Tree Nut–Free Diet

The list on pages 75–79 is set up to mimic the organization of a grocery store, with fresh foods arranged around the outside walls and processed foods in the inner aisles. The list is not exhaustive. **Please read the food label every time.**

Common Tree Nuts

- Almonds
- Brazil nuts
- Cashews (anacardium nuts)
- Chestnuts
- Hazelnuts (filberts, cob nuts)
- Macadamia nuts (Queensland nut, candle nuts)
- Pecans

- Pine nuts (pignoli or pignolia nuts, piñon nuts)
- Pistachio nuts
- Walnuts

Tree nuts found in other foods and as food ingredients:

- Beechnuts
- Butternuts
- Hickory nuts
- Mixed nuts
- Nut butters
- Nut oils
- Praline

Foods to Enjoy, Question, and Exclude if You Have a Tree Nut Allergy

Aisle by Aisle	Foods to Enjoy	Foods to Question	Foods to Exclude
Produce section	• All fresh fruits and vegetables • All pure fruits and fruit juice • Fresh, frozen, or canned fruit juices • Freshly cut ready-to-eat fruits • Freshly cut ready-to-eat vegetables • Water chestnuts • Packaged salads	• Dried fruits — check for cross-contamination with tree nuts	• Fruit and nut mixes • Date rolls • Fruit pie toppings containing tree nuts • Salad toppings containing tree nuts • Dried fruit and nut trail mixes
Bakery and crackers	• Homemade breads and baked goods (e.g., doughnuts, muffins, pancakes) prepared without tree nut ingredients • Commercial breads (French, Italian, rice, rye, Kamut, whole wheat) made without tree nut–derived ingredients, in a nut-free facility • Soda crackers • Rye crackers and rye crisps • Lavash • Meringues	• Pastries • Seasoned croutons • Seasoned crackers • Angel or sponge cake • Party wafers	• Almond croissants • Brownies • Fruit and nut cakes • Cakes • Sweet rolls • Fruit and nut or morning glory muffins containing tree nuts • Breads, biscuits, pancakes, and pies made with tree nut ingredients • Nut and grain crackers

Aisle by Aisle	Foods to Enjoy	Foods to Question	Foods to Exclude
Dairy/dairy alternatives and eggs section	• All fresh milk, cheese, yogurt, cottage cheese, aged cheese • Coconut milk • Soy beverages • Rice milk • Hemp milk • Oat milk • Potato-based milk • Non-dairy creamers • Vegan margarine • Fresh eggs (boiled, fried, poached) • Liquid egg product	• Cheese spreads • Flavored yogurts • Nut-flavored coffee whiteners	• Yogurts with muesli mix • Almond milk • Cheese balls covered with tree nuts • Dairy foods made with tree nut–derived ingredients
Deli section	• All processed deli meats made without tree nut–based ingredients (e.g., chicken breast, turkey breast, ham)	• Seasoned hummus with pine nuts • Marinated olives • Cheese complements or jelly	• Mortadella (may contain pistachios) • Olives stuffed with tree nuts • All deli products made with undeclared tree nut–derived ingredients
Meat, poultry, and fish section	• All fresh or frozen meat, poultry, fish and seafood		• Nut roast • Fish canned in undisclosed oil
Aisle 1 Breakfast cereals, hot cereal, jam, peanut butter, canned fruit, syrup	• All plain boxed cereals, cooked or ready-to-eat cereals, grain flours, and starches made without tree nuts in a nut-free facility • All plain canned fruit • All jams, jellies, preserves • All plain canned fruit • Honey • Maple syrup • Pancake syrup	• Seed butters — ensure no cross-contamination with tree nuts • Soy butter — ensure no cross-contamination with tree nuts • Cereal bars • Pancake or waffle mixes • Hot chocolate • Mixed hot cereal	• Honey nut cereals • Fruit and nut cereals • Granola bars • Muesli • Nut butters (e.g., cashew, hazelnut) • Chocolate hazelnut spread (e.g., Nutella) • Hot cereal with tree nut ingredients

Aisle by Aisle	Foods to Enjoy	Foods to Question	Foods to Exclude
Aisle 2 Cookies, confectionery, crackers, potato chips, snacks, popcorn, nuts and seeds, desserts	• Plain popcorn • Plain corn tortilla chips • Rice crackers • Rice cakes • Plain candies clearly labeled nut-free • Plain potato chips • Hard candy • Plain or flavored gelatins • Homemade cookies, cakes, and pies made without tree nut ingredients	• Chocolate bars • Candy • Seasoned rice crackers • Seasoned potato or corn chips • Roasted seeds — ensure no cross-contamination with tree nuts	• Plain or seasoned roasted tree nuts • Brownies • Chocolate bars • Cookies made with tree nut ingredients • Callison (marzipan-like candy) • Giandula (chocolate blended with hazelnuts) • Nougat • Marzipan • Pralines • Trail mix • Turkish delight • Almond popcorn • Fudge
Aisle 3 Spices, flour, baking supplies, sugar and other sweeteners	• All pure spices and herbs • All single plain grain flours • Sugar • Molasses • Artificial sweeteners	• Imitation/artificial flavoring • Seasoning mixes • Herb mixtures • Baking mixes — ensure no cross-contamination with tree nuts	• Pure almond essence • Pure almond extract • Almond paste • Black walnut hull extract (flavoring) • Natural nut extract • Walnut hull extract • Natural wintergreen extract • Baking mixes containing tree nut ingredients

Aisle by Aisle	Foods to Enjoy	Foods to Question	Foods to Exclude
Aisle 4 Oils, vinegars, sauces, salad dressings, condiments	• All vegetable oils except tree nut oils • All animal fats • All vinegar products • Mustard, ketchup, soy sauce, relish, pickles • Pickled vegetables (e.g., sauerkraut) • Oil-based salad dressings made without tree nut oil • Homemade gravy without tree nut oil • Mayonnaise	• Barbecue sauce • Gravy • Salad dressings — check for undeclared tree nut ingredients • Dried salad dressings • Vegetables packed in oil — check for undisclosed oil	• Almond oil • Pesto sauce • Nut oils (cold-pressed)
Aisle 5 Soup, canned vegetables, pasta, pasta sauce, Mexican rice and other side dishes	• Homemade, prepared, canned, or refrigerated soups made without tree nut ingredients • Pasta sauce made without tree nut ingredients • Salsa • All plain dried or canned beans, peas, lentils • Plain macaroni and other pasta • Plain rice or mixed rice • Guacamole • Plain whole grains (e.g., quinoa, barley, millet)	• Seasoned rice pilaf — may contain nuts • Canned chili • Pasta sauce with tree nut ingredients (e.g., tomato pesto)	• Thai dishes (e.g., pad Thai) • Vietnamese dishes • Indonesian dishes • Nutted couscous • Trout amandine
Aisle 6 Water, soft drinks, sport drinks, fruit juices, alcoholic beverages	• All fruit juices and shelf-stable juices • Regular coffee and tea • Water, flavored water • Soft drinks • Alcoholic beverages made without tree nut ingredients		• Flavored specialty coffee containing almond or hazelnut flavor • Nut-flavored liqueurs (e.g., Amaretto, Frangelico) • Nut distillates/alcoholic extracts

Aisle by Aisle	Foods to Enjoy	Foods to Question	Foods to Exclude
Aisle 7 Frozen fruits and vegetables, frozen meals and desserts	• All plain frozen fruits and vegetables • Sorbet or sherbet manufactured in a tree nut–free facility • Fruit ice • Frozen yogurt made without tree nuts in a tree nut–free facility	• Ice cream from parlors — cross-contact occurs with shared scoops • Frozen pancakes • Frozen waffles • Frozen french fries • Frozen scalloped potatoes • Frozen muffins	• Ice cream or frozen yogurt flavored with hazelnuts, almonds, or other tree nuts (e.g., maple walnut) • Frozen meals containing tree nuts • Frozen muffins containing tree nut topping
Other		• Face creams • Body creams • Shampoo • Sunscreen • Suntan lotion	• Bath oils containing tree nuts • Lotions made with tree nut oils • Soaps containing tree nut oil

Nutritional Profile of Peanuts, Tree Nuts, and Substitutes

Peanuts and tree nuts are often thought of as nutritional powerhouses, delivering heart-healthy nutrients, such as fiber and mono- and polyunsaturated fats, that can help lower cholesterol levels. Peanuts, as legumes, are good sources of folate and, together with other nuts, they are excellent sources of niacin, vitamin B_6, pantothenic acid (vitamin B_5), vitamin E, magnesium, manganese, and chromium. Nuts are also a concentrated source of calories and should not constitute a major source of caloric intake.

Excluding nuts from the diet should not lead to any significant nutrient deficiencies, although if you are following a strict vegan diet, you may depend on nuts and seeds for high-quality protein and other nutrients. For this group, a thorough evaluation of alternative nutrient intake is strongly advised.

Did You Know?

Cross-Contamination
The high risk of cross-contamination between peanuts and tree nuts during the food manufacturing process warrants strict monitoring and, in some cases, complete avoidance of peanuts and tree nuts.

Alternative Sources of Nutrients

Nutrient	Alternative Food Sources
High-quality protein	Milk and milk products, meat, fish, poultry, legumes (as tolerated)
Folate	Fortified wheat flour, fortified pasta, bread, spinach, broccoli, dark green leafy vegetables
Niacin	Beef, pork, fortified flour, eggs, milk
Pantothenic acid	Chicken, beef, potatoes, tomato products, yeast, egg yolk, broccoli, whole grains
Vitamin E	Plant oils (except peanut and tree nut oils), meat, poultry, dairy
Magnesium	Dark green leafy vegetables, grains, milk and milk products, red meat
Manganese	Green vegetables, cereals, whole grains
Chromium	Whole grains, legumes (as tolerated), spices

Fish, Shellfish, and Crustacean Allergy

Seafood allergy has been increasing around the world, mostly due to increased consumption. The three largest consumers of fish and shellfish are China, Japan, and the United States. Indeed, a survey of anaphylactic events in the United States reported that shellfish were the most frequently implicated food in persons ages 6 years and older.

Crustacean and shellfish allergies commonly affect adults rather than young children. In fact, approximately 60% of people with this type of seafood allergy and 40% of those with allergy to fish had their first allergic experience as an adult. Children are most often affected in countries where fish is a dietary staple.

The major allergenic protein responsible for reactions to seafood (mostly crustaceans and shellfish) is the muscle protein tropomyosin. Interestingly, similar amino acid sequences have also been found in mites, such as house dust mites, and cockroaches, which may explain why patients allergic to seafood are frequently reported to also have allergic reactions to mites and insects.

Kinds of Seafood

To understand seafood allergy, we need to distinguish between the different categories of seafood:

- *Fish:* vertebrate animals with gills and fins that live entirely in water. They are grouped into three major classes: jawless fish, cartilaginous fish, and bony fish.
- *Shellfish (mollusks):* clams, mussels, oysters, scallops, and various types of octopus, snails, and squid.
- *Crustaceans:* aquatic animals with jointed legs, a hard shell, and no backbone; includes crab, crayfish, lobster, prawns, and shrimp.

Food ingredients classified as or containing fish and shellfish:

- *Fish:* anchovy, basa, bass, bluefish, bream, carp, catfish (channel cat, mudcat), char, chub, cisco, cod, eel, flounder, grouper, haddock, hake, halibut, herring, mackerel, mahi-mahi, marlin, monkfish (angler fish, lotte), orange roughy, perch, pickerel (dore, walleye), pike, plaice, pollock, pompano, porgy, rockfish, salmon, sardine, shark, smelt, snapper, sole, sturgeon, swordfish, tilapia (St. Peter's fish), trout, tuna (albacore, bonito), turbot, whitefish, whiting.
- *Shellfish:* abalone, clam, cockle, conch, limpet, mussel, octopus, oyster, periwinkle, quahaug, scallop, land and sea snail (escargot), squid (calamari), whelk.
- *Crustaceans:* crab, crayfish (crawfish, écrevisse), lobster (langouste, langoustine, coral, tomalley), prawn, shrimp (crevette).

Other forms of seafood protein:

- Unfertilized fish eggs, also known as caviar or roe.
- Imitation crab and lobster meat, also known as kamboko or surimi.
- Salted carp roe in sushi and tarama.
- Gelatin derived from fish and used as an ingredient in food products.

Did You Know?

Histamine Poisoning
When some species of fish start decomposing, dangerous levels of histamine start being produced, which may lead to a reaction called histamine poisoning. The symptoms are similar to those of allergy — development of a rash, nausea, vomiting, diarrhea, headache, dizziness, burning throat, stomach pain, itchy skin, or tingling — but the mechanism is different. If you experience these symptoms immediately after consuming fish, seek emergency medical treatment.

Q I have an allergy to fish. Is it safe to take omega-3 fish oils?

A Most fish oils on the market are highly refined, which means they are free of protein residues. However, if you have a severe allergic reaction to fish, you will need to consult with your allergy specialist before consuming any products containing fish-derived omega-3 fatty acids. In this case, you may be advised to avoid all varieties of fish-derived oils or omega-3 supplements. Also contact the manufacturer to inquire about the extraction and purification process and whether they can guarantee the purity and quality of their product.

Examples of fish oils include:

- Omega-3 fatty acid supplements
- Cod liver oil
- Halibut liver oil
- Salmon oil
- Menhaden oil

Alternatively, you may find other ways to supplement your intake of omega-3 fatty acids from flax seeds, chia seeds, walnuts, and canola and soy oils. These contain ALA (alpha-linolenic acid), of which only a small amount converts to the more beneficial DHA (docohexanoic acid) and EPA (eicosapentaenoic acid). Algae oils are a vegetarian source of DHA.

Q I have an allergy to shellfish and I ordered a vegetable stir-fry at a restaurant. I still experienced a reaction. How come?

A Airborne fish or shellfish particles, such as those produced from frying fish in a pan, steaming lobster in a pot, or even touching fish, have been reported to trigger an allergic reaction.

Seafood-Free Diet

The list on pages 83–87 is set up to mimic the organization of a grocery store, with fresh foods arranged around the outside walls and processed foods in the inner aisles. The list is not exhaustive. **Please read the food label every time.**

Foods to Enjoy, Question, and Exclude if You Have a Seafood Allergy

Aisle by Aisle	Foods to Enjoy	Foods to Question	Foods to Exclude
Produce section	• All fresh fruits and vegetables • All pure fruits and fruit juice • Freshly cut ready-to-eat fruits • Freshly cut ready-to-eat vegetables • Packaged salads • Fresh, frozen, or canned fruit juices	• Fruits or vegetable dishes prepared with gelatin (check source of the gelatin) • Fruit wax coatings — check for the use of chitosan (derived from crustaceans)	• Salad dressings containing anchovies (fish) • Vegetable dips containing anchovies (fish)
Bakery and crackers	• Homemade breads and baked goods (doughnuts, muffins, pancakes) • Commercial breads made from all grains (e.g., French, Italian, rice, oatmeal, rye, Kamut, whole wheat) • Soda crackers • Rye crackers and rye crisps • Lavash • Angel or sponge cake • Fudge • Meringues	• Baked goods (check for use and source of gelatin) • Asian-style crackers (check for fish- or seafood-derived flavoring)	• Caesar-style croutons • Caesar- or ranch-style crackers

Aisle by Aisle	Foods to Enjoy	Foods to Question	Foods to Exclude
Dairy/dairy alternatives and eggs section	• All fresh milk, aged cheese • Coconut milk • Soy beverages • Rice milk • Nut milks (e.g., almond milk) • Potato-based milk • Hemp milk • Non-dairy creamers • Vegan margarine • Fresh eggs (boiled, fried, poached) • Omega-3 eggs • Plain or seasoned egg white product	• Yogurt (check for the use and source of gelatin) • Sour cream (check for the use and source of gelatin) • Cottage cheese (check for the use and source of gelatin) • Margarines fortified with omega-3 fatty acids (check source of omega-3 fats) • Mousse (check source of gelatin) • Soy milk fortified with omega-3 fatty acids (check the source of omega-3 fat)	• Liquid egg product fortified with fish oil (e.g., omega-3 liquid eggs) • Fish-flavored cream cheese (smoked salmon)
Deli section	• All processed deli meats made without fish- or seafood-derived ingredients	• Bologna • Hot dogs • Wieners	• Imitation crab meat • Seafood salad • Tuna salad • Gefilte fish
Meat, poultry, and fish section	• All fresh or frozen meat, poultry		• All fresh or frozen fish and seafood • Smoked fish • Fish mixtures • Seafood salads • Surimi • Caviar • Roe • Sushi • Sashimi • Tempura • Fresh, ready-to-eat fish chowder • Canned seafood (tuna, salmon, sardines, crab) • Mussels, clams, escargot

Aisle by Aisle	Foods to Enjoy	Foods to Question	Foods to Exclude
Aisle 1 Breakfast cereals, hot cereal, jam, peanut butter, canned fruit, syrup	• All plain boxed cereal, grains flours, starches • All plain cooked or ready-to-eat cereals • Peanut or nut or seed butters • All plain canned fruit • All plain jams, jellies • Fruit preserves • Honey • Maple syrup • Pancake syrup	• Fruit snacks (check for the use and source of gelatin)	
Aisle 2 Cookies, confectionery, crackers, potato chips, snacks, popcorn, nuts and seeds, desserts	• Plain popcorn • Plain corn tortilla chips • Rice crackers • Rice cakes • Plain potato chips • Plain nuts and seeds • Hard candy • Caramel candy • Pudding • Custard	• Seasoned crackers (teriyaki flavor, Asian-style) • Seasoned nuts and seeds • Plain or flavored gelatin • Marshmallows (check source of gelatin) • Candy bars (check for the use and source of gelatin)	• Taro cake • Daikon cake • Prawn or shrimp chips • Cuttlefish seaweed snack • Seasoned dried fish and/or meat crackers
Aisle 3 Spices, flour, baking supplies, sugar and other sweeteners	• All pure spices and herbs • All pure grain flours • Sugar • Molasses • Artificial sweeteners • Baking mixes • Icings • Glazes • Fruit pie fillings		

Aisle by Aisle	Foods to Enjoy	Foods to Question	Foods to Exclude
Aisle 4 Oils, vinegars, sauces, salad dressings, condiments	• All vegetable oils • All animal fats • All vinegar products • Mustard • Ketchup • Soy sauce • Relish • Pickles • Hot sauce • Oil-based salad dressings made without fish ingredients (e.g., anchovies) • Mayonnaise	• Antipasto spreads • Pizza toppings • Salad dressing — check for the presence of fish- or seafood-derived ingredients, such as anchovies (e.g., Caesar salad dressings) • Steak sauce • Chili sauce • Barbecue sauce (may contain anchovy paste)	• Fish sauce • XO sauce • Oyster sauce • Anchovy paste • Kamaboko (imitation crab or lobster meat) • Caponata (Sicilian relish) • Caviar • Roe • Tarama (salted carp roe) • Taramasalata spread (fish roe salad) • Worcestershire sauce • Satay sauce
Aisle 5 Soup, canned vegetables, pasta, pasta sauce, Mexican rice and other side dishes	• Homemade or packaged soups without seafood-derived ingredients • All plain dried or canned beans, peas and lentils • Salsa • Guacamole • Plain rice or mixed rice • Plain macaroni and other pasta • Plain whole grains (e.g., quinoa, barley, millet)	• Fried foods (check for contamination in frying oil) • Tomato- or cream-based pasta sauce (check for fish- or seafood-derived ingredients) • Congee (check for seasoning with fish or seafood ingredients)	• Paella, fried rice • Gumbo • Kedgeree • Spring rolls • Fish soup or broth • Fish and shrimp balls • Nuoc mâm (fish sauce) • Bouillabaisse • Seafood chowder • Putanesca or Neapolitan tomato sauce (contains anchovies) • Shrimp noodles • Thai dishes using fish- or seafood-derived ingredients • Chinese dishes using fish- or seafood-derived ingredients • Vietnamese dishes • Japanese dishes • Shrimp salad roll • Sui mai (pork and shrimp dumplings)

Aisle by Aisle	Foods to Enjoy	Foods to Question	Foods to Exclude
Aisle 6 Water, soft drinks, sport drinks, fruit juices, alcoholic beverages	• Coffee, tea, decaffeinated coffee • Carbonated beverages • All milks • Cocoa • Water, flavored water • Fresh fruit juices • Shelf-stable juices • Soft drinks	• Wine, beer, whisky (check for the use of fish-derived fining agent)	• Orange juice fortified with fish oil (omega-3 orange juice) • Fruit juice fortified with fish oil
Aisle 7 Frozen fruits and vegetables, frozen meals and desserts	• All plain frozen fruits, vegetables, or mixed vegetables • Waffles • Pancakes • All frozen meals made without seafood-derived ingredients • Ice cream • Frozen yogurt • Sorbet	• Frozen cakes (check for the use and source of gelatin) • Sherbet (check source of gelatin)	• Frozen appetizers containing fish and seafood • Frozen seafood dumplings • Frozen breaded fish sticks • Frozen meals made with seafood (e.g., fried fillet of sole)
Other		• Glucosamine supplements • Vitamin and mineral supplements (check for the use and source of gelatin) • Lip balm • Lip gloss • Pet food • Compost or fertilizer	• Fish food

Omega-3-Fortified Foods

Omega-3 fatty acids are known as essential fatty acids because the body cannot produce them, so they must be derived from our diet. They are best known for their cardiovascular benefits and are being added to many food products because they may reduce the risk of heart disease. All fish contain at least some omega-3 fatty acids, including EPA (eicosapentanoic acid) and DHA (docohexaenoic acid). If you have an allergy to fish, reading the label should uncover the source of omega-3 fatty acids. If you cannot find information about the source of omega-3 fatty acids, call the manufacturer.

Sources of omega-3 fatty acids used to fortify foods:

- *Flax seeds:* Flax seeds are rich in ALA (alpha-linolenic acid), which the body converts to EPA and DHA fatty acids. Examples of foods containing omega-3 fatty acids derived from flax seeds are omega-3 eggs and some brands of omega-3-fortified yogurt and milk.
- *Fish oil (menhaden oil):* This oil is added directly to the product. Examples of foods containing omega-3 fatty acids derived from fish oil are liquid egg products and fortified orange juice. These products are not safe for those with allergy to fish.
- *Krill oil:* This oil is derived from krill, a type of crustacean. Products fortified with krill oil are not safe for those with allergy to seafood.
- *Algal DHA:* This is DHA derived from algae. Examples of foods containing algal DHA are fortified soy milk and some brands of omega-3-fortified yogurt and infant formulas.

Nutritional Profile of Fish, Shellfish, and Crustaceans and Substitutes

Fish and shellfish deliver high-quality protein. Most notably, fatty fish are known as a rich source of fat-soluble vitamins, such as vitamin A and vitamin D, along with heart-healthy omega-3 polyunsaturated fatty acids. Fish muscle contains a variety of minerals, including iodine. And fish bones (such as those found in sardines and canned salmon) are a good source of calcium, phosphorus, and fluoride.

Nutrient	Alternative Food Sources
High-quality protein	Milk and milk products, meat, poultry, legumes
Omega-3 fatty acids	Flax seeds, chia seeds, pumpkin seeds, sunflower seeds, sesame seeds, tree nuts (e.g., almonds, hazelnuts, Brazil nuts), dark green leafy vegetables, beans
Niacin (Vitamin B_3)	Beef, pork, fortified flour, eggs, dairy
Vitamin B_6	Chicken, beef liver, pork, eggs, milk, wheat germ, brewer's yeast, brown rice, soybeans, oats, peanuts, walnuts
Vitamin B_{12}	Meat (lean ground beef), dairy (cottage cheese, yogurt), fortified non-dairy milks, eggs
Vitamin E	Plant oils (soy, corn, and olive), meat, poultry, dairy products
Calcium	Milk and milk products, fortified soy products, dark green leafy vegetables, tree nuts (e.g., almonds, hazelnuts, Brazil nuts)
Phosphorus	Red meats, dairy products, poultry, whole grains (including gluten-free grains)
Selenium	Eggs, Brazil nuts, sunflower seeds, whole grains (e.g., barley, brown rice, oats)

Milk Allergy and Lactose Intolerance

Milk allergy develops as a result of an IgE- or non-IgE-mediated hypersensitivity reaction of the immune system to one or more proteins in cow's milk. Cow's milk protein allergy (CMPA) typically develops in the first year of life in both exclusively and partially breastfed babies when cow's milk protein is introduced into the feeding regimen either through breast milk or cow's milk–based formula. The overall estimated prevalence of CMPA in young children is 2% to 3%.

Casein and Whey

Cow's milk protein is composed of two large fractions: casein (80%) and whey (20%). In turn, casein consists of five protein fractions (αs1-, αs2-, β-, κ-, and γ-casein), and whey fractions contain two large proteins called α-lactalbumin and β-lactoglobulin. The specific allergen potency of each fraction remains unclear, but it is well established that both casein and whey components trigger significant reaction in atopic individuals.

Milk Proteins

Protein	Concentration in Cow's Milk (mg/mL)
α_{s1}-casein	11.6
β-casein	9.6
κ-casein	3.6
α_{s2}-casein	3.0
β-lactoglobulin	3.0
γ-casein	1.6
α-lactalbumin	1.2
Immunoglobulins	0.6
Serum albumin	0.4
Lactoferrin	0.3
Lyzozyme	Trace

Keep in mind that research performed on other mammalian milks, such as sheep, goat, water buffalo, and horse, have similar protein structures to those found in cow's milk. For this reason, they are not suitable as alternatives for individuals with cow's milk protein allergy.

Onset

Symptoms of CMPA can occur within minutes or hours of contact with milk and can range from mild to severe. In a selected group of 100 children with CMPA, with a mean age of 16 months, 27% developed symptoms within 45 minutes of ingesting cow's milk protein. This would represent an IgE-mediated response, and the symptoms included urticaria (itching) and angioedema (swelling). About half the children in this group showed paleness and gastrointestinal symptoms (vomiting and diarrhea) between 45 minutes and 20 hours after ingestion. The final 20% developed atopic dermatitis (eczema) after more than 20 hours and up to several days after the ingestion of milk. This latter reaction would represent a non-mediated-IgE reaction. Note that some estimates of the percentage of children displaying early or late reaction, or positive or negative for IgE, may vary depending on the criteria for selection of study subjects.

Lactose Intolerance

Lactose intolerance is the condition that results from the body's inability to break down and absorb the milk sugar called lactose. Lactose is a disaccharide, meaning it is a larger sugar made up of two smaller sugars called monosaccharides. The agent responsible for splitting lactose into its individual components and making them available for absorption into the body is the enzyme lactase, which resides in the microvilli of intestinal cells.

When lactose cannot be properly broken down into its individual components, it remains in the intestine undigested, attracting water and causing bloating, abdominal discomfort, and diarrhea — the main symptoms of lactose intolerance. The lactose also becomes food for intestinal bacteria residing in the colon, which multiply and produce irritating acid and gas, further contributing to the discomfort and diarrhea. Symptoms typically occur 30 minutes to 2 hours after consuming milk, dairy products, or meals prepared with these ingredients.

Causes of Lactase Deficiency

When lactose intolerance develops, three causes are usually explored:

1. *Primary lactase deficiency:* This is the most common cause of lactase deficiency, affecting as many as 75% of adults throughout the world. As we age, there is a natural decline in the amount of lactase enzyme available to break down lactose, causing decreased tolerance of dairy products. This natural decline is genetically determined and occurs at different rates in different ethnic groups. In fact, the frequency of primary lactase deficiency can range from as little as 5% in Scandinavian and northern European populations to as much as 90% in groups of African, Jewish, or Asian descent. In North American adults, the prevalence rate follows a similar pattern depending on their ethnic origin.

2. *Secondary lactase deficiency:* This is usually environmentally induced and temporary in nature, meaning that individuals can usually recover and slowly regain the ability to tolerate milk and dairy products. This type of lactase deficiency

Did You Know?

Outgrowing Milk Allergy

Fortunately, most children eventually "outgrow" this allergy, but in severe cases, it may persist, depending on the child's age and the concentration of specific IgE antibodies at the time of diagnosis. In adults, however, IgE-mediated CMPA is very rare. It is estimated that only 0.7% of adults with other allergies have a positive skin prick test to cow's milk protein. The most common reactions in adulthood are non-immune-mediated, with a small percentage of adults reporting abdominal bloating, pain, and diarrhea.

Did You Know?

Cross-Contamination at the Deli Counter

While some deli meats may not contain any milk or milk ingredients, they may become contaminated while being sliced at the deli counter if meat slicers are used for both cheese and deli products.

results from injury to the small intestine caused by certain types of medical treatments, such as chemotherapy, or it may occur because of gastrointestinal infections or inflammatory bowel disease, such as Crohn's disease. Celiac disease is another cause of secondary lactase deficiency. Once the disease or injury resolves, lactase reappears on the surface of the intestinal mucosa and proper lactose digestion resumes.

3. *Congenital lactase deficiency:* This type of lactase deficiency occurs because of a congenital absence (absence from birth) of lactase due to a mutation in the gene that is responsible for producing it. This is a very rare but severe case of lactose intolerance and the symptoms begin shortly after birth.

Excluding Cow's Milk

Individuals with a known allergy to cow's milk protein need to exclude the following foods from their diet:

Did You Know?

Nisin

Nisin is a food preservative derived by fermentation using active bacterial cultures. Beware — it may contain residual milk protein.

- All milk and milk-containing foods, including liquid and evaporated milks
  - Whole or homogenized (3.8%), 2%, 1%, or skim milk
  - Acidophilus milk
  - Chocolate milk or other flavored milks
  - Lactaid/Lacteeze milk
  - Malted milk
  - Condensed milk
  - Evaporated milk
  - Light (5%), half-and-half (10%), table (18%), or heavy or whipping (35%) cream
  - Sour cream
  - Yogurt
- All forms of fermented milks (yogurt, kefir, kumiss, buttermilk)
- All cheeses
  - Hard aged cheese

- Cottage cheese
- Cream cheese
- Cheese curds
- Feta cheese
- Mascarpone
- Processed cheese
- Quark
- Ricotta
- Cultured soft cheese (blue cheese, Brie, Stilton, Oka, Camembert)
- Butter
- Clarified butter (ghee)
- Chocolate
- Ice cream, ice milk, frozen yogurt, sherbet
- Lactic acid starter cultures and other active bacterial cultures
- Nisin
- Any foods containing milk solids, such as cream, butter, and margarine containing whey

Comparisons Between Milk Allergy and Lactose Intolerance

	Milk Allergy	**Lactose Intolerance**
Trigger	Reaction of the immune system to the protein in milk; the body produces antibodies of the IgE class that are specific to one or more proteins in milk.	Inability to digest the sugar lactose, found in milk and milk products; the immune system is not involved in this reaction.
Age	Develops within the first year of life; very rare in adulthood.	Develops at any age but is very rare in the first 2 years of life.
Onset of symptoms	Can be immediate (within 45 minutes of contact with milk) or delayed (ranging from 45 minutes to 20 hours or even days after exposure).	Symptoms occur within 30 minutes to 2 hours after ingesting milk or a meal containing milk products.
Types of symptoms	Gastrointestinal: • Nausea, vomiting, diarrhea, stomach cramps Skin manifestations: • Hives, eczema, swelling Respiratory manifestations: • Runny nose, nasal congestion, wheezing, coughing • In rare cases, anaphylaxis; can be life-threatening	Gastrointestinal: • Abdominal bloating, gas, stomach cramps • In very sensitive individuals, diarrhea and/or vomiting
Diagnosis	• Skin prick test • Blood test: total IgE or RAST (radioallergosorbent test) • Open or double-blind food challenge	• Hydrogen breath test • Stool acidity test (for infants)
Treatment	• Avoidance of all foods containing milk protein. For infants: • Breastfeed as long as possible (mother may have to limit her own intake of milk products). • Milk-allergic children can become allergic to soy and goat's milk protein. • Test the tolerance for hypoallergenic formulas made with predigested protein (casein hydrolysates).	• No need to avoid all milk products — hard aged cheese (which is lactose-free) is well tolerated. • Some individuals may tolerate a small amount of yogurt and even up to ½ cup (125 mL) regular milk. • Use lactase enzyme supplements when consuming meals or foods containing lactose.

Food ingredients that may indicate milk protein:

- Casein or any ingredients derived from casein (look for the word "casein" or "caseinate")
  - Ammonium caseinate
  - Calcium caseinate
  - Caseinate
  - Hydrolyzed casein
  - Magnesium caseinate
  - Potassium caseinate
  - Rennet casein
  - Sodium caseinate
- Butter
  - Artificial butter flavor
  - Butter acid
  - Butter ester(s)
  - Butter-flavored oil
  - Butter fat
  - Butter solids
  - Ghee
- Buttermilk solids
- Whipped butter
- Lactalbumin
- Lactalbumin phosphate
- Lactoferrin
- Lactoglobulin
- Lactose (this is the sugar in milk; you need only avoid if extremely allergic to milk)
- Lactulose
- Milk and any other ingredients derived from milk (look for the word "milk")
  - Dried milk
  - Dry milk solids
  - Hydrolyzed milk protein
  - Milk derivative
  - Milk fat
  - Milk ingredients
  - Milk powder
  - Milk protein
  - Milk solids
  - Modified milk ingredients
  - Sour milk solids
- Whey and any other ingredients containing whey
  - Delactose whey
  - Demineralised whey
  - Whey protein concentrate
  - Whey syrup sweetener
- Yogurt
- Simplesse (fat replacer)
- Sour cream solids

Other ingredients that may contain milk protein:

- Flavoring
- Brown sugar flavoring
- Natural flavoring
- High-protein flour
- Caramel color
- Caramel flavoring

You need to check the ingredient list or contact the manufacturer to ensure that a product is free of milk protein.

Ingredients that do not contain milk protein:

- Calcium and sodium lactate
- Calcium and sodium stearoyl lactylate
- Cocoa butter
- Cream of tartar
- Oleoresin

Although these ingredients have names similar to those of milk components, they are not actually related to milk and are therefore safe for consumption by those with milk allergies and lactose intolerance.

Milk-Free Diet

The list on pages 95–100 is set up to mimic the organization of a grocery store, with fresh foods arranged around the outside walls and processed foods in the inner aisles. The list is not exhaustive. **Please read the food label every time.**

Foods to Enjoy, Question, and Exclude if You Have a Milk Allergy

Aisle by Aisle	Foods to Enjoy	Foods to Question	Foods to Exclude
Produce section	• All fresh fruits and vegetables • All pure fruits and fruit juice • Freshly cut ready-to-eat fruits • Freshly cut ready-to-eat vegetables • Packaged salads • Fresh fruit juices	• Dried fruits (ensure no cross-contamination with milk or milk products) • Fruit and vegetable wax coatings (check the source of protein)	• Any fruit or vegetable salads with cream, milk, or butter toppings or sauces • Yogurt-covered dried fruit • All fruit juice smoothies made with milk or milk ingredients • Fruit dips containing milk or milk ingredients • Veggie dips • Salad dressings made with milk or milk ingredients

Aisle by Aisle	Foods to Enjoy	Foods to Question	Foods to Exclude
Bakery and crackers	• Homemade breads and baked goods (e.g., doughnuts, muffins, pancakes) made without milk or milk products • Soda crackers • Rye crackers and rye crisps • Lavash • Meringues	• French or Italian bread • Rye, Kamut, or whole wheat breads • Crackers or rusks • Bread crumbs • Nut and rice crackers	• Baked products (e.g., breads, biscuits, muffins, pancakes, or cakes) made with milk or milk products • Croissants • Crispy baguette • Fudge • Angel or sponge cake • Cookies
Dairy/dairy alternatives and eggs section	• Soy milk • Rice milk • Coconut milk • Nut milks (e.g., almond milk) • Oat milk • Potato-based milk • Hemp milk • Vegan margarine (whey- and casein-free) • Fresh eggs (boiled, fried, poached, prepared without milk or milk ingredients) • Casein-free tofu • Vegan butter • Vegan shortening • Soy-based coffee creamer (casein-free)	• Whipped cream substitutes • Margarine	• All cow's milk and cow's milk products • Other animal-based milks: goat, sheep, mare, deer, buffalo • All flavored chocolate milks and specialty coffee-based drinks • Eggnog • Ghee • Battered vegetable bites • All yogurt • All sour cream • Any dairy or non-dairy products containing ingredients to be excluded • Whipped cream • Low-fat whipped cream products • Eggs cooked with milk or milk products • Cheez Whiz • Coffee whiteners (contain casein)

Aisle by Aisle	Foods to Enjoy	Foods to Question	Foods to Exclude
Deli section	• Processed meats made without milk ingredients (chicken, turkey, ham, roast beef, prosciutto, bacon)	• Corned beef • Salami • Pepperoni • Sopressata • Kielbasa • Seasoned hummus (may contain cheese)	• Mortadella • Bologna • Ready-to-eat scalloped potatoes • Ready-to-eat mashed potatoes
Meat, poultry, and fish section	• All fresh or frozen meat, poultry, or fish prepared without milk or milk ingredients	• Sausages • Hot dogs • Weiners • Fresh or frozen meatballs • Liver pâté • Frozen beef, chicken, turkey, or hamburgers	• Commercially prepared meat, poultry, or fish that is breaded, battered, or creamed • Meatloaf • Fritters
Aisle 1 Breakfast cereals, hot cereal, jam, peanut butter, canned fruit, syrup	• All plain boxed cereal, grain flours, and starches • All plain cooked or ready-to-eat cereal • All jams, jellies, preserves • Peanut, nut, and seed butters • All plain canned fruit • Honey • Maple syrup • Pancake syrup	• Hot cereal mixes • Flavored oatmeal • Granola bars	• Yogurt-flavored cereal • Cereals containing milk or milk solids • High-protein cereal • Buttermilk pancake mix • Pancake and waffle mix • Caramel spread • Chocolate hazelnut spread (e.g., Nutella) • Yogurt- or chocolate-covered granola bars • Hot chocolate mixes • Malt drink mixes

Aisle by Aisle	Foods to Enjoy	Foods to Question	Foods to Exclude
Aisle 2 Cookies, confectionery, crackers, potato chips, snacks, popcorn, nuts and seeds, desserts	• Plain popcorn made without butter, butter flavor, cheese, or margarine • Plain corn tortilla chips • Plain rice crackers • Plain rice cakes • Plain candies made without milk ingredients • Plain potato chips • Plain nuts and seeds • Hard candy • Plain or flavored gelatin • Fruit bites or snacks	• Seasoned potato chips, tortilla chips, corn chips, rice crackers, rice cakes • Fudge • Nougat	• Chocolate cookies • Chocolate chip cookies • Cream-based cookies • Soft cookies (e.g., ladyfingers) • Toffee or creamy caramel candies • Yogurt- or chocolate-covered nuts • Bavarian cream • Pudding • Custard • Junket • Mousse • Dessert shells
Aisle 3 Spices, flour, baking supplies, sugar and other sweeteners	• All pure spices and herbs • All pure grain flours • Sugar • Molasses • Artificial sweeteners made without lactose • Fruit pie filling • Glazes	• High-protein flour • Icing	• Seasoning mixes made with milk ingredients (e.g., Greek, Caesar, ranch) • Sugar substitutes containing lactose (e.g., tagatose, lactitol) • Baking mixes containing milk or milk ingredients • Dessert toppings

Aisle by Aisle	Foods to Enjoy	Foods to Question	Foods to Exclude
Aisle 4 Oils, vinegars, sauces, salad dressings, condiments	• All vegetable oils • All animal fats • All vinegar products • Mustard • Ketchup • Soy sauce • Relish • Pickles • Hot sauce • Oil-based salad dressings made without milk or milk ingredients • Vegan mayonnaise • Bruschetta • Salsa • Guacamole	• Gravy • Seasoning mixes • Olive tapenade (may contain feta cheese) • Vegetable tapenade (may contain Asiago cheese) • Dried sauces • Horseradish sauce (may contain cream)	• Mayonnaise containing milk or milk solids • Cream-based marinating or seasoning sauces • Salad dressings containing milk, butter, or cheese • Pesto sauce (contains cheese) • Margarine containing whey or milk ingredients
Aisle 5 Soup, canned vegetables, pasta, pasta sauce, Mexican rice and other side dishes	• Homemade, canned, or refrigerated soups made without milk or milk ingredients • Pasta sauce made without milk or milk products • Salsa • All plain dried or canned beans, peas and lentils • Plain macaroni and other pasta • Plain rice or mixed rice • Plain whole grains (e.g., quinoa, barley, millet)	• Seasoned rice • Seasoned canned beans • Seasoned pasta • Seasoned canned tuna, salmon, or shellfish (check for the presence of casein protein) • Broth • Bouillon	• Cream-based canned soups (bisques, chowder, cream soups) • Dried soups containing milk ingredients • Pasta sauces made with cream, butter, cheese, or other milk ingredients • Risotto • Stuffing containing milk ingredients
Aisle 6 Water, soft drinks, sport drinks, fruit juices, alcoholic beverages	• Coffee, tea, decaffeinated coffee • Carbonated beverages • Water, flavored water • Fresh fruit juices • Shelf-stable juices • Soft drinks	• Sport drinks containing milk-based ingredients (lactalbumin) • Wine, beer, or whisky (may use milk-derived clarifying agents)	• Alcoholic beverages or cocktails made with cream (e.g., Bailey's Irish Cream) • Peanut punch

Aisle by Aisle	Foods to Enjoy	Foods to Question	Foods to Exclude
Aisle 7 Frozen fruits and vegetables, frozen meals and desserts	• Plain frozen fruits and vegetables • Sorbet	• Frozen broth-based soups • French fries made from potato mixes or mashed potatoes • Sherbet	• Frozen meals containing milk or milk ingredients • Frozen yogurt • Ice cream • Frozen scalloped potatoes • Scalloped vegetables prepared with milk or milk ingredients
Other		• Cosmetics • Medication • Pet food	• Simplesse (fat replacer) • Recaldent (used in tooth-whitening gum)

Lactose-Free Diet

The list on pages 100–105 is set up to mimic the organization of a grocery store, with fresh foods arranged around the outside walls and processed foods in the inner aisles. This list is not exhaustive. **Please read the food label every time.**

Foods to Enjoy, Question, and Exclude if You Have Lactose Intolerance

Aisle by Aisle	Foods to Enjoy	Foods to Question	Foods to Exclude
Produce section	• All fresh fruits and vegetables • All pure fruits and fruit juice • Freshly cut ready-to-eat fruits and vegetables • Packaged salads • Fresh, frozen, or canned fruit juices • Dried fruit		• Salads with cream, milk, or butter sauces • Yogurt-covered dried fruit • Fruit juice smoothies made with milk or milk ingredients • Fruit or veggie dips containing milk or milk ingredients • Salad dressings made with milk or milk ingredients

Aisle by Aisle	Foods to Enjoy	Foods to Question	Foods to Exclude
Bakery and crackers	• Homemade breads and baked goods (e.g., doughnuts, muffins, pancakes) made without milk or milk ingredients • Soda crackers • Rye crackers and rye crisps • Lavash • Meringues	• French or Italian bread • Rye, Kamut, or whole wheat breads • Crackers or rusks • Bread crumbs • Nut and rice crackers	• Baked products (e.g., breads, biscuits, muffins, pancakes) made with milk or milk products • Angel or sponge cake
Dairy/dairy alternatives and eggs section	• Lactose-free milk (e.g., Lactaid or Lacteeze) • Hard aged cheese (e.g., Cheddar, Parmesan, Swiss) • Lactose-free sour cream • Lactose-free yogurt • Lactose-free chocolate milk • Lactose-free cottage cheese • Soy-based creamers • Tofu • Coconut milk • Soy beverages • Rice milk • Nut milks (e.g., almond milk) • Potato-based milk • Hemp milk • Vegan margarine • Fresh eggs (boiled, fried, poached) prepared without milk or milk ingredients • Butter • Soy-based spreads	• Yogurt — check for tolerance to the content of lactose • 90% lactose-free yogurt • Whipped cream substitutes • Margarine • Coffee whiteners (contain milk protein but are lactose-free)	• All regular cow's milk and milk from other ruminants: goat, sheep, mare, buffalo, deer • Eggnog • Milkshakes • Fresh cheese (e.g., cottage cheese, ricotta, mascarpone, cream cheese) • Cottage cheese • Sour cream • Whipped cream • Low-fat whipped cream • All flavored chocolate milks and specialty coffee–based drinks • Battered vegetable bites • Eggs cooked with milk or milk products • Cheese spreads

Aisle by Aisle	Foods to Enjoy	Foods to Question	Foods to Exclude
Deli section	• Processed meats made without milk ingredients (e.g., chicken, turkey, ham, roast beef, prosciutto) • Lactose-free salami, pepperoni, sopressata	• Corned beef • Liver pâté	• Mortadella • Bologna • Ready-to-eat scalloped potatoes • Ready-to-eat mashed potatoes
Meat, poultry, and fish section	• All fresh or frozen meat, poultry, or fish • Canned tuna • Canned crab • Canned sardines • Canned mussels	• Sausages • Hot dogs • Frankfurters • Frozen beef, chicken, turkey, or hamburgers	• Commercially prepared meat, poultry, or fish that is breaded, battered, or creamed • Meatloaf • Fritters
Aisle 1 Breakfast cereals, hot cereal, jam, peanut butter, canned fruit, syrup	• All plain boxed cereal, grains, flours, and starches • All plain cooked or ready-to-eat cereal • All jams, jellies, preserves • Peanut, nut, or seed butters • All plain canned fruit • Honey • Maple syrup • Pancake syrup	• Hot cereal mixes • Flavored oatmeal • Granola bars • High-protein cereal	• Yogurt-flavored cereal • Cereals containing milk or milk solids • Yogurt- or chocolate-covered granola bars • Buttermilk pancake mix • Pancake and waffle mix • Caramel spread • Chocolate hazelnut spread (e.g., Nutella) • Hot chocolate mixes • Malt drink mixes

Aisle by Aisle	Foods to Enjoy	Foods to Question	Foods to Exclude
Aisle 2 Cookies, confectionery, crackers, potato chips, snacks, popcorn, nuts and seeds, desserts	• Plain popcorn • Plain tortilla chips • Plain rice crackers • Plain rice cakes • Plain candies made without milk ingredients • Plain potato chips • Plain nuts and seeds • Hard candy • Caramel candy • Plain or flavored gelatins • Fruit bites or snacks	• Seasoned potato chips, tortilla chips, corn chips, rice crackers, rice cakes, popcorn • Dark chocolate • Fudge	• Chocolate • Chocolate chip or cream-based cookies • Soft cookies (e.g., ladyfingers) • Toffee or creamy caramel candies • Yogurt- or chocolate-covered nuts or seeds • Bavarian cream • Pudding • Custard • Junket • Mousse • Dessert shells • Appetizer shells
Aisle 3 Spices, flour, baking supplies, sugar and other sweeteners	• All pure spices and herbs • All single plain grain flours • Sugar • Molasses • Artificial sweeteners made without lactose • Fruit glazes • Fruit pie filling	• Seasoning mixes • Icing	• Seasoning mixes made with milk ingredients (e.g., Greek, Caesar, ranch) • Sugar substitutes containing lactose (e.g., tagatose, lactitol) • Baking mixes containing milk or milk ingredients • Dessert toppings

Aisle by Aisle	Foods to Enjoy	Foods to Question	Foods to Exclude
Aisle 4 Oils, vinegars, sauces, salad dressings, condiments	• All vegetable oils • All animal fats • All vinegar products • Mustard, ketchup, soy sauce, relish, pickles • Hot sauce • Oil-based salad dressings made without milk or milk ingredients • Homemade gravy made without milk or milk ingredients • Mayonnaise	• Gravy • Dried sauces	• Cream-based marinating or seasoning sauces • Salad dressings containing milk, butter, or cheese
Aisle 5 Soup, canned vegetables, pasta, pasta sauce, Mexican rice and other side dishes	• Homemade, canned, or refrigerated soups made without milk or milk ingredients • Pasta sauce made without milk or milk ingredients • Salsa • All plain dried or canned beans, peas and lentils • Plain macaroni and other pasta • Plain rice or mixed rice • Plain whole grains (e.g., quinoa, barley, millet) • Guacamole	• Seasoned rice • Seasoned canned bean salads • Seasoned pasta • Broths • Bouillons	• Cream-based canned soups (e.g., bisques, chowder, cream soups) • Dried soups containing milk ingredients • Pasta sauces made with cream, butter, cheese, and other milk ingredients • Risotto • Stuffing made with milk ingredients
Aisle 6 Water, soft drinks, sport drinks, fruit juices, alcoholic beverages	• Coffee, tea, decaffeinated coffee • Carbonated beverages • Water, flavored water • Fresh fruit juices • Shelf-stable juices • Soft drinks		• Cream-based alcoholic beverages or cocktails (e.g., Bailey's Irish Cream) • Peanut punch

Aisle by Aisle	Foods to Enjoy	Foods to Question	Foods to Exclude
Aisle 7 Frozen fruits and vegetables, frozen meals and desserts	• Plain frozen fruits and vegetables • Sorbet	• Frozen broth-based soups • French fries made from mashed potatoes or potato mixes	• Frozen meals containing milk or milk ingredients • Frozen yogurt • Ice cream • Sherbet • Frozen scalloped potatoes • Scalloped vegetables or vegetable meals prepared with milk or milk ingredients
Other			• Simplesse (fat replacer) • Recaldent (used in tooth-whitening gum)

Nutritional Profile of Lactose Intolerance Supplements and Substitutes

Over-the-counter lactase enzyme supplements are available in tablet or liquid format. The supplements have no systemic effect; in other words, they are not absorbed into your bloodstream and are very safe. Their role is to supplement the lack of lactase enzymes produced by your own intestine and to help break down lactose in milk products or meals that may contain milk or milk products. Use them any time you anticipate consuming a meal that may contain milk or milk ingredients or when you crave foods that are listed as foods to exclude. Being lactose intolerant does not require complete avoidance of dairy products. Because avoidance of milk and milk ingredients is absolutely critical in milk allergy, however, finding suitable alternatives that can provide the necessary calcium and vitamin D becomes essential.

Food Sources of Calcium

Fortunately, many non-dairy foods can provide adequate intake of calcium. To meet the recommendations, take into account your overall daily intake of calcium.

Recommended Calcium Intake by Age Group

Age Group	Dietary Reference Intakes (mg/day)
0–6 months (boys and girls)	210
7–12 months (boys and girls)	270
1–3 years (boys and girls)	500
4–8 years (boys and girls)	800
9–18 years (men)	1300
9–18 years (women)	1300
19–50 years (men)	1000
19–50 years (women)	1000
51–70+ years (men and women)	1200
Pregnancy, 14–18 years	1300
Pregnancy, 19–50 years	1000
Lactation, 14–18 years	1300
Lactation, 19–50 years	1000

Adapted by permission from *Dietary Reference Intakes.* Institute of Medicine, National Academy of Sciences, 2004.

Tips for Maintaining Healthy Bones

- Get your recommended intake of calcium from acceptable foods first; if this doesn't work, your doctor will prescribe calcium and vitamin D supplements along with bone-building drugs.
- Keep active. Weight-bearing exercises, such as jogging, hiking, stair-climbing, and resistance training, help maintain bone mass.
- Eat your veggies. Studies show that fruits and vegetables may protect bone by making the urine more alkaline, but diets high in grains and protein foods generate more acid residues, forcing the body to neutralize it by using calcium from the bones. Fruits and vegetables are also a great source of potassium and vitamin K, which help protect the bone matrix.
- Cut back on salt. A high salt intake causes further calcium loss from bones.

- Moderate your caffeine intake. Caffeine also leads to calcium being lost in the urine.
- Alcohol intake and smoking are additional risk factors for osteoporosis.
- Take vitamin D (1000 IUs daily) to assist calcium and to prevent rickets and osteomalacia.

Calcium Content, from Highest to Lowest, in Common Foods

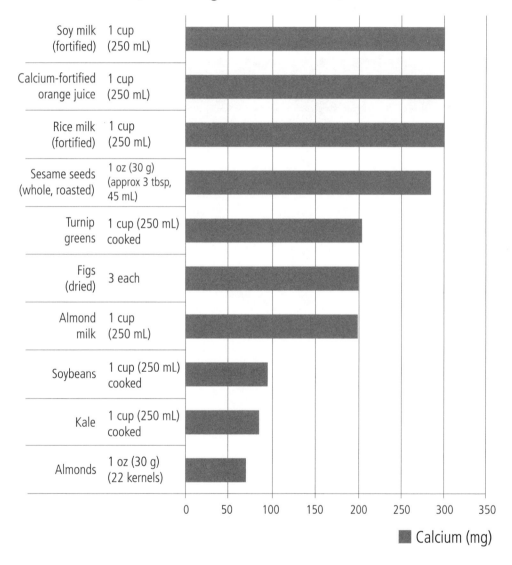

Calcium (mg)

Egg Allergy

Egg allergy is one of the most prevalent food allergies in children, estimated to affect 1.6% to 3.2%. As in the case of milk allergy, egg allergy is much less common in older children and in the adult population. In many cases, egg allergy resolves itself by age 16.

Eggs are composed of 56% to 61% egg white and 27% to 32% yolk. Both components can trigger immune responses, but allergy to egg white is more commonly seen.

Egg Allergy Triggers

Protein	Commonly Triggers Reactions in Children	Commonly Triggers Reactions in Adults
Egg white		
Ovoalbumin (54% of egg white)	✓	✓
Ovotransferrin (12% of egg white)		✓
Ovomucoid (11% of egg white)	✓	✓
Ovomucin (3.5% of egg white)	✓	
Lysozyme (3.4% of egg white)	✓	✓
Egg yolk		
Apovitellenins I, VI	✓	
Phosvitin	✓	
α-livetin		

Symptoms of Egg Allergy

- Atopic dermatitis (rash)
- Urticaria (itching)
- Angioedema (swelling of the face, lips, and tongue)
- Acute vomiting
- Violent diarrhea
- Anaphylaxis (IgE-mediated)

Family History

Parents who have a history of any food allergy are advised to ask a doctor or an allergy specialist when to introduce eggs to the baby's diet. If there is no family history of food allergies, cooked egg yolk may be introduced at 6 months of age and cooked egg white at about 12 months. Baby's first birthday is a good time to introduce the whole egg.

Food ingredients that contain egg protein:
The only way to treat egg allergy is to avoid all eggs and egg products. This is often easier said than done because you may not be aware of what kinds of foods contain these ingredients. Egg-derived ingredients are not always clearly labeled or may appear under different names. Here is a list of terms and ingredients that may indicate the presence of eggs. If you are uncertain, contact the food manufacturer.

- Albumin (also spelled albumen)
- Conalbumin
- Apovitellenins I and VI
- Eggs of all species (e.g., duck, turkey, goose, quail)
  - Egg white
  - Egg yolk
  - Egg solids
  - Egg powder
  - Dried egg
  - Pasteurized egg
  - Egg substitutes made of egg whites (e.g., Egg Beaters)
- Globulin
- Lecithin
- Livetin
- Lysozyme
- Ovalbumin
- Ovoglobulin
- Ovomucin
- Ovomucoid
- Ovotransferrin
- Ovovitelin
- Phosvitin
- Silico-albuminate
- Simplesse
- Surimi

Eggs may also be used in food formulations as:

- Binders
- Emulsifiers
- Coagulants

Read labels carefully!

Egg-Free Diet

The list on pages 110–115 is set up to mimic the organization of a grocery store, with fresh foods arranged around the outside walls and processed foods in the inner aisles. The list is not exhaustive. **Please read the food label every time.**

Foods to Enjoy, Question, and Exclude if You Have an Egg Allergy

Aisle by Aisle	Foods to Enjoy	Foods to Question	Foods to Exclude
Produce section	• All fresh fruits and vegetables • All pure fruits and fruit juice • Freshly cut ready-to-eat fruits • Freshly cut ready-to-eat vegetables • Packaged salads • Fresh, frozen, or canned fruit juices • Dried fruit	• Fruit dips • Veggie dips	• Fruit whips • Any fruit prepared in a sauce that contains egg or egg ingredients (e.g., custard sauce) • Battered fried vegetables • All vegetable dishes prepared in casseroles with sauces containing egg (e.g., hollandaise sauce) • Salads containing egg • Yogurt-covered or glazed fruit products • Salad dressings containing egg (e.g., Caesar or ranch)

Aisle by Aisle	Foods to Enjoy	Foods to Question	Foods to Exclude
Bakery and crackers	• Breads, buns, and baked goods made without egg or egg ingredients • Plain rye crackers • Plain rice crackers • Plain rice cakes • Rye crackers and rye crisps • Lavash	• French or Italian bread • Seasoned rice crackers • Bread crumbs • Soda crackers • Seasoned croutons	• Glazed breads and buns (glaze may contain egg white) • Cookies • Doughnuts • French toast • Waffles • Toaster pastries • Cakes, breads, and other baked goods with egg-based glaze • Dessert shells • Appetizer shells • Fruit whips • Confectioneries containing egg, (e.g., fondants, cupcakes, mousse, soufflés)
Dairy/dairy alternatives and eggs section	• Homogenized (3.8%), 2%, 1%, or skim milk • Cream • Plain cream cheese • Sour cream • Yogurt and kefir • Buttermilk • Fresh cheese • Tofu (plain) • Tempeh (plain) • Egg-free breading (specialty allergen-free breaded products)	• Gelatin desserts (check ingredient list) • Aged cheese (some brands may contain egg white lysozyme)	• All eggs (chicken, duck, quail, etc.) • Liquid egg products • Egg white products • Egg nog • Novelty milk beverages containing egg ingredients • Cocomalt • Malted beverages • Foam or milk topping on coffee • Ovaltine • Egg custard or pudding
Deli section	• Deli meats made without egg ingredients (e.g., bacon, prosciutto, salami, plain chicken or turkey breast, ham) • Ready-to-eat mashed or scalloped potatoes	• Hot dogs • Sausages • Liver pâté • Ready-to-eat seasoned chicken breast strips • Seasoned deli meats (e.g., Tandoori-style chicken)	• Meatloaf • Meatballs • Processed deli meats made with egg ingredients

Aisle by Aisle	Foods to Enjoy	Foods to Question	Foods to Exclude
Meat, poultry, and fish section	• All pure fresh meat, fish, and poultry prepared without eggs	• Sausages • Meatless burgers • Veggie hot dogs • Frozen chicken or turkey burgers	• Meat, fish, or poultry in batter • Meat, fish, or poultry preparations using egg as a binding agent (e.g., meatloaf, meatballs) • Croquettes • Soy-based veggie snacks
Aisle 1 Breakfast cereals, hot cereal, jam, peanut butter, canned fruit, syrup	• Ready-to-eat cereal made without egg-derived ingredients • Plain oatmeal • Plain cream of wheat • Rice and other gluten-free hot cereals made without egg-derived ingredients • All pure fruit jams, marmalade, and preserves • Peanut, nut, and seed butters • All canned fruit • Honey • Maple syrup • Pancake syrup	• Flavored hot cereal or oatmeal	• Baked products (e.g., waffles, pancakes, toaster pastries, muffins, fritters, and doughnuts) • Pancake or waffle mix • Angel or sponge cake • Cereal bars or granola bars containing egg ingredients

Aisle by Aisle	Foods to Enjoy	Foods to Question	Foods to Exclude
Aisle 2 Cookies, confectionery, crackers, potato chips, snacks, popcorn, nuts and seeds, desserts	• Jell-O • Plain popcorn • Plain potato chips • Plain corn chips or tortilla chips • Rice cakes or crackers made without egg-ingredients • Fruit crisps • Homemade desserts made without egg or egg-derived ingredients • Hard candy	• Seasoned popcorn, potato chips, tortilla or corn chips, crackers • Seasoned rice cakes or crackers • Cream-filled candies • Chocolate • Pretzels (some are dipped in egg white prior to seasoning) • Marzipan	• Bavarian creams • Biscuits • Custards • Cakes • Cookies • Dessert mixes • Fritters • Cream pies • Puddings • Doughnuts • Junkets • Meringue, meringue powder • Marshmallow cream (contains egg white) • Fudge • Nougat
Aisle 3 Spices, flour, baking supplies, sugar and other sweeteners	• All single plain spices and herbs • All pure grain flours • Sugar • Molasses	• Lecithin (often derived from soy, but may sometimes be derived from egg) • Glazed preparations • Pie fillings	• Royal icing mixes using egg ingredients • Frosting • Baking mixes containing egg • Pie crusts brushed with egg white

Aisle by Aisle	Foods to Enjoy	Foods to Question	Foods to Exclude
Aisle 4 Oils, vinegars, sauces, salad dressings, condiments	• All vegetable oils • All vinegars • Plain mustard • Honey mustard • Ketchup • Pickles • Oil-and-vinegar-based dressings • Lard • Vegetable shortening • Vegan mayonnaise (egg-free)	• Some specialty mustards (e.g., Hellman's Dijonnaise) • Gravy (egg may be found in some brands of dried gravy powder)	• Cream sauces (e.g., béarnaise, hollandaise or Newburg) • Mayonnaise • Tartar sauce • Salad dressings containing egg (e.g., Caesar or Ranch) • Low-fat mayonnaise
Aisle 5 Soup, canned vegetables, pasta, pasta sauce, Mexican rice and other side dishes	• Any soup prepared without egg-derived ingredients or egg noodles • All plain canned beans, peas and lentils • Salsa • Bruschetta • Plain rice or mixed rice • Plain whole grains (e.g., quinoa, barley, millet)	• Macaroni (check for cross-contamination with egg) • Pasta (check for cross-contamination with egg) • Seasoned pasta (e.g., Hamburger Helper) • Seasoned rice • Dried soups	• Soups clarified with eggshell (e.g., consommé, broth, bouillon) • Egg drop soup • Matzo balls in chicken broth • Egg noodle soup • Turtle or mock turtle soup • Egg pasta or noodles • No-yolk pasta (contains egg white) • Fried rice containing egg
Aisle 6 Water, soft drinks, sport drinks, fruit juices, alcoholic beverages	• Tea • Decaffeinated coffee • Carbonated beverages • Water, flavored water • Fresh fruit juices • Shelf-stable juices • Soft drinks	• Beers, coffee, or wine (check for egg-derived clarifying agents) • Vegetable cocktail juice	• Alcoholic cocktails and ingredients (e.g., sweet Marsala) • Orange Julius • Some root beers • Protein drinks containing egg or egg products

Aisle by Aisle	Foods to Enjoy	Foods to Question	Foods to Exclude
Aisle 7 Frozen fruits and vegetables, frozen meals and desserts	• All plain frozen fruits and vegetables • Frozen french fries • Frozen scalloped potatoes • Sorbet • Popsicles • Fruit ice	• Ice cream (some flavors) • Frozen yogurt (some flavors) • Sherbet (may contain egg white)	• Frozen meals containing egg-derived ingredients (e.g., fried rice) • Frozen appetizers containing egg-derived ingredients • Frozen waffles, pancakes, muffins, and cookie dough • Frozen pastry dough containing egg • Frozen quiche • Frozen egg rolls • Dumplings made with egg-derived ingredients
Other		• Crafts and some artist paints (may contain eggshell) — check with manufacturer • Vaccines or flu shots — check with your doctor	• Simplesse (fat replacer) • Egg shampoo • Anesthetics (e.g., Diprivan and Propofol)

Nutritional Profile of Eggs and Substitutes

Eggs are an excellent source of high-quality protein, as well as essential vitamins and minerals, including folate, vitamin B_{12}, zinc, iron, and phosphorus. For individuals with egg allergy or sensitivity, many foods can be consumed to replace these important nutrients (see chart, page 116).

Egg Alternatives

Nutrient	Alternative Food Sources
High-quality protein	Milk and milk products, meat, fish, poultry, legumes
Folate	Beans and peas (romano beans, black-eyed peas), spinach, broccoli, dark green leafy vegetables
Vitamin B_{12}	Fish (salmon, light canned tuna), meat (lean ground beef), dairy (cottage cheese, yogurt), fortified dairy-free milks (soy, rice)
Iron	Shellfish (clams, mussels), seeds (pumpkin seeds), beans (romano beans, white kidney beans), gluten-free grains (teff, Job's tears)
Phosphorus	Milk and milk products (milk, yogurt, cottage cheese), meat, fish, poultry, tofu

Baking without Eggs

Following an egg-free diet does not mean that baking is off limits. Here are some tips for substituting for eggs in a baking recipe. For each egg that the recipe calls for, try substituting with *one* of the following options:

- 1 tsp (5 mL) baking powder, $1\frac{1}{2}$ tbsp (22 mL) water, and $1\frac{1}{2}$ tbsp (22 mL) oil
- 5 mL (1 tsp) baking powder, 1 tbsp (15 mL) water, and 1 tbsp (15 mL) vinegar
- 5 mL (1 tsp) yeast dissolved in $\frac{1}{4}$ cup (60 mL) warm water
- 1 packet ($\frac{1}{4}$ oz/7 g) unflavored gelatin and 2 tbsp (30 mL) warm water (do not combine until ready to use)
- $\frac{1}{2}$ medium banana, mashed

Commercial egg substitutes, such as Kingsmill Foods Egg Replacer, Celimix Brand Egg Replacer, and Ener-g Egg Replacer, can be ordered directly from the company. They can also be found in some health food stores or the natural food section of some grocery stores.

Cross-Contamination

Cross-contamination is a reality that is frequently the cause of allergic reactions. You need to be alert and always ask questions:

- *Food product manufacturers:* If you are uncertain about the presence of egg in a food product, call the manufacturer or avoid using the product.
- *Grocery stores:* Avoid purchasing meats from the deli section because the meat slicers are frequently used for deli meats containing egg.
- *Restaurants:* Speak to the chef or sous chef about your egg allergy. Inquire about the presence of eggs in any of the ingredients used in a meal and also about using fresh utensils, pots, and pans when preparing your meal.
- *Home:* Ensure that soaps, shampoos, body creams, artist paints, and certain crafts do not have egg-derived ingredients (eggshell is used in certain crafts).
- *Doctor's office:* Certain children's vaccines and flu shots may contain egg. Ask your doctor about alternatives.

Q Can someone who is allergic to raw eggs tolerate a cooked egg?

A When egg allergy develops, all forms, raw or cooked, should be avoided. When the allergy is disappearing, however, a person may tolerate cooked eggs but still have a reaction to raw eggs. The severity of the allergy can also affect the tolerance for cooked eggs: Some individuals with a mild form of egg allergy may tolerate small amounts of cooked egg. Consult your allergist before you try to introduce any new foods containing eggs.

Q Can someone be allergic only to egg white or egg yolk?

A Both parts of the egg, the white and the yolk, are allergenic, but the proteins in egg white are responsible for the more severe reactions. The proteins in yolk are also more readily broken down by heat, making cooked egg yolk more easily tolerated by some. Regardless, it is usually very hard to separate the two without having some components combine, and very small amounts of egg protein, from either the white or the yolk, may trigger severe reactions. Avoidance of the whole egg is highly advised.

Soy Allergy

Soy allergy is an abnormal immunologic reaction to proteins found in soybeans. Soy foods are the second most prevalent legume allergen worldwide next to peanuts. Soy allergies are most common in infants and usually develop at 3 months of age. Most infants outgrow their allergy by the age of two, but in some cases, the allergy may persist throughout a lifetime. Individuals who are allergic to soy may also develop allergies to other legumes. The only treatment for soy allergy is complete avoidance of soy and soy-derived ingredients.

Food ingredients containing soy protein:

- Edamame
- Kinako
- Kouridofu
- Kyodofu
- Miso
- Monodiglyceride
- Natto
- Nimame
- Okara (soy pulp)
- Shoyu, shoyu sauce
- Sobee
- Soya, soja, soybean
- Soy flour
- Soy protein (isolate/ concentrate)
- Supro
- Tamari
- Tempeh
- Textured (or texturized) soy flour (TSF), textured (or texturized) soy protein (TSP)
- Tofu (soybean curds)
- Yuba

Soy can also be found in other foods, such as:

- Vegetable protein
- Hydrolyzed vegetable protein
- Vegetable gum
- Soy lecithin
- Soy (or soybean) oil
- Vegetable broth
- Vegetable gum
- Vegetable starch
- Natural flavoring
- Flavorings
- Vitamin E
- Seasonings (may contain soy-derived ingredients, such as lecithin or hydrolyzed soy protein)
- Monosodium glutamate (MSG)
- Emulsifiers (when source is not listed)
- Stabilizers (when source is not listed)
- Sprouts (when source is not listed)

If not specified in the food label, contact the manufacturer to find out:

- Whether soy is used as a carrier for natural flavoring.
- Whether seasoning mixes may contain hydrolyzed soy protein or other soy-derived ingredients.
- Whether vitamin E contains soybean oil.
- Whether soy is the source of "vegetable" in the following ingredients: hydrolyzed vegetable protein, texturized vegetable protein, or vegetable gum.

Soy Oil

Most highly refined soy oil does not contain soy protein, which causes soy allergy, because the protein is removed during processing. Both Health Canada and the FDA recognize, however, that although highly refined soybean oil may not pose a threat to all soy-allergy sufferers, it is best to consult your allergist before eating anything made with soy oils. Cold-pressed, expeller, or extruded soy oil may still carry minute amounts of protein and are not recommended.

As with all allergens, food processing may affect the allergenic potential of a food. Heating, for example, may decrease the allergen potential of some proteins in egg yolk, and refining soybean oil removes all the protein content from the final product. However, other processes, such as fermentation, will have no effect, making a product such as soy sauce as allergenic as soybean products.

 Q What is soy lecithin?

A Soy lecithin is an emulsifier used in many foods. It prevents foods from breaking apart and gives a consistent texture to creamy products, such as soups, sauces, and dressings. Soy lecithin is produced through extraction during the processing of soybean oil. Research shows that some of the soybean proteins are included in the extract and are therefore present in small amounts in soy lecithin, but the allergenic potential of these proteins has been found to be very small. Nevertheless, there is a small subset of highly allergic individuals who may still react to soy lecithin. For this reason, it is highly recommended that you speak to your allergy specialist before consuming foods that contain soy lecithin.

Soy-Free Diet

The list on pages 120–124 is set up to mimic the organization of a grocery store, with fresh foods arranged around the outside walls and processed foods in the inner aisles. The list is not exhaustive. **Please read the food label every time.**

Foods to Enjoy, Question, and Exclude if You Have a Soy Allergy

Aisle by Aisle	Foods to Enjoy	Foods to Question	Foods to Exclude
Produce section	• All fresh, ready-to-eat fruits and fruit juices • All fresh, ready-to-eat vegetables and their juices • Packaged salads • Freshly squeezed juices and smoothies • Salad dressings made without soy ingredients	• Salad dressings • Vegetable and fruit dips	• Soybeans • Soybean sprouts • Edamame (soybeans) • Breaded vegetables • Fruit sauce • Whipped cream substitute (e.g., Nutriwhip, Cool Whip) • Vegetable and fruit dips containing soy ingredients
Bakery and crackers	• Breads made without soy-derived ingredients • Plain rye crackers • Plain rice crackers • Plain rice cakes • Homemade pastries and baked goods made without soy-derived ingredients	• Enriched whole wheat or white bread • Dinner rolls	• Multigrain or enriched breads containing soy protein • Bread crumbs • Baked goods (e.g., sweet rolls, muffins, Danish, croissants) • Cake mixes • Sponge cakes • Turnovers • Multigrain crackers • Soy crackers or crisps • Corn chips • Panko-style bread crumbs or flakes • Stuffing

Aisle by Aisle	Foods to Enjoy	Foods to Question	Foods to Exclude
Dairy/dairy alternatives and eggs section	• Milk, buttermilk, cream, yogurt, plain hard aged cheese, fresh cheese, plain cream cheese • Chocolate milk • Fresh, boiled, poached, fried eggs prepared without any soy ingredients • Plain liquid egg • Butter • Soy-free buttery spread or margarine	• Seasoned liquid eggs	• Soy milk • Soy cream cheese • Cheese substitutes made with soy: tofu/bean curd, natto, miso • Soy yogurt • Tofu • Margarine • Miso • Tempeh • Lactose-free coffee whitener
Deli section	• Deli meats made without soy-based ingredients (e.g., prosciutto, bacon, sopressata, chorizo, kielbasa)	• Seasoned deli meats • Hummus (may contain soybean oil)	• Deli meats containing soy: corned beef, Montreal smoked meat, ham, bologna, hot dogs, wieners, sausages • Deli meat substitutes that contain soy: soy-based chicken breast, turkey breast, hot dogs, sausages • Ready-to-eat mashed or scalloped potatoes • Edamame hummus
Meat, poultry, and fish section	• All fresh lean cuts of beef, veal, pork, and lamb • All fresh poultry • All fresh or frozen fish • All fresh or frozen seafood: shrimp, scallops, lobster, clams, mussels	• Flavored or plain canned tuna in water or oil (may contain hydrolyzed soy protein) • Flavored or plain canned sardines in water or oil • Minced ham • Meat pâté • Meat pies • Frozen beef burgers	• Meatballs (fresh or frozen) • Meat substitutes (e.g., vegetarian hamburgers, hot dogs, patties, and sausages) • Surimi • Imitation crabmeat • Imitation fish • Imitation bacon bits • Canned ham

Aisle by Aisle	Foods to Enjoy	Foods to Question	Foods to Exclude
Aisle 1 Breakfast cereals, hot cereal, jam, peanut butter, canned fruit, syrup	• Most plain hot cereal (e.g., oatmeal, cream of wheat, cream of buckwheat) made without soy • Most plain cold cereals made without soy • All pure jams, jellies and preserves • Canned fruit • Honey • Maple syrup • Pancake syrup	• Multigrain cereals (may contain soy grits) • Mixed hot cereals • Peanut, nut, and seed butters — check the source of the oil	• Pancake, waffle, and biscuit mixes • English muffins • Multigrain hot cereal containing soy • Multigrain cold or high-protein cold cereal containing soy ingredients • Granola containing soy ingredients • Caramel spread
Aisle 2 Cookies, confectionery, crackers, potato chips, snacks, popcorn, nuts and seeds, desserts	• Rice crackers, corn chips, tortilla chips, and vegetable crisps made without soy-derived ingredients • Homemade cookies, cakes, and desserts made without soy-derived ingredients • Plain sugar candies • Nuts and seeds roasted in sunflower or canola oil	• Potato chips and popcorn cooked in soy oil (check with your doctor before consuming these) • Seasoned nuts or seeds • Seasoned potato, corn, or rice chips • Chewing gum • Chocolate • Granola bars • Snack bars	• Soy nuts (roasted soybeans) • Soy butter • Roasted soybeans • Soy crisps • Soy crackers • Hard candies, nut candies, and fudge made with soy-derived ingredients (e.g., soy flour) • Cookies made with soy-derived ingredients • Nut mixes with soybeans

Aisle by Aisle	Foods to Enjoy	Foods to Question	Foods to Exclude
Aisle 3 Spices, flour, baking supplies, sugar and other sweeteners	• Individual spices (e.g., cinnamon, pepper, cloves, allspice, ginger, paprika) • Individual herbs (e.g., thyme, basil, sage, savory) • All plain grain flours except soy flour: amaranth, arrowroot, barley, corn, corn bran, cornmeal, potato flour, quinoa, millet, rice, brown rice, rye, sorghum, spelt, sago, wheat • Molasses • Sugar • Artificial sweeteners	• Legume flour (e.g., fava, gram, besan, garbanzo, chickpea, lentil) — check for cross-contamination with soy flour • Spice mixtures • Seasoning mixes • Baking mixes — check for cross-contamination with soy • Fruit pie filling	• Soy flour • Textured (or texturized) soy flour • Soy grits • Caramel sauce • Baking mixes containing soy ingredients • Cake icing containing soy ingredients
Aisle 4 Oils, vinegars, sauces, salad dressings, condiments	• Sunflower, olive, grapeseed, corn, and canola oils • Vinegars • Mustard • Pickles • Ketchup • Relish • Tomato paste • Hot sauce • Roasted red peppers	• Cooking sprays • Vegetable shortening • Vegetable oil • Highly refined soybean oil — check with your doctor • Imitation bacon bits (may contain hydrolyzed soy protein) • Salsa • Bruschetta • Barbecue sauce • Olives	• Soy sauce • Shoyu sauce • Tamari sauce • Teriyaki sauce • Worcestershire sauce • Dressings, gravies, and marinades made with soy-derived ingredients • Vegan mayonnaise • Low-fat or seasoned mayonnaise

Aisle by Aisle	Foods to Enjoy	Foods to Question	Foods to Exclude
Aisle 5 Soup, canned vegetables, pasta, pasta sauce, Mexican rice and other side dishes	• Homemade or packaged soups made without soy-derived ingredients • Canned or dried chickpeas, black peas, white or red kidney beans • Pasta • Macaroni (soy-free) • Gluten-free pasta (rice, quinoa, potato) • Plain rice or mixed rice • Plain whole grains (e.g., quinoa, barley, millet)	• Canned or packaged soups, mixes, broths, bouillon • Seasoned rice mixes • Pasta sauce • Commercial risotto	• Soy pasta • Dry, canned or frozen soybeans • Mixed canned beans (e.g., 9-bean salad may contain soybeans) • Dry bean soup mixes • Commercial pasta and rice in sauces
Aisle 6 Water, soft drinks, sport drinks, fruit juices, alcoholic beverages	• Coffee, tea, decaffeinated coffee • Carbonated beverages • Water, flavored water • Fresh fruit juices • Shelf-stable juices • Soft drinks	• Fruit beverage mixes (e.g., powdered lemonade mix containing soy lecithin) • Vegetable cocktail juice (may contain soy lecithin)	• Hot cocoa mixes • Malt beverages • Coffee substitutes made with soy (e.g., soy coffee)
Aisle 7 Frozen fruits and vegetables, frozen meals and desserts	• All plain frozen fruits, vegetables, or mixed vegetables • Sorbet • Sherbet • Fruit ice	• Ice cream (some flavors)	• Frozen edamame • Frozen waffles, pancakes, and muffins • Frozen vegetables in sauce and vegetarian meals • Frozen french fries or scalloped potatoes • Frozen Asian-style meals • Frozen desserts • Ice cream substitutes
Other		• Cosmetics and soaps • Craft materials • Glycerine • Pet food • Vitamins • Energy bars	• Soy protein concentrate • Soy protein isolate • Nutritional supplements containing soy protein

Nutritional Profile of Soybeans and Substitutes

Soybeans are a great source of fiber and phytosterols (healthy plant fats), along with antioxidant compounds. Soybeans also provide very high-quality protein for vegetarian diets. If adults only need to eliminate soybeans but tolerate other members of the legume family — such as chickpeas, lentils, and red kidney beans — then the risk of developing nutritional deficiencies is not as great.

Soy Alternatives

Nutrient	Alternative Food Sources
High-quality protein	Milk and milk products, meat, fish, poultry, legumes
Calcium	Milk, lactose-free milk, cheese, other dairy products, dark green leafy vegetables (kale, Swiss chard), nuts (almonds, Brazil nuts), seeds (sesame seeds)
Thiamine (vitamin B_1)	Wheat germ, brewer's yeast, meat, sunflower seeds, green peas, split peas, asparagus, legumes
Riboflavin (vitamin B_2)	Milk products (yogurt, ricotta cheese), eggs, enriched flour, enriched rice, mushrooms, spinach
Vitamin B_6 (pyrodixine)	Chicken, fish, organ meats, eggs, milk, wheat germ, brewer's yeast, brown rice, peanuts, walnuts
Zinc	Shellfish (clams, mussels), meat, fortified cereals
Folate	Beans and peas (romano beans, black-eyed peas), spinach, broccoli, dark green leafy vegetables
Vitamin B_{12}	Fish (salmon, light canned tuna), meat (lean ground beef), dairy (cottage cheese, yogurt), fortified dairy-free milks (not made with soy-derived ingredients)
Iron	Shellfish (clams, mussels), seeds (pumpkin seeds), beans (romano beans, white kidney beans), gluten-free grains (teff, Job's tears)
Phosphorus	Milk and milk products (milk, yogurt, cottage cheese), meat, fish, poultry, tofu
Magnesium	Whole grains, nuts, dairy products, meat

Wheat Allergy and Celiac Disease

Allergy to wheat involves the production of IgE antibodies to the proteins found in this grain and its relatives. The symptoms are very similar to those found with allergies to other foods. Celiac disease is the immune system's reaction to gluten, a protein found in wheat, rye, barley, spelt, Kamut, and triticale. In this case, gluten damages the lining of the small intestine, robbing the individual of the ability to absorb nutrients from foods. This can lead to diarrhea, weight loss, malnutrition, and a host of other symptoms.

Comparisons Between Wheat Allergy and Celiac Disease

	Wheat Allergy	**Celiac Disease**
Trigger	• Reaction of the immune system to the protein in wheat. The body produces antibodies of the IgE class that are specific to one or more proteins in wheat and other grains related to wheat.	• The body's immune system mounts a response against gluten, the protein found in wheat, barley, rye, spelt, Kamut, triticale, and contaminated oats. The site of damage is the lining of the small intestine.
Age	• Develops early in life and is usually outgrown. Wheat allergy is very rare in adults.	• May develop at any age, but the majority of individuals diagnosed are 50 and older.
Onset of symptoms	• Can be immediate (within 45 minutes of contact) or delayed (ranging from 45 minutes to 20 hours or even days after exposure).	• Varies widely, from asymptomatic (silent celiac disease) to appearance of symptoms immediately upon ingestion of gluten.
Types of symptoms	• See table (opposite).	• See table (opposite).
Diagnosis	• Skin prick test. • Blood test: Total IgE or RAST. • Open or double-blind food challenge.	• IgA-EMA/IgA-TTG. • Small bowel biopsy is the gold standard for diagnosis.
Treatment	• Avoidance of wheat and its derivatives. Because allergy may be outgrown, adults may eventually tolerate wheat-based products.	• Complete avoidance of gluten for life. • Celiac disease is never outgrown.

Symptoms of Wheat Allergy and Celiac Disease

Symptoms of Wheat Allergy	Symptoms of Celiac Disease
Swelling, itching of the mouth and throat	Gastrointestinal: Chronic diarrhea, constipation, bloating, abdominal pain, gastroesophageal reflux
Hives, itchy rash, swelling of the skin	Weight loss (although individuals may be overweight or have a normal weight when diagnosed)
Nasal congestion	Dermatitis herpetiformis (skin rash), easy bruising
Itchy, watery eyes	Anemias and deficiencies in iron, folic acid, vitamins A, B$_{12}$, D, E, K
Difficulty breathing	Extreme weakness and fatigue
Cramps, nausea, vomiting	Abnormalities of liver enzyme
Anaphylaxis	Mouth ulcers, dental enamel defects
	Bone and joint pain, swelling of hands and ankles
	Amenorrhea, infertility, miscarriages
	Headaches, including migraines; mood swings, depression; tingling in the hands and feet; gait disturbance

Remember! A wheat-free diet is not necessarily gluten-free. If you are allergic to wheat, you may consume barley (contains gluten), rye (contains gluten), and oats (pure, uncontaminated) along with amaranth, corn, rice, quinoa, and other gluten-free grains. Make sure to consult with your allergy specialist. If you have celiac disease, you need to avoid gluten in grains such as wheat, barley, rye, spelt, Kamut, triticale, and commercial oats (which may be contaminated).

Wheat by any other name:

- Atta
- Bulgur
- Couscous
- Durum wheat
- Einkorn
- Emmer
- Enriched/white/whole
- wheat flour (all-purpose, bread, cake, instant, pastry, self-rising, soft wheat, steel-ground, stone-ground)
- Farina
- Gluten

Did You Know?

WDEIA

Wheat allergy in adults is very rare and most commonly associated with wheat-dependent exercise-induced anaphylaxis (WDEIA). Allergy to wheat means that all products made from wheat and wheat derivatives must be avoided.

- Graham flour
- High-gluten flour, high-protein flour
- Kamut
- Seitan
- Semolina
- Spelt (dinkel, farro)
- Triticale (a cross between wheat and rye)
- *Triticum aestivum*
- Wheat bran/flour/germ/starch/gluten/grass/malt/sprouts

Other foods and food ingredients to exclude:

- Bread crumbs
- Cereal extract
- Cracker meal
- Gelatinized starch derived from wheat
- Glucose syrup derived from wheat
- Hydrolyzed wheat protein
- Imitation crabmeat (often contains wheat flour)
- Pasta
- Matzoh (also spelled as matzo, matzah, or matza), matzoh meal
- Seitan
- Soy sauce
- Surimi
- Modified wheat starch
- Wheat germ hydrolysate
- Wheat germ oil
- Wheat protein isolate
- Whole wheat berries

Food ingredients that may be derived from wheat:

- Modified food starch
- Hydrolyzed plant protein
- Hydrolyzed vegetable protein

When the label does not clearly state the source of the "food," "plant," or "vegetable" in the ingredients listed above, you need to contact the manufacturer.

Wheat-Free Diet

The list on pages 129–35 is set up to mimic the organization of a grocery store, with fresh foods arranged around the outside walls and processed foods in the inner aisles. The list is not exhaustive. **Please read the food label every time.**

Foods to Enjoy, Question, and Exclude if You Have a Wheat Allergy

Aisle by Aisle	Foods to Enjoy	Foods to Question	Foods to Exclude
Produce section	• All fresh, ready-to-eat fruits and fruit juices • All fresh, ready-to-eat vegetables and their juices • Packaged salads	• Some dried fruit (dried dates may contain wheat flour)	• Strained fruit with added cereal • Breaded or floured vegetables
Bakery and crackers	• Rye crisps made with rye flour only • Plain rice crisps, crackers, or cakes • Rice, barley, or rye bread made without wheat flour • Corn or polenta chips • Corn tostadas	• Seasoned rice crisps, crackers, or cakes	• Whole wheat, enriched, or white bread • Wheat rolls • Bread crumbs • Croissants • Graham crackers • Doughnuts • Sweet rolls • Muffins or popovers • Rusks • Stuffing
Dairy/dairy alternatives and eggs section	• Milk, buttermilk, yogurt, plain hard aged cheese, fresh cheese, plain cream cheese • Fresh, boiled, poached, fried eggs prepared without any wheat ingredients • Plain liquid egg • Plain tofu	• Seasoned shredded cheese (may contain hydrolyzed wheat protein) • Cheese sauce or spreads • Flavored cream cheese • Seasoned liquid egg products • Soy-based dairy products (may contain wheat starch)	• Malted milk • Flavored yogurt containing multigrain granola or other wheat-derived ingredients • Tofu seasoned with soy sauce or teriyaki sauce

Aisle by Aisle	Foods to Enjoy	Foods to Question	Foods to Exclude
Deli section	• All deli meats made without wheat-based ingredients (e.g., hydrolyzed wheat protein, wheat starch)	• Bacon (most bacon is gluten-free, but some may be seasoned with soy sauce, which contains wheat) • Ham (most brands are wheat- and gluten-free, but some may contain wheat starch) • Kielbasa • Wieners • Salami (most brands are gluten- and wheat-free, but some may contain hydrolyzed wheat protein)	• Sausages made with wheat-derived ingredients (e.g., wheat flour, wheat starch) • Meatloaf • Stuffing • Liver pâté
Meat, poultry, and fish section	• All fresh lean cuts of beef, veal, pork, lamb • All fresh poultry (chicken and turkey) • All fresh or frozen fish • All fresh or frozen seafood: shrimp, scallops, lobster, clams, mussels • Canned tuna in water or oil • Canned sardines in water or oil	• Sausages (may contain hydrolyzed wheat protein, wheat starch) • Meatballs (made with bread crumbs) • Dried meats such as beef jerky (may contain soy sauce or wheat flour) • Frozen hamburgers (may contain wheat starch or flour or hydrolyzed wheat protein) • Canned tuna in vegetable broth (may contain hydrolyzed wheat protein) • Canned sardines in vegetable broth (may contain hydrolyzed wheat protein)	• All breaded meat • Frozen turkey or pork roasts with bread stuffing • Frozen patties or croquettes • Seasoned frozen turkey or chicken breasts (may contain hydrolyzed wheat protein) • Breaded fish sticks • Breaded or battered shrimp • Seasoned fish in pouches • Imitation crabmeat (contains wheat flour) • Surimi (contains wheat flour)

Aisle by Aisle	Foods to Enjoy	Foods to Question	Foods to Exclude
Aisle 1 Breakfast cereals, hot cereal, jam, peanut butter, canned fruit, syrup	• Pure, uncontaminated oats • Puffed rice (wheat-free) • Corn, quinoa, flax, amaranth, or rice cereal to which no wheat-derived ingredients have been added • Gluten-free granola • Hot cereals: cream of buckwheat, quinoa flakes, cream of brown rice, millet grits, cornmeal, mixed hot cereal made with wheat-free grits (amaranth, barley, buckwheat, corn, quinoa) • All pure fruit jams, jellies, preserves, and marmalades • Honey • Maple syrup	• Peanut butter (most brands are gluten-free, but some may contain wheat germ) • Nut butters (most brands are gluten-free, but some may contain wheat germ)	• Cream of wheat • Cold cereal made with wheat or whole wheat flour, farina, semolina, spelt, Kamut, einkorn, emmer (shredded wheat, bran buds) • Granola • Hot cereal made with wheat, wheat flour, wheat germ, wheat bran, spelt, Kamut, triticale • Graham crackers
Aisle 2 Cookies, confectionery, crackers, potato chips, snacks, popcorn, nuts and seeds, desserts	• Plain rice cakes • Corn tacos, chips, nachos • Gluten-free corn- or rice-based cookies • Plain potato chips • Rye crackers made without wheat flour (e.g., Finn crisps) • Plain popcorn • Hard candy	• Seasoned nuts or seeds (may be contaminated with wheat flour) • Seasoned potato chips (seasoning may contain wheat-derived ingredients) • Seasoned taco chips • Seasoned rice cakes	• Pretzels • Crackers and cookies made with wheat flour • Licorice candy (contains wheat flour) • Matzoh • Melba toast • Trail mixes • Chocolate bars made with wheat ingredients

Aisle by Aisle	Foods to Enjoy	Foods to Question	Foods to Exclude
Aisle 3 Spices, flour, baking supplies, sugar and other sweeteners	• Individual spices (e.g., cinnamon, pepper, cloves, allspice, ginger, paprika) • Individual herbs (e.g., thyme, basil, sage, savory) • Amaranth flour (not to be confused with arrowroot biscuits made with wheat flour and arrowroot flour) • Corn flour, cornmeal, corn bran, corn starch • Potato starch • Quinoa flour • Flax seeds, ground flax seeds (flaxseed meal) • Millet flour and grits • Legume flours (e.g., fava, gram, besan, garbanzo, chickpea, lentil) • Sorghum flour • Brown rice flour, whole-grain rice flour, glutinous rice flour • Rye flour, sago flour • Soy flour, tapioca flour • Indian rice grass (Montina) • Inulin (dietary fiber found in artichokes, leeks, and chicory root) • Psyllium husks • Nut flours (e.g., almond, hazelnut, chestnut) • Potato flour • Pure, uncontaminated (wheat-free, gluten-free) oat flour, oat bran	• Spice mixtures • Buckwheat flour (may sometimes be mixed with wheat flour in a product, and there is a high risk of cross-contamination) • Baking powder (generally made with cornstarch, but some brands may contain wheat starch) • Icing mixes and prepared frosting (may contain wheat starch or wheat flour)	• Atta, or chapatti, flour (from low-gluten wheat used to make chapatti flatbreads, a specialty of Indian cuisine) • Wheat flour • Wheat starch • Wheat germ • Semolina flour • Durum wheat flour • Plain cake and pancake mixes • Buckwheat pancake mixes containing wheat flour • Ice cream cones and wafers made from wheat flour

Aisle by Aisle	Foods to Enjoy	Foods to Question	Foods to Exclude
Aisle 3 (continued)	• Salba (oil seed derived from an ancient plant species belonging to the Chia family, grown in Peru) • Sago (starchy food derived from palm trees) • Soy flour, teff flour • Taro flour • Sweet potato flour • Gluten-free pancake mixes • Gluten-free bread mixes • Baking soda • Active dry yeast • Baker's yeast • Nutritional yeast • Xanthan gum, guar gum • Vanilla extract (pure or artificial) • Rum extract • Food coloring • Baking chocolate chips • Carob chips • Pure cocoa powder • Cream of tartar • Shredded coconut • Baking chocolate • Agave nectar • Corn syrup • Molasses • Granulated or brown sugar • Raw sugar • Confectioners' (icing) sugar		

Aisle by Aisle	Foods to Enjoy	Foods to Question	Foods to Exclude
Aisle 4 Oils, vinegars, sauces, salad dressings, condiments	• All vegetable oils • Vinegars • Mustard bran • Mustard flour • Pickles • Ketchup • Relish • Olives • Tomato paste • Hot sauce • Gluten-free soy sauce • Real bacon bits • Roasted red peppers • Roasted tomatoes	• Specialty mustards (may contain wheat flour as a thickener) • Mustard pickles (may contain wheat flour) • Prepared dry mustard • Cooking sauces (may contain wheat flour or wheat starch) • Creamy salad dressings (e.g., Caesar; may contain wheat flour or wheat starch) • Imitation bacon bits (may contain hydrolyzed wheat protein)	• Soy sauce (usually contains wheat, but some brands are gluten-free) • Tamari sauce (contains wheat, but some brands are gluten-free) • Teriyaki sauce (contains soy sauce) • Gravy containing wheat flour • Suet (contains wheat starch)
Aisle 5 Soup, canned vegetables, pasta, pasta sauce, Mexican rice and other side dishes	• All dried or canned peas, beans, lentils, and pulses • Pasta made from rice, quinoa, soy, beans, lentils, or potato • Soup broth labeled gluten-free • Ready-to-eat soups made with wheat-free ingredients • Wheat-free whole grains (e.g., rice, quinoa, millet, buckwheat) • Plain rice or mixed rice • Guacamole	• Buckwheat noodles — ensure pure buckwheat flour is used • Seasoned rice (e.g., chicken wild rice, chicken vegetable) • Soup mixes • Bean soup mixes including seasonings • Canned soups • Bouillon cubes • Some brands of baked beans • Soft tortillas made with corn flour — ensure corn flour is gluten-free and is not mixed with wheat flour • Cheese sauces • Creamy pasta sauces — ensure no wheat flour, wheat starch	• Couscous • Orzo • Regular pasta • Whole wheat pasta • Multigrain pasta • Durum semolina pasta • Udon noodles • Potato gnocchi • Soft tortillas made with a combination of corn and wheat flours • Commercial powdered mashed potatoes made with wheat starch or wheat flour • Scalloped potatoes containing wheat flour

Aisle by Aisle	Foods to Enjoy	Foods to Question	Foods to Exclude
Aisle 6 Water, soft drinks, sport drinks, fruit juices, alcoholic beverages	• Coffee, tea, decaffeinated coffee • Carbonated beverages • All milks • Cocoa • Water • Flavored water • Fresh fruit juices • Shelf-stable juices • Soft drinks • Alcoholic beverages: wine, bourbon, gin, port, rye whisky, Scotch whisky, vodka, liqueurs (e.g., amaretto), gluten-free beers (e.g., sorghum- or buckwheat-based beers)	• Sport drinks — check to ensure gluten-free ingredients are used • Flavored herbal teas • Flavored coffees • Chocolate drinks • Alcoholic beverages: flavored coolers, flavored vodka mixes (e.g., Bloody Mary; the seasoning may contain wheat starch)	• Malted drinks • Coffee substitutes made with wheat-derived ingredients • Alcoholic beverages: beer, ale
Aisle 7 Frozen fruits and vegetables, frozen meals and desserts	• All plain frozen fruits, vegetables, or mixed vegetables • Frozen gluten-free foods (e.g., gluten-free pizza, gluten-free chili) • Gluten-free waffles • Gluten-free pancakes	• Frozen french fries (wheat starch or hydrolyzed wheat protein may be used in the seasoning) • Restaurant-made frozen french fries • Frozen meals	• Frozen waffles • Frozen pancakes • Battered frozen vegetables • Frozen pies, pizza • Frozen pasta dishes • Frozen dumplings
Other		• Medications — check with your pharmacist for wheat starch or modified wheat starch • Lipstick, lip balm, lip gloss — check for the presence of wheat starch	• Playdough

Nutritional Profile of Wheat and Substitutes

Wheat and wheat-related grains are a very good source of B vitamins, such as thiamine and riboflavin, as well as iron, calcium, and calories (energy). Products made from wheat and whole wheat are high in protein and fiber. If you need to avoid wheat, you may be at risk of lower intakes of these nutrients. Fortification is a feature of most wheat-based flours, particularly when it comes to folic acid and other B vitamins such as niacin, riboflavin, and thiamine.

Wheat Alternatives

Nutrient	Alternative Food Sources
High-quality protein	Milk and milk products, meat, fish, poultry, legumes
Thiamin (vitamin B_1)	Brewer's yeast, meat, sunflower seeds, green peas, split peas, asparagus, legumes
Niacin (vitamin B_3)	Beef, pork, corn flour, eggs, cow's milk
Riboflavin (vitamin B_2)	Milk products (yogurt, ricotta cheese), eggs, some lean meats, spinach, mushrooms
Folate	Beans and peas (romano beans, black-eye peas), spinach, broccoli, dark leafy green vegetables
Vitamin B_{12}	Fish (salmon, light canned tuna), meat (lean ground beef), dairy (cottage cheese, yogurt), fortified dairy-free milks (not made with wheat- or gluten-derived ingredients)
Iron	Shellfish (clams, mussels), seeds (pumpkin seeds), beans (romano beans, white kidney beans), gluten-free grains (teff, Job's tears)
Phosphorus	Milk and milk products (milk, yogurt, cottage cheese), meat, fish, poultry, tofu

Sesame Seed Allergy

Allergy to sesame seed is increasing in North America and Europe, as reflected in the rise in reported anaphylactic reactions. This may be due to an increased consumption of sesame seeds and the use of sesame oil in processed foods. In some parts of the world, such as Australia, sesame seed allergy is more common than tree nut allergy and represents a major allergen, ranked in the top five. And in Israel, sesame seed allergy is second to cow's milk protein allergy as a cause of anaphylaxis. It is thought that the heavy consumption and early exposure to sesame seed may be blamed for the high prevalence in this part of the world.

Unlike refined soybean oil, very few sesame oils on the market are refined enough to remove all the protein that causes allergic reaction. If you are allergic to sesame seed, you must avoid sesame oil.

Food ingredients that contain sesame seed protein:

- Benne, benne seed, benniseed
- Gingelly, gingelly oil
- Sesame seeds
- Sesamol, sesamolina
- *Sesamum indicum*
- Sim sim
- Tahini, tahina (sesame seed butter)
- Til
- Vegetable oil (check source of oil)

Imported Products

Imported food products and products purchased through mail order or over the Internet are not produced using the same manufacturing and labeling standards as in North America. Cross-contamination is a risk that may not be mentioned on the label.

Eating Out

Several international cuisines use sesame seeds and other products derived from them on a regular basis. Check with the restaurant to see whether the chef cooks with sesame oil or uses sesame seeds.

- Middle Eastern cuisine (hummus, shish kebabs)
- Turkish cuisine
- Asian cuisine: Sushi topped with sesame seeds, salads and meals made with sesame oil, sesame-topped meals

---

Did You Know?

Resolution
Data are limited on the resolution of sesame seed allergy, but it has been reported that only 15% of children diagnosed at age 10 to 12 months outgrew their sesame allergy within 18 and 24 months. Similar to occupational wheat allergy, inhalation of sesame seed dust can also cause occupational respiratory allergy (asthma, hay fever) to sesame.

Did You Know?

Cross-Reactions
Individuals who experience allergy to sesame seeds have also reported similar allergic reactions to poppy seed, hazelnut, and rye grain. There are also cross-reactions between sesame seeds and members of the nut family, namely Brazil nuts, almonds, walnuts, and pistachios.

Sesame-Free Diet

The list on pages 138–141 is set up to mimic the organization of a grocery store, with fresh foods arranged around the outside walls and processed foods in the inner aisles. The list is not exhaustive. **Please read the food label every time.**

Foods to Enjoy, Question, and Exclude if You Have a Sesame Allergy

Aisle by Aisle	Foods to Enjoy	Foods to Question	Foods to Exclude
Produce section	• All fresh fruits, vegetables, and their juices		• Packaged ready-to-eat salads with toppings including sesame seeds • Sesame seed sprouts
Bakery and crackers	• Plain white, whole wheat, rye, potato, sourdough, and other breads made without sesame seed products	• Melba toast (check for sesame topping and traces of sesame seed) • Baked goods: buns, bagels, croissants, crackers (check for sesame seeds or oil as ingredients) • Oven-ready breads • Seasoned croutons	• Hamburger buns topped with sesame seeds • Baked goods (e.g., pastries, buns, bagels) topped with sesame seeds or made with sesame oil • Bread crumbs • Bread sticks and seasoned crackers topped with sesame seeds
Dairy/dairy alternatives and eggs section	• Milk, yogurt, cheese, cream • Fresh eggs prepared without sesame oil or seeds • Seasoned egg whites • Seasoned liquid eggs	• Margarine (check source of vegetable oil)	• Tempeh • Vegetarian snacks
Deli section	• All deli meats made without sesame-derived ingredients • Liver or meat pâté	• Dips • Spreads • Chutneys	• Hummus • Baba ganoush (eggplant spread or "caviar")

Aisle by Aisle	Foods to Enjoy	Foods to Question	Foods to Exclude
Meat, poultry, and fish section	• All fresh meat, poultry, fish	• Sausages • Vegetarian burgers, meat substitutes, vegetarian sausages, and hot dogs • Turkey or chicken burgers (some brands may contain sesame oil) • Hamburgers (check the source of oil) • Seasoned meats (e.g., seasoned pork)	• Sesame-flavored meat alternatives (e.g., tempeh burger)
Aisle 1 Breakfast cereals, hot cereal, jam, peanut butter, canned fruit, syrup	• Plain hot cereal: cream of wheat, oatmeal, cream of buckwheat • All pure fruit jams, jellies, preserves, and marmalades • Maple syrup • Pancake syrup • Honey • Canned fruit	• Muesli • Peanut, almond, hazelnut, and seed butters (check for traces of sesame) • Granola	• Multigrain cold cereals containing sesame seeds • Hot cereal mixes containing sesame seeds • Granola containing sesame seeds • Tahini
Aisle 2 Cookies, confectionery, crackers, potato chips, snacks, popcorn, nuts and seeds, desserts	• Plain hard candy • Plain potato chips • Plain nuts or seeds without traces of sesame seeds • Rice crackers, corn chips, tortilla chips, and vegetable crisps that are free of sesame • Homemade cookies, cakes, and desserts that are free of sesame	• Seasoned potato chips, popcorn, and corn chips • Cookies • Bagel or pita chips	• Nut- or grain-based halvah (halva) • Trail mixes • Sesame-topped pretzels • Sesame-topped rice cakes • Sesame snap bars • Sesame balls (Chinese dessert) • Sesame seed cake

Aisle by Aisle	Foods to Enjoy	Foods to Question	Foods to Exclude
Aisle 3 Spices, flour, baking supplies, sugar and other sweeteners	• All pure grain flours without risk of cross-contamination with sesame seeds or sesame seed flour • Plain herbs and spices • Baking powder • Baking soda • Sugar • Molasses • Artificial sweeteners	• Mixed spices • Seasoning mixes • Baking mixes — check for cross-contamination with sesame	• Sesame seed flour • Sesame salt (gomasio) • Sesame seeds • Baking mixes containing sesame ingredients
Aisle 4 Oils, vinegars, sauces, salad dressings, condiments	• Olive, canola, soy, grapeseed, and corn oil • All animal fats • All plain vinegar products • Mustard • Ketchup • Soy sauce • Relish • Pickles • Barbecue sauce • Oil-based salad dressings without sesame oil • Homemade gravy without sesame-derived ingredients	• Vegetable oil (may contain traces of sesame seed oil) • Seasoned rice vinegar • Asian-style sauces and marinades • Salad dressings • Marinated olives • Marinated vegetables • Mayonnaise (check source of oils used)	• Sesame oil • Salad dressing using sesame ingredients • Japanese-style vinaigrette with sesame oil or seeds • White sauce containing sesame seeds • Tahini sauce • Satay sauce • Hoisin sauce
Aisle 5 Soup, canned vegetables, pasta, pasta sauce, Mexican rice and other side dishes	• All plain dried or canned beans, peas, and lentils • Plain macaroni and other pasta • Plain rice or mixed rice • Plain whole grains (e.g., quinoa, barley, millet) • Guacamole • Salsa	• Soups • Risotto • Seasoned couscous • Seasoned rice • Seasoned pasta • Pasta sauce	• Falafel topped with tahini sauce • Japanese meals (with sesame seed topping) • Thai meals (e.g., curries) • Vietnamese meals (with sesame seed topping) • Spring rolls • Satays

Aisle by Aisle	Foods to Enjoy	Foods to Question	Foods to Exclude
Aisle 6 Water, soft drinks, sport drinks, fruit juices, alcoholic beverages	• Coffee, tea, decaffeinated coffee • Carbonated beverages • All milks • Cocoa • Water, flavored water • Fresh fruit juices • Shelf-stable juices • Soft drinks • Alcoholic beverages		• Aqua Libra
Aisle 7 Frozen fruits and vegetables, frozen meals and desserts	• All plain frozen fruits, vegetables, or mixed vegetables • Ice cream • Frozen yogurt • Sorbet • Sherbet	• Frozen waffles • Frozen pancakes • Frozen baked goods (e.g., muffins) • Frozen french fries • Frozen scalloped potatoes • Frozen appetizers (check for sesame topping and sesame-derived ingredients)	• Frozen waffles or pancakes containing sesame-derived ingredients • Frozen meals (e.g., stir-fries, stews, burritos) • Frozen muffins with sesame seed topping
Other		• Adhesive bandages • Cosmetics: lipstick, lip balm, face creams • Body oils • Moisturizing creams • Topical creams and oils • Hair care products • Perfumes • Soaps • Sunscreen • Drugs	

Nutritional Profile of Sesame Seeds and Substitutes

Sesame seeds are very nutritious and a good source of calcium — 1 ounce (28 g) of whole roasted sesame seeds provides 33% of the daily recommended intake of calcium. They are also a very good source of trace minerals, including copper and manganese, as well as a good source of iron, phosphorus, vitamin B_1, selenium, and zinc.

Sesame Seed Alternatives

Nutrient	Alternative Food Sources
Calcium	Milk, lactose-free milk, cheese, other dairy products, dark green leafy vegetables (e.g., kale, Swiss chard)
Thiamine (vitamin B_1)	Brewer's yeast, sunflower seeds, wheat germ, red meat, legumes, seafood
Selenium	Seafood, red meat, grains harvested from selenium-rich soil
Zinc	Shellfish (clams, mussels), meat, fortified cereals
Iron	Shellfish (clams, mussels), seeds (pumpkin seeds), beans (romano beans, white kidney beans), gluten-free grains (teff, Job's tears)
Phosphorus	Milk and milk products (milk, yogurt, cottage cheese), meat, fish, poultry, tofu

Sulfite Sensitivity

Sulfites are substances found naturally in foods. They are also added to foods to preserve color, prolong shelf life, prevent browning, and reduce spoilage. In some cases, sulfites are used to remove color from starches, such as potato flour and corn grits.

Sensitivity to sulfites is thought to affect as many as 1% of the American population. Asthma sufferers are more likely to be affected — up to 4% of asthmatics are also sensitive to sulfites. However, the reverse is not necessarily true — there is no evidence that avoiding all dietary sources of sulfites improves asthma. What puzzles researchers is that sulfites are not protein entities, so it is unknown how they may cause allergic-like symptoms.

Food ingredients that contain sulfites:

- Sodium sulfite
- Sulfur dioxide
- Sodium bisulfite/ dithionite/metabisulfite/ sulfite
- Potassium bisulfite/ metabisulfite
- Sulfiting agents
- Sulfurous acid

Regulations

In most countries, the use of sulfites in foods is highly regulated. In Canada, the government prohibits the spraying of fresh fruits and vegetables with sulfites, with two exceptions: fresh grapes, which are fumigated with sulfur dioxide gas or stored in packaging material that slowly emits sulfur dioxide gas; and fresh peeled or precut potatoes that are destined for further processing (to make french fries or potato chips). These foods must be labeled as treated with sulfites. In America, Canada, and the European Union, sulfite must be listed on the label of a food product if the concentration exceeds 10 parts per million (ppm). This greatly simplifies the avoidance of sulfites for sensitive individuals, but consumption of large amounts of foods with undeclared sulfite (less than 10 ppm) could still trigger reactions.

Did You Know?

Reliable Testing
The most reliable method for diagnosing sulfite sensitivity is an oral challenge in a hospital setting. The skin prick test is not reliable enough for measuring reaction to sulfites.

Did You Know?

Caution
Do not consume a food or food product if there is no ingredient list or if there is a risk the product might have been in contact with sulfites. When in doubt, call the food manufacturer, and when dining out, ask the chef or sous chef for information on sulfite content.

Sulfite-Free Diet

The list on pages 144–147 is set up to mimic the organization of a grocery store, with fresh foods arranged around the outside walls and processed foods in the inner aisles. The list is not exhaustive. **Please read the food label every time.** Avoid any product whose ingredient list warns "may contain" or "may contain traces of" sulfites. If you are uncertain about the presence of sulfites in a product, call the manufacturer to confirm.

Foods to Enjoy, Question, and Exclude if You Have a Sulfite Allergy

Aisle by Aisle	Foods to Enjoy	Foods to Question	Foods to Exclude
Produce section	• All fresh fruits and vegetables without added sulfites (except for those listed under Foods to Question or Foods to Exclude)	• All fruits and vegetable juices, domestic or imported • Dried prunes • Prewashed packaged salads and greens • Packaged fruit salads • Lettuce	• Apple cider (nonalcoholic) • Citrus peel • Fresh grapes • Fresh mushrooms • Grape juice • Peeled and precut potatoes • Glazed or glacéed fruit • Most dried fruit (apricots, coconut, figs, raisins) • Canned fruits • Bottled lemon juice or concentrate • Bottled lime juice or concentrate • Maraschino cherries (sulfite is added as bleaching agent) • Fruit toppings • Dried vegetables (e.g., sun-dried tomatoes)

Aisle by Aisle	Foods to Enjoy	Foods to Question	Foods to Exclude
Bakery and crackers	• Plain fresh breads, buns, biscuits, or pizza dough made with allowed ingredients • Plain crackers made without sulfites	• Crispy baguette-style crackers • Bread crumbs • Seasoned multigrain or multi-seed crackers • Multigrain bagels • Tea biscuits • Doughnuts • Oven-ready breads and buns	• Any baked goods with dried or glacéed fruit, molasses, coconut, dehydrated vegetables, frozen apple slices, or icing (e.g., carrot cake, sponge cake) • Mincemeat • Garlic bread • Tart shells
Dairy/dairy alternatives and eggs section	• Milk, buttermilk, cream, sour cream • Plain yogurt • Cheese • Plain cottage cheese • Processed cheese • Kefir • Quark cheese • Butter • Fresh eggs prepared without sulfites • Seasoned egg whites • Seasoned liquid eggs	• Flavored yogurt • Flavored cottage cheese	• Tofu • Tempeh • Prepared dairy products made with sulfites (e.g., yogurt with dried fruit or muesli topping)
Deli section	• Deli meats made without sulfites	• Deli meats • Sausages • Hot dogs • Kielbassa • Seasoned hummus	• Olive tapenade • Vegetable tapenade • Marinated vegetables • Marinated olives
Meat, poultry, and fish section	• All unprocessed fresh meat, poultry, and fish • Fresh crab, lobster, prawns, shrimp, and squid without sulfite wash	• Seasoned meats (e.g., sun-dried tomato chicken burgers) • Crustaceans • Canned tuna • Canned salmon • Canned crab	• Dried fish • Canned clams • Clam juice • Ready-to-eat tuna

Aisle by Aisle	Foods to Enjoy	Foods to Question	Foods to Exclude
Aisle 1 Breakfast cereals, hot cereal, jam, peanut butter, canned fruit, syrup	• Cold breakfast cereals without dried fruit • Plain crackers without sulfites • Honey	• Cold cereals • Jams, jellies, marmalades, and preserves • Canned fruit • Maple syrup • Pancake syrup	• Muesli containing dried fruit or coconut • Granola containing dried fruit or coconut • Seasoned oatmeal (flavors may contain sulfites) • Fruit snacks • Cinnamon spread
Aisle 2 Cookies, confectionery, crackers, potato chips, snacks, popcorn, nuts and seeds, desserts	• Homemade cookies and sweets made without sulfites • All nuts and seeds • Popcorn • Plain rice crackers, chips, and cakes	• Candy • Chocolate • Fruit bars • Tortilla chips	• Trail mix • Multigrain cereal bars • Granola bars with dried fruit or coconut • Potato chips • Vegetable chips • Candy with dried fruit
Aisle 3 Spices, flour, baking supplies, sugar and other sweeteners	• All single plain grain flours • Baking powder • Baking soda • Sugar • Artificial sweeteners • Baking mixes made without added sulfites	• Dried herbs • Spices • Spice mixtures • Seasoning mixtures • Pectin • Fruit filling • Corn syrup • Glucose and dextrose • Cornstarch • Cornbread mix • Corn muffin mix	• Potato starch • Potato flour • Molasses
Aisle 4 Oils, vinegars, sauces, salad dressings, condiments	• All vegetable oils • Margarine • Shortening • Homemade salad dressing made without sulfite-containing ingredients	• Gravy • Sauces and marinades • Tomato paste, pulp, and purée • Prepared salad dressings • Malt vinegar • White vinegar • Barbecue sauce • Olives	• Pickled cocktail onions • Horseradish (plain or creamy) • Mustard • Cider vinegar • Wine vinegar • Steak sauce • Pickled peppers • Sauerkraut • Coleslaw • Marinated vegetables • Mustard pickles

Aisle by Aisle	Foods to Enjoy	Foods to Question	Foods to Exclude
Aisle 5 Soup, canned vegetables, pasta, pasta sauce, Mexican rice and other side dishes	• Canned potatoes • All plain dried or canned beans, peas, and lentils • Plain macaroni or other pasta • Plain rice or mixed rice • Plain whole grains (e.g., quinoa, barley, millet)	• Canned vegetables • Dried pasta side dishes • Canned pasta dishes • Seasoned rice • Salsa • Guacamole • Dips	• Clam chowder • Dried potato side dishes
Aisle 6 Water, soft drinks, sport drinks, fruit juices, alcoholic beverages	• Coffee, tea, decaffeinated coffee, carbonated beverages, all milks, cocoa • Water • Flavored water	• Fruit juice (domestic or imported, fresh or shelf-stable) • Coconut water • Soft drinks • Beer (alcoholic and nonalcoholic	• Wine (especially white wine) • De-alcoholized wine • Alcoholic fruit cordial (e.g., lime cordial) • Apple cider (alcoholic and nonalcoholic) • Coolers
Aisle 7 Frozen fruits and vegetables, frozen meals and desserts	• Plain frozen waffles • Plain frozen pancakes • Ice cream • Frozen yogurt • Sorbet • Sherbet	• Frozen fruits • Frozen vegetables (e.g., mushrooms, peas, peppers) • Flavored waffles and pancakes • Frozen pizza • Frozen hamburgers or chicken burgers	• Frozen french fries • Frozen cookie dough • Frozen apple pie • Frozen baked goods with dried fruit (e.g., frozen muffins)

Mustard Allergy

Widely consumed but often hidden in many food products, mustard is a spice that can trigger life-threatening IgE-type mediated reactions. In France, mustard seed allergy is the fourth most prevalent allergy and is estimated to affect 1.1% of children and 0.84% of adults. Mustard seed is now listed as one of the top 10 allergens in Canada and is one of the top 14 allergens included in the European Union food labeling laws list. Canada accounts for about 35% of the world's mustard production and 50% of global exports.

In addition to being used as a spice and condiment, mustard is used as an emulsifier because it helps stabilize oil-and-water preparations, such as mayonnaise, salad dressings, and many sauces, and as a binding agent in meats to allow for easier slicing.

Mustard-derived products include:

- Mustard seeds
- Ground mustard
- Mustard bran
- Dry mustard powder
- Mustard flour
- Mustard oil
- Prepared mustard
- Prepared mustard powder

Source of Antioxidants

Mustard belongs to the Brassicaceae family, the same botanical family that includes cabbage, cauliflower, Brussels sprouts, turnips, radishes, and broccoli. This family is well known for its nutritional benefits. Mustard provides cancer-fighting antioxidants — called glucosinolates — that help enzymes detoxify the body and change the way the body protects itself against cancer. Mustard is also a good source of protein, dietary fiber, and omega-3 fatty acids, as well as providing healthy amounts of minerals, such as calcium, magnesium, and potassium. It is an excellent source of selenium — a trace mineral that has antioxidant properties and may slow down or prevent the rate of cancer. Luckily, because the intake of mustard is variable and small on a daily basis, developing nutritional deficiencies as a result of its exclusion is highly unlikely.

Mustard-Free Diet

The list on pages 149–152 is set up to mimic the organization of a grocery store, with fresh foods arranged around the outside walls and processed foods in the inner aisles. The list is not exhaustive. **Please read the food label every time.**

Foods to Enjoy, Question, and Exclude if You Have a Mustard Allergy

Aisle by Aisle	Foods to Enjoy	Foods to Question	Foods to Exclude
Produce section	• All fresh, ready-to-eat fruits and fruit juices • All fresh vegetables except those listed under Foods to Exclude)	• Packaged ready-to eat salads with dressing that may contain mustard • Vegetable juices (check for mustard greens)	• Sprouted mustard seeds • Mustard greens
Bakery and crackers	• All breads (e.g., wheat, whole wheat, rye, pumpernickel, rice, potato) • Plain crackers • Melba toast • Bread sticks • Croissants	• Seasoned crackers (check seasoning for mustard) • Seasoned croutons • Oven-ready breads and buns • Baked goods (e.g., buns, hamburger buns)	
Dairy/dairy alternatives and eggs section	• Milk, buttermilk, cream, sour cream • Yogurt • Cheese • Plain cottage cheese • Processed cheese • Kefir • Quark cheese • Butter • Fresh eggs prepared without mustard ingredients • Seasoned egg whites • Seasoned liquid eggs • Plain tofu	• Seasoned tofu • Seasoned tempeh • Flavored cheese spreads	• Cheese spreads containing mustard ingredients

Aisle by Aisle	Foods to Enjoy	Foods to Question	Foods to Exclude
Deli section	• All deli products made without mustard (e.g., oven-roasted chicken breast, turkey breast, ham)	• Seasoned hummus • Seasoned, ready-to-eat chicken breast strips • Hot dogs • Weiners • Liver pâté	• Deli meats containing mustard (e.g., pepperoni, salami, sausages)
Meat, poultry, and fish section	• All fresh lean cuts of beef, veal, pork, lamb • All fresh poultry (chicken and turkey) • All fresh or frozen fish • All fresh or frozen seafood: shrimp, scallops, lobster, clams, mussels • Canned tuna or sardines in water or oil	• Hamburgers • Sirloin burgers • Chicken or turkey burgers	• Prepared meats, poultry, and fish coated with or prepared in a sauce containing mustard • Vegetarian meats containing mustard (e.g., sausages, hot dogs, burgers)
Aisle 1 Breakfast cereals, hot cereal, jam, peanut butter, canned fruit, syrup	• All hot or cold cereals • All pure fruit jams, jellies, preserves, and marmalades • All nut and seed butters • All canned fruit • Pancake syrup • Maple syrup • Honey		
Aisle 2 Cookies, confectionery, crackers, potato chips, snacks, popcorn, nuts and seeds, desserts	• Candy • Cookies • Chocolate • Plain crackers • Plain potato chips, corn chips, rice crackers • Plain popcorn • Plain peanuts and tree nuts • Plain seeds	• Seasoned potato chips, corn chips, rice chips (check seasoning for mustard) • Seasoned popcorn (check seasoning for mustard) • Seasoned nuts and seeds (check seasoning for mustard)	• All seasoned nuts, seeds, and chips containing mustard

Aisle by Aisle	Foods to Enjoy	Foods to Question	Foods to Exclude
Aisle 3 Spices, flour, baking supplies, sugar and other sweeteners	• Individual spices (e.g., cinnamon, pepper, cloves, allspice, ginger, paprika) except mustard and mustard-related spice products • Individual herbs (e.g., thyme, basil, sage, savory) • All single plain grain flours • Baking mixes • Sugar • Molasses • Corn syrup • Artificial sweeteners	• Spice blends • Seasoning mixes	• Spices: whole mustard seeds, ground mustard, dry mustard, mustard bran
Aisle 4 Oils, vinegars, sauces, salad dressings, condiments	• All vegetable oils • Plain vinegars (e.g., apple cider, balsamic, rice, wine, malt) • Olives • Tomato paste • Ketchup • Hot sauce • Soy sauce • Real bacon bits • Roasted red peppers • Roasted tomatoes	• Pickled beets • Seasoned vinegar • Salad dressings • Gravy • Marinating or basting sauces • Stir-fry sauces • Seasoning mixes • Chutney • Relish • Garlic sauce • Olive tapenade	• Prepared mustard (e.g., plain, Dijon, honey) • Pickles with mustard seeds • Gerkins • Pickled onions • Barbecue sauce • Mayonnaise • Horseradish • Mayonnaise products (e.g., Miracle Whip) • Vegan mayonnaise • Low-fat, seasoned mayonnaise made with Dijon mustard • Béarnaise sauce • Piccalilli sauce • Tartar sauce

Aisle by Aisle	Foods to Enjoy	Foods to Question	Foods to Exclude
Aisle 5 Soup, canned vegetables, pasta, pasta sauce, Mexican rice and other side dishes	• All plain dried or canned beans, peas, and lentils • Plain macaroni and other pasta • Buckwheat (kasha) • Plain rice or mixed rice • Plain whole grains (e.g., quinoa, barley, millet) • Tomato-based pasta sauce	• Soup broths • Dried soup powders • Seasoned bean salads • Seasoned potato side dishes (may contain mustard) • Creamy pasta sauces • Seasoned rice side dishes (check seasoning for mustard)	• Falafel mix
Aisle 6 Water, soft drinks, sport drinks, fruit juices, alcoholic beverages	• Water • Coffee • Tea • Juice • Carbonated beverages • Alcoholic beverages	• Cocktail seasoning mixes (e.g., Bloody Mary seasoning)	
Aisle 7 Frozen fruits and vegetables, frozen meals and desserts	• All plain frozen fruits and vegetables • Ice cream • Frozen yogurt • Sorbet • Sherbet • Frozen waffles and pancakes • Frozen baked goods	• Frozen beef burgers	• Prepared frozen dishes containing mustard ingredients
Other		• Prepared ready-to-eat baby food	

Corn Allergy

Corn, or maize, allergy is relatively rare and there are very few studies that document it. Questions about its mechanisms, symptoms, prevalence in both children and adults, allergens involved, and useful diagnostic tests still need to be answered. When it occurs, however, the reactions can be quite severe and include anaphylaxis, urticaria (itching), conjunctivitis (itchy eyes), rhinorrhea (runny nose), edema (swelling), and wheezing.

In a small North American study, out of 52 individuals with previous reported reactions to corn and positive skin prick tests, only 5 developed allergic reactions when undergoing a double-blind, placebo-controlled food challenge that confirmed their true allergy to corn. Corn allergy has been more frequently reported in southern Europe and Mexico, where corn is commonly consumed.

Managing a corn-free diet can prove to be difficult because corn and corn products are found as components of so many food products. In addition, corn is not considered one of the most common allergens in either North American or EU labeling laws.

Ingredients that contain corn include:

- Baking powder
- Corn flour, cornstarch, cornmeal, corn alcohol
- Corn sweeteners — high-fructose corn syrup, corn syrup solids
- Dextrins, dextrates
- Caramel flavoring, as well as other natural and artificial flavorings
- Grits
- Hominy
- Maize
- Marshmallows
- Confectioners' (icing) sugar
- Modified corn starch

Allergy to Fruits and Vegetables

Allergy to fruits and vegetables is thought to be quite prevalent, at 5%. There are two kinds of these allergies:

1. An allergic reaction to a specific allergen in the plant food. Examples include allergy to strawberries, celery, and apple. This allergy involves a group of allergens known as non-specific lipid transfer proteins (nsLTPs). This type of allergy is not very common.

2. A secondary reaction caused by cross-reaction between a plant food allergen and an antibody to pollen or latex. This type of IgE-mediated reaction is far more common than the first kind.

Fruits

Primary allergy to fruit includes apples, peaches, grapes, and kiwifruit. Grapes contain allergenic proteins that also cause reactions to raisins, grape juice, wine vinegar, and wine. Case reports of allergies to fruit have also been reported for banana, lychees and longans, mandarins, blueberries, and mango.

Vegetables

Primary allergy to vegetables, such as celery and carrot, is widely recognized in some parts of Europe, where these two vegetables are listed as common allergens. In particular, celery can cause severe anaphylactic reactions either through ingestion of celery spice or celery root — both of which maintain allergen potential even after extended heat treatment. Allergies to cabbage, coriander, eggplant, garlic, lettuce, and zucchini have been documented as triggering anaphylactic reactions.

Monosodium Glutamate Sensitivity

Monosodium glutamate (MSG) is also known as the single salt of glutamate. Glutamate is a non-essential amino acid — a protein building block the body can produce on its own — found naturally in free form in tomatoes, Parmesan cheese, and soy sauce or in bound form in yeast extracts and hydrolyzed protein, all of which are used as flavor enhancers. It can also appear as a byproduct of metabolism and can be found in considerable amounts in body tissues and organs.

Symptoms

MSG appears to produce a wide variety of symptoms, including headache, neck pain, nausea, tingling, flushing, and chest heaviness. First described in 1968 as the "Chinese restaurant syndrome," this collection of symptoms was attributed to consumption of meals containing MSG. Some reports have also linked MSG to the development of asthma, urticaria (itching), and angioedema (swelling). Despite concerns raised by early reports, subsequent studies have failed to demonstrate a clear and consistent relationship between MSG ingestion and the development of these conditions.

MSG Consumption

The glutamate added to foods for flavor represents only a small fraction of the total amount of glutamate consumed in the average daily diet. The average person consumes between 10 and 20 grams of glutamate daily. The average intake of glutamate from MSG added to foods is estimated at 0.5 to 1.5 grams daily. This represents a small fraction of the amount of free glutamate available in common foods.

MSG Dietary Sources

Food	Free Glutamate (mg)	Bound Glutamate (mg)
Parmesan cheese	1200	9.85
Tomato	246	0.26
Soy sauce	782	
Corn	130	0.5

Other Food Additives Causing Food Intolerance

Food additives are ubiquitous in our food supply. Some are used to preserve the freshness of food, others to impart color and taste. There is currently no useful blood or skin test to identify reactions to any of these additives. If you suspect intolerance to any of them, you may identify it by eliminating all foods containing these substances for up to 30 days, followed by a food challenge. Some people may be able to tolerate small amounts of additives upon reintroduction. There are no nutritional deficiencies expected from eliminating foods containing additives.

Did You Know?

MSG Intolerance
MSG intolerance is not mediated by IgE antibodies and it is not an allergic reaction. There are no skin tests or blood tests for detecting reactions to MSG. If you suspect an intolerance to MSG, the only way to diagnose it is through elimination of all foods containing MSG for up to 30 days and follow-up with a food challenge of products containing MSG. Test doses for MSG may range between 2.5 and 2500 mg and may be obtained as MSG powder mixed into foods and meals that do not contain MSG. Speak to your registered dietitian or allied health practitioner about a protocol for testing your tolerance to MSG.

Common Food Additives

While hundreds of food additives are used, only a limited number have been implicated in triggering both immune-mediated and non-allergic reactions.

- **Tartrazine:** This orange-yellow food coloring may be found in soft drinks, candy, jams, cereals, and packaged soups.
- **Sunset yellow:** This yellow food coloring may be found in cereals, baked goods, candy, ice cream, soft drinks, and medication.
- **Annatto:** This yellowish to reddish orange color additive is obtained from the seed coating of the tropical achiote tree. It is often found in sausages, cheese products, margarine, shortening, cereals, and snack foods.
- **Cochineal/carmine:** This red food coloring may be found in meat, sausages, processed deli meats, marinades, pie fillings, jams, jellies, sauces, and some alcoholic drinks.
- **Benzoates:** These substances are used to prevent yeast and mold growth in acidic foods and are often used in soft drinks, salad dressings, jams, canned fruits, and pickled vegetables.

CHAPTER 6
Food Label Regulations

Managing food allergies requires complete avoidance of the food allergens that trigger a reaction. In many cases, identifying these allergens is quite simple — an egg is an egg. In other cases, the allergens are hidden in processed and packaged foods. Governments in the Western world now demand that ingredient labels list the content of most processed foods, and they have begun to demand that manufacturers also identify the allergens in the packaged food. Being able to read labels is one of the most important strategies you can use to manage food hypersensitivities. You can avoid reaction to foods by reading the food label every time you purchase a food product. You also need to avoid food products that do not have an ingredient listing.

Canadian Regulations

Starting in August 2012 in Canada, the labels on all packaged food products must declare the presence of any of the 10 key allergens discussed in this book:

- Peanut
- Tree nut
- Seafood (fish, crustaceans, and shellfish)
- Egg
- Milk
- Wheat
- Soy
- Sesame seed
- Sulfites (to be declared when added to foods or when the total amount — exceeds 10 parts per million or more)
- Mustard

Gluten Sources

In addition, in Canada, the following grains are recognized as gluten sources and must be declared as allergens:

- Wheat
- Barley
- Oats
- Rye
- Triticale
- Kamut
- Spelt
- A hybridized strain of any of these cereals

Exemptions

A few types of foods are exempted from these labeling requirements:

- Products packaged from bulk on retail premises, except packaged products that are a mixture of nuts.
- Packaged individual portions of food (such as soda crackers or single servings of peanut butter) that are served with meals or snacks by a restaurant or other commercial enterprise.
- Packaged individual servings of food that are prepared by a commissary and sold by automatic vending machines or mobile canteens.
- Packaged meat and meat byproducts that are barbecued, roasted, or broiled on the retail premises.
- Packaged poultry, poultry meat, or poultry meat byproducts that are barbecued, roasted, or broiled on the retail premises.
- One-bite confectionery, such as candy or a stick of chewing gum, sold individually.
- Fresh fruit or vegetables packaged in a wrapper or confining band less than $1/2$ inch (1 cm) in width.

Did You Know?

Beer

Beer is considered a standardized food and is also exempt from ingredient declaration. For those with wheat allergy or celiac disease, be aware that most beers are brewed with a large proportion of wheat in addition to malted barley. Of course, there are also gluten-free beers made from sorghum, millet, or buckwheat available on the market.

Fining Agents for Alcoholic Beverages

Fining agents are used in the manufacture of standardized alcoholic beverages, particularly wine and beer, to achieve clarity and to improve color, flavor, and physical stability. Fining agents may be derived from milk, eggs, or fish. Manufacturers of alcoholic beverages must declare these allergens whenever the protein, modified protein, or protein fraction from the allergen source is found in standardized alcoholic beverages.

Wax Coatings on Fruit and Vegetables

Wax coatings on fresh fruit and vegetables are used to extend the shelf-life of produce. Wax coatings may contain ingredients derived from milk, soy, and crustaceans. Manufacturers of wax coatings and produce growers, packers, and importers using them will need to declare these allergens on the label of prepackaged fruits and vegetables.

American Regulations

In the United States, the Food Allergen Labeling and Consumer Protection Act (FALCPA) requires that manufacturers declare on ingredient labels the presence of eight major allergens:

- Milk
- Egg
- Peanut
- Tree nut
- Fish
- Crustacean
- Seafood
- Wheat
- Soy

The allergens must be listed within the ingredient list, next to the ingredient that bears the source of the allergen or in a separate statement (for example, "Contains..."), usually found at the end of the list of ingredients. FALCPA applies to foods manufactured in the United States as well as foods imported.

European Regulations

The European Union UK regulations require manufacturers to list all top 12 allergens and their derivatives on the label regardless of the amount used:

- Cereals containing gluten — wheat, rye, barley, oats, spelt, kamut
- Crustaceans
- Egg
- Fish
- Peanuts
- Milk
- Nuts
- Soy
- Sesame
- Celery
- Mustard
- Sulphur dioxide (Sulfites)

CHAPTER 7

Living with Food Allergies and Intolerances

There are several common practical and psychological problems associated with allergies. With the knowledge you now have of allergies, you can cope with these challenges.

Practical Strategies

Managing Cross-Contamination

Cross-contamination occurs when food allergens or food particles inadvertently come in contact with other foods. Cross-contamination may occur:

- During the food manufacturing process
- When preparing foods as part of a recipe
- When foods are sold together as part of a buffet
- When foods are sold in a bulk-barn setting

The food manufacturing process is out of your control, but do not hesitate to call the manufacturer to find out what allergens may be hiding in the ingredients they use. Be careful not to cross-contaminate food while preparing recipes. Replace any allergenic foods with foods containing similar nutritional value. Simply swear off eating at buffets and avoid shopping at bulk food stores.

Managing Personal Contact

Pay particular attention to personal contact. Be aware of:

- Touching a surface where the allergen may be found, such as a table, desk, door knob or even a water fountain.
- Playing cards.
- Inhaling dust containing the allergen, as in the case of sitting next to a person opening a bag of peanuts.
- Kissing a person who just consumed an allergen-containing food. Kissing puts those with allergies at risk because even trace amounts of an allergen may trigger an anaphylactic

reaction. This is especially difficult for teenagers and young adults who may not be comfortable asking a partner they have recently met to disclose whether they had consumed an offending substance. But it is a hard truth that needs to be dealt with.

Managing Food Allergy at Work

You deserve a safe working environment. Your health and safety cannot be compromised and you need to be up front about your needs. Here are some strategies to help you manage a new working environment:

- Let your immediate supervisor and colleagues know about your allergies as quickly as possible. Wear your MedicAlert bracelet or necklace.
- Inform your managers and colleagues of where you keep the auto-injector and how to use it. Otherwise, make sure that you have an emergency plan that lists your allergies, the location of your auto-injector, and directions for how to use it, when needed.
- Be careful with catered food at work meetings. If there are no suitable options for you or if you are not satisfied with the allergy information you receive from the caterer, keep some suitable snacks at the office or bring your own food to the meeting. Make sure you carry food in a sealed container or a wrapper.
- When going out, ensure you research the restaurant ahead of time to find out if they can accommodate your allergy.
- Check if your workplace has an anaphylaxis policy in place. If it does not, you may help the human resources department craft one by suggesting that areas in the kitchen be designated as places you can store your food, that caterers supply non-allergenic food options, and that cross-contamination be prevented. This would be an ideal way to educate coworkers about how serious allergies are and what can be done to minimize risks.

Managing Food Allergy in Restaurants

Dining out is probably the most difficult aspect of managing a food allergy. In fact, most allergic reactions, including anaphylaxis, occur when eating away from home. Restaurants have come a long way in how they manage patrons with food allergies, but gaps clearly still exist. Here are some tips for managing an allergic reaction at a restaurant:

- Check the restaurant's website or call ahead of time. Many food establishments have food allergen listings available on-line or on-site.
- Call ahead and speak to the chef or the restaurant manager. Choose a quiet time in the day — for example, mid-afternoon — to ensure the owner is available to speak to you. Let them know of your planned visit and the list of your allergies. Ask them what specific meals they would recommend. This is the best time to also ask about how the kitchen staff avoids cross-contamination and to request the use of fresh utensils and pots/pans when preparing your food. The ideal situation would be visiting the restaurant by appointment and speaking directly to the chef — this is the best way to explain your needs and have the chef's full attention.
- Do not forget the grill! For example, in case of a seafood allergy, you need to ensure that the grill used to prepare your chicken breast or steak is designated fish/seafood-free. Otherwise, you will need to opt for a fried or sautéed version where a clean pan will be used.
- When traveling to other countries and if you do not speak the native language, use translated restaurant cards available from national allergy support groups.

Managing Family Gatherings

Even more sensitive is the issue of dining at family gatherings. Those situations can become emotional landmines because those preparing the meal may have the best intentions but may not be aware of ingredients and cross-contamination issues. Dealing with invitations to attend family gatherings — birthday parties, wedding anniversaries, and simple family dinners — requires some advance planning and considerable tact when you have a food allergy.

- The week before the party, speak to the host and ask how you may help. Offer to bring a meal or side dish for everyone to enjoy. If the host is interested in more information about your allergy, you may direct her to reliable sources of information. There is a lot of goodwill out there, and your family and friends can be the most receptive people because they want to help out. You can ensure that they get the right information about food allergies and how serious anaphylactic reactions may be.

- When in doubt, politely decline: If you are uncertain about the food or meal you are being offered, acknowledge and express gratitude for the good intention and simply say, "No, thank you."
- If someone mistakenly offers you a food to which you are allergic, try not to make the person feel bad. You may turn it around and make a light remark without getting personal.

Managing Food Allergies While Traveling

Traveling should be an exciting and fulfilling experience! A restricted diet should not take away from it. Again, preparation and planning ahead are crucial in helping you manage your allergies with as little stress as possible.

While flying:

1. Wear your MedicAlert bracelet or necklace and identification, and carry at least two doses of auto-injector medication with you.
2. Inform the airline staff (check-in attendants, flight attendants) about your allergy. You should also inform the gate attendant so that you may have a chance to pre-board and wipe down the seats, tray, and armrests.
3. Security may require a special physician note that documents the need for you to carry auto-injectors. Have it ready to show to security personnel. They may argue that there is suitable medication on-board, but this is not appropriate.
4. Eating food offered by the airline is not recommended. Bring your own food and have extra snacks available in case of delays.
5. Have a chat with your in-flight travel companion and inform them of your allergy. Keep in mind that they may also have chosen to self-cater, in which case you may extend the offer to purchase a snack suitable for them.

Managing Food Allergy in Your Kitchen

The home should be a safe and relaxed environment in which to enjoy foods and experiment with new foods and recipes. Studies have shown that families of allergy sufferers are more closely knit and communication rated higher than in families of non-allergic individuals. The supportive family should be positive and offer encouragement toward the new diet — this can make a tremendous difference to the allergy sufferer's outlook and long-term management of the diet. A positive attitude can improve and lower the stress and anxiety that usually comes with a diagnosis of food allergy.

Food Allergen Ban

Depending on the severity of the allergy, the allergic food may have to be banned entirely from the house. If this is not a strategy accepted by every member of the family, then the following precautions will need to be taken:

1. Have separate pots and pans.
2. Have separate cutting boards.
3. Have separate cooking utensils.
4. Have a designated allergen-free food preparation area. If available, a separate cleaning area, such as a separate sink, would be ideal.

Kitchen Hygiene

Keeping a kitchen free of allergenic foods is not easy, but try these strategies.

Hands

Conventional cleaning methods using liquid soap, bar soap, or commercial wipes are effective at removing food protein, such as peanut, from hands. Plain water and antibacterial hand sanitizer are not.

Wash your hands:

- Before meals.
- Before serving the allergen-free meal.
- After meals.
- After consuming the allergen, if you are eating a meal that is different than that of the allergic family member.

Surfaces and Utensils

To remove protein from surfaces, such as tables, cutting boards, spatulas and plates, wash with soap and water — simply wiping off food crumbs will not be enough. Common household cleaning agents with bleach have been found to effectively remove food protein from surfaces. Dishwashing liquid soap alone (as part of the dishwasher cleaning method) has not been shown to be effective at removing food protein allergens from surfaces. Be aware of the risk of cross-contamination when an unclean utensil, such as a knife that had been dipped in peanut butter, is placed in the dishwasher by a non-allergic family member and exposes the allergic individual to the risk of contact. It is best to clean all dishes that have been in contact with an allergen by hand using dish detergent and water.

While preparing and serving food:

- Thoroughly clean the surface areas and pots/pans before preparing an allergen-free meal.
- Prepare the allergen-free meal first to avoid inadvertently cross-contaminating.
- If you are cooking a side dish intended for the use of all family members, make sure you keep the pot/pan covered to avoid any food splattering from adjacent pots.
- Do not share cooking utensils or food containers.

Refrigerator

To prevent spilling and contamination, keep jars and food containers sealed. If using jars for foods commonly used by the family, such as jam, honey, or condiments, keep a separate jar labeled with the name of the allergic family member. This prevents accidental contamination. It would be ideal to store these labeled food containers on a designated shelf in the refrigerator. Some families have found that colored tags work well for easier identification.

Organizing Your Kitchen

- Designate specific containers to be used by the allergic person only and label them clearly.
- Dedicate a pantry shelf to foods that are allergen-free and that will be for the use of the allergic person only.
- Designate an allergen-free food preparation area, which will minimize the risk of accidental contamination.

Psychological Challenges

Studies have shown over and over again that adults and children suffering from food sensitivities are dealing with higher levels of stress and anxiety and lower quality of life. In the words of one patient: "One of the toughest things for me is to watch my friends eat something I can't have; it makes me feel left out."

Did You Know?

Perceived Food Intolerance
Some people perceive that they have food intolerance when in fact they may not. A study of 300 patients with perceived food intolerance reported higher absenteeism from work compared to healthy controls. Approximately 17% of the study group also reported that daily activities, such as traveling and participating in sports, were greatly affected.

Managing Anaphylactic Fear

The burden of living with anaphylaxis and food allergy is a taxing one for both the individual involved and the supporting family. Those who suffer from severe allergies are at risk of potentially fatal reactions. Sufferers of food sensitivities may not be exposed to the same risk as food allergy sufferers, but they have a wide range of issues to deal with, including depression, feelings of anxiety and stress, and feelings of being misunderstood.

With all anaphylactic reactions and other severe food intolerances, the first experience often takes you by surprise and you feel threatened. Fear sets in and persists throughout the diagnostic process, and continues later on, through managing the avoidance diet. Food allergic patients live in a constant state of vigilance and fear as they try to prevent accidental ingestion and manage emergency situations.

Managing Psychological Effects

There is an interplay between the reality of the physical reaction — the body's immune system reaction — and the psychological one, that is, the impact on mood, behavior, and outlook that also need to be assessed. While it may be a relief to have a clear diagnosis of a food allergy as a way of identifying and explaining symptoms, it is very difficult to immediately switch gears and start avoiding the allergen-causing food without 'taking in' the reality and the impact on one's quality of life, especially if the person has never encountered the concept of allergy. Even subjective food hypersensitivity — that is, perceived reactions to foods — can have negative consequences in day-to-day life. If you feel any of these psychological effects, be sure to consult your doctor to arrange for counseling.

Involve Your Family

Once you have cleared out the pantry and the fridge and labeled your own jars, boxes, and bags, take the opportunity to gather your family members and explain to them what the diagnosis means to you and to them. Don't try to manage your food allergy on your own. Enlist your family for support:

- Enlist their help to craft an anaphylaxis emergency plan, explaining how to reduce risks of accidental ingestion of allergen and how to treat reactions.
- Show them how to use the auto-injector and emphasize the importance of checking the expiry date.

- Explain to them why you need your own food jars/containers or your own labeled jar of peanut butter or jam.
- Take them on a tour of the kitchen and the pantry and explain to them where everything is and why.

It may be easier if, at first, you keep a book on food allergies on the kitchen counter or in the family room as a reminder to everyone of your diagnosis. Keeping the Aisle-by-Aisle Guides found in this book on the refrigerator door in plain view might also make it easier for everyone to remember that you need their support.

Meal Planning with Food Allergies

Ensuring that you eat a balanced diet while excluding allergenic foods can be a challenge, but it cannot be overlooked. Achieving and maintaining general good health will give you the strength to manage your allergies.

Nutritional Status

Begin by determining your current nutritional status. For those following an elimination diet to identify food sensitivity, the assessment of your nutritional status before you start the diet is very important because it will help identify the nutritional gaps that may exist. This will act as a baseline for all other dietary interventions. For example, if you suspect an intolerance to dairy products and you are already calcium-deficient, counseling regarding appropriate intakes of calcium, riboflavin (vitamin B_2), vitamin D, magnesium, and phosphorus is critical at the beginning of the testing period. If the diet continues in the long-term, controlling dairy intake from all sources — food and supplementation — will be necessary. Your nutritional status will also need to be reassessed on a regular basis while you're following the exclusion diet.

How to

Assess Nutritional Status

In adults, there are a number of methods to assess nutritional status:

1. Anthropometric measurements: weight, height, waist circumference, and body mass index (BMI) can be simple markers of nutritional status in some cases.
2. Blood tests may assess your levels of important nutrients, such as iron, folate, vitamin B_{12}, and vitamin D.
3. Bone mass density testing can indicate the health of your bones and can signal osteopaenia or osteoporosis.
4. A food diary kept over a number of days (usually 5 to 7 days) that includes weighed meal portions, recipes, and fluid intake can be a useful tool to assess both caloric intake and approximate nutrient intake through a detailed analysis. This can help determine if nutrients are missing from the diet.

Dietary Constraints

In some cases of multiple food sensitivities or allergies, it may be very difficult to obtain all needed nutrients from foods, despite best intentions. This may happen for several reasons:

1. The range of alternatives is too limited to ensure nutritional adequacy.

2. The individual food preferences may further limit the range of foods.

3. The exclusion diet becomes monotonous — boring — as individuals search for new solutions and may find it difficult to be compliant.

4. Product availability and cost can be a limiting factor.

Food Guides

To achieve a balanced diet without nutritional deficiencies, follow one of the daily food guides published by government health agencies to ensure:

- Adequate intake of all nutrients
- Balance of essential vitamins and minerals
- Calorie control
- Consumption of nutritionally dense foods
- Moderation
- Variety

It may be useful to consider using a single-nutrient supplement to ensure consistent daily intake. Again, a doctor or dietitian with experience in dealing with food allergies and sensitivities can help you determine your nutrient requirements for optimal health.

Meal Planning

In planning your daily meals, consult the MyPlate food guide, issued by the United States Department of Agriculture (USDA), and Canada's Food Guide to Eating Well, issued by Health Canada. Health Canada also issues a food guide for vegetarians. These guides must be tailored to your specific food allergies or sensitivities. A dietitian can help you ensure you have a nutritionally balanced diet while excluding the foods that cause your allergy or sensitivity.

You will find many meal ideas in the recipe section in this book. Some of these meals are allergen-free, while others may contain one or two of the top 10 allergens. In those cases, allergen-free alternatives are offered. All the meals are delicious.

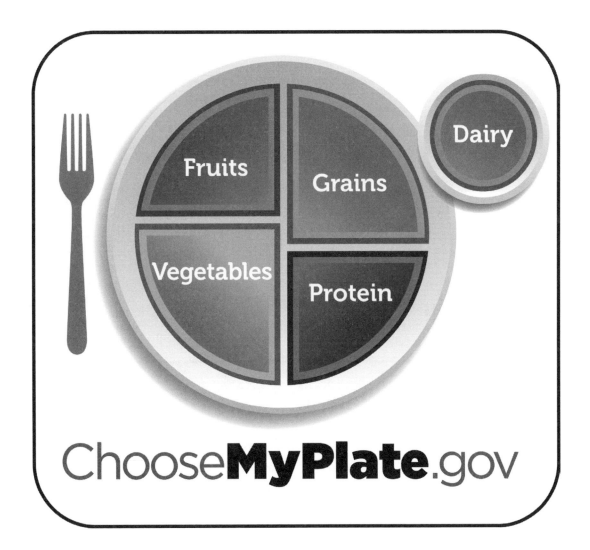

Balancing Calories
- Enjoy your food, but eat less.
- Avoid oversized portions.

Foods to Increase
- Make half your plate fruits and vegetables.
- Make at least half your grains whole grains.
- Switch to fat-free or low-fat (1%) milk.

Foods to Reduce
- Compare sodium in foods like soup, bread, and frozen meals and choose the foods with lower numbers.
- Drink water instead of sugary drinks.

Eating Well with Canada's Food Guide

Recommended Number of *Food Guide Servings* per Day

	Children			Teens		Adults			
Age in Years	2-3	4-8	9-13	14-18		19-50		51+	
Sex	Girls and Boys			Females	Males	Females	Males	Females	Males
Vegetables and Fruit	4	5	6	7	8	7-8	8-10	7	7
Grain Products	3	4	6	6	7	6-7	8	6	7
Milk and Alternatives	2	2	3-4	3-4	3-4	2	2	3	3
Meat and Alternatives	1	1	1-2	2	3	2	3	2	3

What is One Food Guide Serving?
Look at the examples below.

Fresh, frozen or canned vegetables
125 mL (½ cup)

Bread
1 slice (35 g)

Bagel
½ bagel (45 g)

Milk or powdered milk (reconstituted)
250 mL (1 cup)

Cooked fish, shellfish, poultry, lean meat
75 g (2 ½ oz.)/125 mL (½ cup)

The chart above shows how many Food Guide Servings you need from each of the four food groups every day.

Having the amount and type of food recommended and following the tips in *Canada's Food Guide* will help:

• Meet your needs for vitamins, minerals and other nutrients.

• Reduce your risk of obesity, type 2 diabetes, heart disease, certain types of cancer and osteoporosis.

• Contribute to your overall health and vitality.

For a full guide, please contact Health Canada or visit their website.

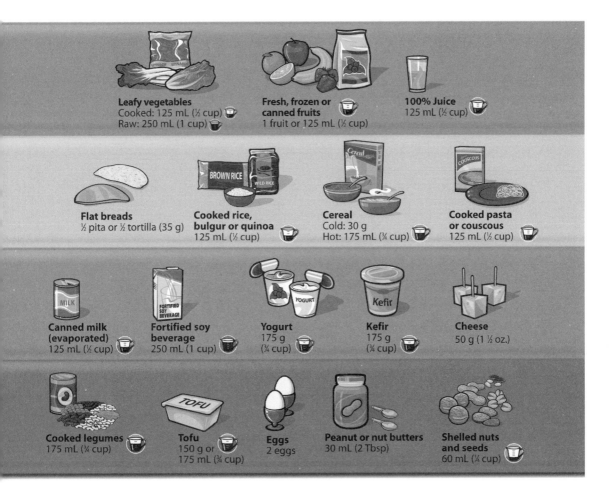

Leafy vegetables
Cooked: 125 mL (½ cup)
Raw: 250 mL (1 cup)

Fresh, frozen or canned fruits
1 fruit or 125 mL (½ cup)

100% Juice
125 mL (½ cup)

Flat breads
½ pita or ½ tortilla (35 g)

Cooked rice, bulgur or quinoa
125 mL (½ cup)

Cereal
Cold: 30 g
Hot: 175 mL (¾ cup)

Cooked pasta or couscous
125 mL (½ cup)

Canned milk (evaporated)
125 mL (½ cup)

Fortified soy beverage
250 mL (1 cup)

Yogurt
175 g (¾ cup)

Kefir
175 g (¾ cup)

Cheese
50 g (1 ½ oz.)

Cooked legumes
175 mL (¾ cup)

Tofu
150 g or 175 mL (¾ cup)

Eggs
2 eggs

Peanut or nut butters
30 mL (2 Tbsp)

Shelled nuts and seeds
60 mL (¼ cup)

Oils and Fats

- Include a small amount – 30 to 45 mL (2 to 3 Tbsp) – of unsaturated fat each day. This includes oil used for cooking, salad dressings, margarine and mayonnaise.
- Use vegetable oils such as canola, olive and soybean.
- Choose soft margarines that are low in saturated and trans fats.
- Limit butter, hard margarine, lard and shortening.

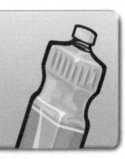

Part 3

The Recipes

Introduction to the Recipes

The recipes that follow were selected to give you as much choice as possible in your meal planning. Whether you suffer from multiple food sensitivities, need to prepare a meal for a family with allergies to different foods, or are entertaining a gathering of people with diverse dietary requirements, you will find a wide variety of recipes that are free of many allergens, including gluten and corn. Where an allergen exists in the original recipe, we have given you suggestions for replacing it with allergen-free ingredients, enabling you to adapt the recipe to your particular food allergies and sensitivities. Many of the recipes also incorporate serving ideas, to help you create complete meals and ensure that you maximize your nutrient intake.

About the Nutrient Analyses

Computer-assisted nutrient analysis of the recipes was prepared using Food Processor® SQL, version 10.10, ©2012, ESHA Research Inc., Salem OR (this software contains over 35,000 food items based largely on the latest USDA data and the Canadian Nutrient File). The database was supplemented when necessary with data from product packaging nutritional information and using the following references: 1. Bob's Red Mill Natural Foods, nutritional information product search, accessed July 2012 from www.bobsredmill.com; 2. Cream Hill Estates, gluten-free oats and oat flour nutritional information product search, accessed July 2012 from www.creamhillestates.com; 3. Turtle Mountain LLC, So Delicious Coconut Milk nutritional information product search, accessed July 2012 from www.sodeliciousdairyfree.com; 4. Earth Balance Natural Spreads, Earth Balance Coconut Spread nutritional information product search, accessed July 2012 from www.earthbalancenatural.com.

The analysis was based on: imperial weights and measures (except for foods typically packaged and used in metric quantities); the smaller ingredient quantity when there was a range; the first ingredient listed when there was a choice of ingredients. Optional ingredients and garnishes, and ingredients that are not quantified, were not included in the calculations. Canola oil was used where the type of fat was not specified. Calculations involving meat and poultry used lean portions without skin and with visible fat trimmed unless otherwise indicated in the recipe. A pinch of salt was calculated as $1/8$ tsp (0.5 mL).

All recipes were analyzed prior to cooking. The method used to prepare the recipe may alter the nutrient content per serving, as may ingredient substitutions and differences among brand-name products.

Breakfasts

Heather's Granola

This recipe offers lots of flexibility, so you can easily adapt it to be free of ingredients you are allergic or sensitive to. Preparing it in large batches makes it a quick, easy and filling breakfast any day. It's an excellent source of iron and fiber, and a good source of calcium.

Tips

To use brown sugar as part of the liquid ingredients, add 2 tbsp (30 mL) water for every $\frac{1}{4}$ cup (60 mL) packed brown sugar.

If you like smaller pieces of fruit in your granola, halve or quarter the larger pieces.

Seeds are typically good sources of non-dairy calcium and magnesium, so it's helpful to incorporate them in recipes as often as you can.

**NUTRIENTS
PER $\frac{1}{2}$ CUP (125 ML)**

Calories	271
Fat	12 g
Carbohydrate	36 g
Fiber	5 g
Protein	7 g
Iron	4.0 mg
Calcium	69 mg

- Preheat oven to 300°F (150°C)
- 10- by 10- by $2\frac{1}{4}$-inch (25 by 25 by 6 cm) casserole dish

7 cups	pure, uncontaminated large-flake (old-fashioned) rolled oats	1.75 L
4 cups	dry ingredients	1 L
2 cups	liquid ingredients	500 mL
3 cups	dried fruit	750 mL

1. In the casserole dish, combine oats and dry ingredients. Set aside.
2. In a 4-cup (1 L) liquid measuring cup, combine liquid ingredients. Pour over oat mixture and stir until combined.
3. Bake in preheated oven for 40 to 50 minutes, stirring every 10 minutes, until toasted and light golden brown. Let cool completely. Stir in dried fruit.
4. Store in an airtight container in the refrigerator for up to 4 weeks.

Variation

Replace half of the oats with any gluten-free flaked grain, such as buckwheat or amaranth flakes.

Dry Ingredients
Quinoa flakes, rice bran, pure, uncontaminated oat bran, ground flax seeds, flaked coconut, seeds (pumpkin, flax, poppy, sunflower)

Optional Dry Ingredients
Peanuts, tree nuts, sesame seeds (where no allergies exist)

Liquid Ingredients
Fruit juices, liquid honey, light (fancy) molasses, pure maple syrup, corn syrup, vegetable oil, frozen orange juice concentrate

Optional Dry Ingredients
Peanut butter, tahini (where no allergies exist)

Dried Fruit
Cranberries, raisins, coarsely chopped or snipped apricots, mango, papaya, apple, dates, figs

Tips

If you have a wheat allergy or celiac disease, ensure that the oat bran is sourced from pure, uncontaminated oats.

If you are sensitive to sulfites, make sure the dried fruits have no added sulfites. Dried cranberries, raisins and some brands of dried apricots available in health food stores are free of added sulfites.

One example of a combination of 4 cups (1 L) dry ingredients includes:

½ cup	pure, uncontaminated oat bran	125 mL
½ cup	ground flax seeds	125 mL
½ cup	cracked flax seeds	125 mL
½ cup	pumpkin seeds	125 mL
½ cup	sunflower seeds	125 mL
½ cup	flaked coconut	125 mL
½ cup	quinoa flakes	125 mL
½ cup	poppy seeds	125 mL

One example of a combination of 2 cups (500 mL) liquid ingredients includes:

1 cup	cranberry juice	250 mL
⅓ cup	pure maple syrup	75 mL
⅓ cup	extra virgin olive oil	75 mL
⅓ cup	frozen orange juice concentrate, thawed	75 mL

One example of a combination of 3 cups (750 mL) dried fruit includes:

¾ cup	dried apricots, quartered	175 mL
¾ cup	dried cranberries	175 mL
½ cup	coarsely chopped dried dates	125 mL
½ cup	raisins	125 mL
¼ cup	coarsely chopped dried mango	60 mL
¼ cup	coarsely chopped dried papaya	60 mL

Breakfast Idea: Combine ½ cup (125 mL) granola with 1 cup (250 mL) milk, lactose-free milk, enriched non-dairy milk alternative or yogurt.

Snack Idea: Combine ¼ cup (60 mL) granola with ½ cup milk, lactose-free milk, enriched non-dairy milk alternative or yogurt.

Homemade Oatmeal

Makes 6 servings

Nothing beats a bowl of good oatmeal. Oats are an excellent source of fiber, B vitamins and iron. There are quick-cooking gluten-free varieties available on the market, which makes oatmeal an excellent choice for busy lifestyles!

3¼ cups	water	800 mL
2 cups	pure, uncontaminated quick-cooking rolled oats	500 mL
¼ cup	pure maple syrup	60 mL
½ tsp	ground cinnamon	2 mL
1 cup	raspberries	250 mL

1. In a medium saucepan, bring water to a boil over high heat. Stir in oats until combined. Reduce heat to medium, cover and simmer for about 7 minutes or until desired consistency.

2. Stir in maple syrup and cinnamon.

3. Divide evenly among individual serving bowls. Fold in raspberries.

> **Breakfast Idea:** Add 1 cup (250 mL) milk, lactose-free milk, enriched non-dairy milk alternative or yogurt to 1 serving of oatmeal. Top with ½ cup (125 mL) fresh or stewed fruit of choice.

NUTRIENTS PER SERVING

Calories	203
Fat	3 g
Carbohydrate	40 g
Fiber	7 g
Protein	7 g
Iron	2.0 mg
Calcium	36 mg

Hot Millet Amaranth Cereal

Millet and amaranth make a delicious combination in this recipe. Don't let the time it takes deter you — prepare it on the weekend and warm it up for a quick weekday breakfast.

Tips

For best results, toast the millet and amaranth before cooking. Stir the grains in a dry skillet over medium heat until fragrant, about 5 minutes.

If you are sensitive to sulfites, make sure the dried fruits have no added sulfites.

Due to their high content of heart-healthy polyunsaturated fats, it is best to store millet and amaranth in airtight containers to prevent them from going rancid.

This hot cereal is an excellent source of manganese, and a good source of calcium, magnesium, phosphorus, iron and zinc. The millet provides good-quality protein.

NUTRIENTS PER SERVING	
Calories	124
Fat	2 g
Carbohydrate	23 g
Fiber	4 g
Protein	4 g
Iron	1.7 mg
Calcium	27 mg

2 1/2 cups	water	625 mL
1/2 cup	millet, toasted (see tip, at left)	125 mL
1/2 cup	amaranth	125 mL
	Honey, pure maple syrup or raw cane sugar	
	Milk, lactose-free milk or enriched non-dairy milk alternative	
	Dried cranberries, cherries or raisins (optional)	
	Toasted chopped nuts (optional)	

Stovetop Method

1. In a saucepan over medium heat, bring water to a boil. Add millet and amaranth in a steady stream, stirring constantly. Return to a boil. Reduce heat to low (see tip, page 253). Cover and simmer until grains are tender and liquid is absorbed, about 25 minutes. Serve hot, sweetened to taste and with milk or non-dairy alternative. Sprinkle with cranberries and nuts (if using).

Slow Cooker Method

1. Use a small (3 1/2-quart) lightly greased slow cooker. Combine ingredients in stoneware, adding 1/2 cup (125 mL) additional water to mixture. Place a clean tea towel, folded in half (so you will have two layers), over top of the stoneware to absorb moisture. Cover and cook on Low for 8 hours or overnight, or on High for 4 hours.

Breakfast Rice

This is a flavorful, comforting breakfast. Using whole-grain brown rice provides you with extra fiber, iron and B vitamins only found in the bran of the rice kernel.

Tip

If you are sensitive to sulfites, make sure the dried fruits have no added sulfites.

Variation

If you are allergic to tree nuts, replace the nuts with roasted pumpkin or sunflower seeds. Sesame seeds are another good option if you're not allergic to them. Whole dried sesame seeds are an excellent source of calcium: 2 tbsp (30 mL) provides 176 mg, almost 20% of the recommended daily intake.

4 cups	vanilla-flavored enriched rice milk	1 L
1 cup	long- or short-grain brown rice, rinsed and drained	250 mL
1/2 cup	dried cherries, cranberries or blueberries	125 mL
	Raw cane sugar, honey or pure maple syrup (optional)	
	Chopped toasted nuts (optional)	

Stovetop Method

1. In a large saucepan over medium heat, bring rice milk to a boil. Gradually stir in rice and cherries. Return to a boil. Reduce heat to low (see tip, page 253). Cover and simmer until rice is tender, about 50 minutes.

Slow Cooker Method

1. Use a small (3 1/2-quart) lightly greased slow cooker. Combine ingredients in stoneware, adding 1/2 cup (125 mL) water or additional rice milk to mixture. (With the quantity of liquid recommended above, it will be a bit crunchy around the edges.) Place a clean tea towel, folded in half (so you will have two layers), over top of the stoneware to absorb moisture. Cover and cook on Low for up to 8 hours or overnight, or on High for 4 hours.

For Both Methods

2. Stir well and serve with your favorite sweetener, if desired. Sprinkle with nuts, if desired.

NUTRIENTS PER SERVING

Calories	220
Fat	2 g
Carbohydrate	45 g
Fiber	1 g
Protein	3 g
Iron	0.1 mg
Calcium	200 mg

Cranberry Quinoa Porridge

Quinoa has become popular for its nutty taste and versatility. It is a great alternative to rice or couscous. This porridge is an excellent source of the trace mineral manganese, and a good source of iron and magnesium. The quinoa provides good-quality protein, folate and fiber.

Tip

If you are sensitive to sulfites, make sure the dried fruits have no added sulfites.

Variations

Substitute dried cherries or blueberries or raisins for the cranberries.

Use red quinoa for a change. Red and black quinoa seeds are higher in antioxidants than regular quinoa.

3 cups	water	750 mL
1 cup	quinoa, rinsed and drained	250 mL
1/2 cup	dried cranberries	125 mL
	Pure maple syrup or honey	
	Milk, lactose-free milk or enriched non-dairy milk alternative (optional)	

1. In a saucepan over medium heat, bring water to a boil. Stir in quinoa and cranberries and return to a boil. Reduce heat to low (see tip, page 253). Cover and simmer until quinoa is cooked (look for a white line around the seeds), about 15 minutes. Remove from heat and let stand, covered, about 5 minutes. Serve with maple syrup and milk or non-dairy alternative (if using).

NUTRIENTS PER SERVING

Calories 137
Fat . . . . .2 g
Carbohydrate . . . . .28 g
Fiber . . . . .3 g
Protein . . . . .4 g
Iron . . . . .1.4 mg
Calcium . . . . 13 mg

Quick Breakfast Fruit Pita

Makes 1 serving

This is a great on-the-go breakfast that is easily adapted for those with wheat allergy, celiac disease or gluten sensitivity.

Tips

To get the full benefits of flax seeds, they should be ground, but whole seeds add great crunch.

If you have celiac disease or a wheat allergy, new gluten-free pita varieties include teff, millet and corn.

½	banana, crushed	½
1 tbsp	flax seeds (ground or whole)	15 mL
1 tsp	pumpkin seeds	5 mL
1	6-inch (15 cm) pita	1
1	strawberry, hulled and thinly sliced	1

1. In a small bowl, combine banana, flax seeds and pumpkin seeds.
2. Toast pita and cut open. Stuff with banana mixture and place slices of strawberry on top. Eat while still warm from the toaster.

This recipe courtesy of Claudette Mayer-Lanthier.

Breakfast Idea: Pair this pita with 1 serving of Just Peachy Blueberry Picnic smoothie (page 334).

NUTRIENTS PER SERVING

Calories	348
Fat	11 g
Carbohydrate	54 g
Fiber	9 g
Protein	11 g
Iron	3.3 mg
Calcium	128 mg

Home-Style Pancakes

These pancakes are delicious topped with fruit and a drizzle of maple syrup.

Tips

If you are allergic to eggs, replace the eggs in this recipe with a mixture of 2 tbsp (30 mL) ground flax seeds (flaxseed meal) and 6 tbsp (90 mL) warm water. Cook for 2 minutes on each side. The yield will be six 4-inch (10 cm) pancakes.

Choose your favorite gluten-free non-dairy milk, such as soy, rice, almond or potato-based milk, or, if you can tolerate lactose, use regular 1% milk.

Combine the dry ingredients and store in an airtight container for up to 2 weeks.

Cook the pancakes the night before and store them in the refrigerator. Toast them in the morning.

½ cup	sorghum flour	125 mL
½ cup	brown rice flour	125 mL
2 tbsp	psyllium husks	30 mL
1 tsp	gluten-free baking powder	5 mL
¼ tsp	baking soda	1 mL
¼ tsp	salt	1 mL
1	egg	1
1 cup	enriched non-dairy milk or lactose-free 1% milk	250 mL
1 tbsp	liquid honey, pure maple syrup or agave nectar	15 mL
2 tsp	grapeseed oil	10 mL
1 tsp	vanilla extract	5 mL
	Grapeseed oil	

1. In a large bowl, combine sorghum flour, brown rice flour, psyllium, baking powder, baking soda and salt.

2. In another bowl, beat egg, milk, honey, oil and vanilla. Pour into flour mixture and whisk for about 1 minute or until smooth.

3. On a griddle or in a nonstick skillet, melt 1 tsp (5 mL) butter over medium heat. For each pancake, pour in ¼ cup (60 mL) batter. Cook for 1 to 2 minutes or until bubbles start to form and edges are firm. Flip over and cook other side for 1 to 2 minutes or until bottom is golden. Transfer to a plate and keep warm. Repeat with the remaining batter, greasing griddle and adjusting heat between batches as needed.

Psyllium Husks: Psyllium husks are the outer part of psyllium seeds, which are from the plantain plant, *Plantago ovato*. Numerous large-scale studies have shown that daily consumption of small amounts of psyllium fiber (3 to 12 grams a day) can help reduce LDL cholesterol ("bad" cholesterol). Other research indicates that when psyllium is incorporated into food, it is more effective at reducing the blood glucose response than a soluble fiber supplement that is taken separately from food.

NUTRIENTS
PER PANCAKE

Calories	150
Carbohydrate	21 g
Fiber	2 g
Protein	4 g
Fat	5 g
Iron	1.0 mg
Calcium	127 mg

Cranberry Banana Loaf

The tartness of the frozen cranberries complements the sweetness of bananas so well in this nutritious banana bread recipe. Enjoy it for breakfast or a mid-afternoon snack.

Tips

If you are allergic to eggs, replace the eggs in this recipe with a mixture of 1/4 cup (60 mL) ground flax seeds (flaxseed meal) and 1/3 cup (75 mL) warm water. Let stand for 5 minutes before combining with liquid ingredients. Increase the amount of baking powder to 2 1/2 tsp (12 mL). Thaw and drain frozen cranberries or use fresh. Bake loaf for 1 hour.

There's no need to wait for the frozen cranberries to thaw; just add them to the batter straight from the freezer.

If you don't have a glass loaf dish, use a metal loaf pan and increase the baking time by 5 to 10 minutes.

NUTRIENTS PER SLICE

Calories	180
Fat	7 g
Carbohydrate	27 g
Fiber	2 g
Protein	3 g
Iron	1.0 mg
Calcium	12 mg

- **Preheat oven to 350°F (180°C)**
- **9- by 5-inch (23 by 12.5 cm) glass loaf dish, greased, bottom lined with parchment paper**

1/2 cup	white rice flour	125 mL
1/4 cup	brown rice flour	60 mL
1/4 cup	quinoa flour	60 mL
2 tsp	gluten-free baking powder	10 mL
1 1/2 tsp	ground cinnamon	7 mL
1/4 tsp	salt	1 mL
1/4 cup	granulated raw cane sugar	60 mL
1/4 cup	butter or non-dairy margarine, softened	60 mL
2	eggs	2
1 cup	mashed ripe bananas	250 mL
1 cup	fresh or frozen cranberries	250 mL

1. In a medium bowl, whisk together white rice flour, brown rice flour, quinoa flour, baking powder, cinnamon and salt.

2. In a large bowl, using an electric mixer, cream sugar and butter until light and fluffy. Beat in eggs, one at a time, until well blended. Stir in bananas. Stir in dry ingredients until combined. Gently fold in cranberries.

3. Pour batter into prepared loaf dish. Bake in preheated oven for 45 to 50 minutes or until a tester inserted in the center comes out clean. Let cool in dish on a wire rack for 10 minutes. Remove from dish and peel off paper. Transfer loaf to rack and let cool completely.

Banana Pumpkin Bread

I am a big fan of this banana bread! Teff flour gives it a nutty, rich texture, and the tart sweetness of the dried apricots complements it well.

Tips

If you are allergic to eggs, replace the eggs in this recipe with a mixture of 3 tbsp (45 mL) ground chia seeds (such as Salba) and $\frac{1}{3}$ cup (75 mL) warm water. Increase the baking time by 2 minutes.

If you don't have a glass loaf dish, use a metal loaf pan and increase the baking time by 5 to 10 minutes.

Teff is a grass native to Ethiopia, where it is used to make the country's staple bread, injera. The grain is a nutritional powerhouse: an excellent source of protein, calcium, zinc, copper, phosphorus and other important nutrients.

If you are sensitive to sulfites, make sure the dried apricots have no added sulfites.

NUTRIENTS PER SLICE

Calories 240
Fat . . . . .13 g
Carbohydrate . . . . .28 g
Fiber . . . . .3 g
Protein . . . . .5 g
Iron . . . . .1.6 mg
Calcium . . . . 28 mg

- **Preheat oven to 350°F (180°C)**
- **9- by 5-inch (23 by 12.5 cm) glass loaf dish, greased, bottom lined with parchment paper**

$\frac{3}{4}$ cup	sorghum flour	175 mL
$\frac{1}{4}$ cup	teff flour	60 mL
2 tsp	gluten-free baking powder	10 mL
1 tsp	baking soda	5 mL
$\frac{1}{4}$ tsp	salt	1 mL
2	eggs	2
$\frac{1}{4}$ cup	granulated raw cane sugar	60 mL
$\frac{1}{3}$ cup	vegetable oil	75 mL
1 cup	mashed ripe bananas	250 mL
$\frac{1}{4}$ cup	chopped dried apricots	60 mL
$\frac{1}{4}$ cup	unseasoned raw pumpkin seeds	60 mL

1. In a large bowl, whisk together sorghum flour, teff flour, baking powder, baking soda and salt.

2. In a medium bowl, whisk together eggs, sugar and oil until well blended. Stir in bananas. Pour over dry ingredients and stir until combined. Gently fold in apricots and almonds.

3. Pour batter into prepared loaf dish. Bake in preheated oven for about 50 minutes or until a tester inserted in the center comes out clean. Let cool in dish on a wire rack for 10 minutes. Remove from dish and peel off paper. Transfer loaf to rack and let cool completely.

Breakfast Idea: Enjoy a slice of this bread with $\frac{3}{4}$ cup (175 mL) low-fat yogurt or a non-dairy alternative, such as soy, rice or coconut milk yogurt.

Snack Idea: Enjoy a slice of this bread with 1 cup (250 mL) milk, lactose-free milk or enriched non-dairy milk alternative.

Applesauce Raisin Muffins

Makes 12 muffins

Whether you use store-bought applesauce or make your own, these comforting muffins will make it hard to stop after just one.

Tip

Other unsulfured dried fruits, such as chopped dried apricots or cherries, may be substituted for the raisins.

- **Preheat oven to 400°F (200°C)**
- **12-cup muffin pan, greased**

2 cups	Brown Rice Flour Blend (see recipe, opposite)	500 mL
2 tsp	gluten-free baking powder	10 mL
1 tsp	ground cinnamon	5 mL
1/2 tsp	ground allspice	2 mL
1/2 tsp	baking soda	2 mL
1/2 tsp	salt	2 mL
1 1/2 cups	unsweetened applesauce	375 mL
1/2 cup	liquid honey or agave nectar	125 mL
1/3 cup	vegetable oil	75 mL
1 tsp	gluten-free vanilla extract	5 mL
1/2 cup	unsulfured raisins	125 mL

1. In a large bowl, whisk together flour blend, baking powder, cinnamon, allspice, baking soda and salt.
2. In a medium bowl, whisk together applesauce, honey, oil and vanilla until blended.
3. Add the applesauce mixture to the flour mixture and stir until just blended. Gently fold in raisins.
4. Divide batter equally among prepared muffin cups.
5. Bake in preheated oven for 25 to 28 minutes or until tops are golden brown and a toothpick inserted in the center comes out clean. Let cool in pan on a wire rack for 5 minutes, then transfer to the rack to cool.

> **Breakfast Idea:** Pair one of these muffins with a Body Builder Smoothie (page 330) for a breakfast that leaves you feeling full for a long time.

NUTRIENTS
PER MUFFIN

Calories 220
Fat .7 g
Carbohydrate . . . . .42 g
Fiber . . . . .1 g
Protein . . . . .2 g
Iron . . . . .0.6 mg
Calcium . . . . 14 mg

Brown Rice Flour Blend

Makes about 3 cups (750 mL)

Tips

You can also make the blend in smaller amounts by using the basic proportions: 2 parts finely ground brown rice flour, $\frac{2}{3}$ part potato starch and $\frac{1}{3}$ part tapioca starch.

You can double, triple or quadruple the recipe to have it on hand. Store the blend in an airtight container in the refrigerator for up to 4 months, or in the freezer for up to 1 year. Let warm to room temperature before using.

2 cups	finely ground brown rice flour	500 mL
$\frac{2}{3}$ cup	potato starch	150 mL
$\frac{1}{3}$ cup	tapioca starch	75 mL

1. In a bowl, whisk together brown rice flour, potato starch and tapioca starch. Use as directed in recipes.

NUTRIENTS
PER 1 CUP (250 ML)

Calories 570
Fat .3 g
Carbohydrate . . . . .130 g
Fiber . . . . .3 g
Protein . . . . .8 g
Iron . . . . .2.0 mg
Calcium . . . . 0 mg

Double Banana Muffins

These fast and easy muffins offer banana two ways — mashed and diced — in a batter spiked with a little nutmeg.

Tip

To maximize your nutrient intake, make sure to select an enriched non-dairy milk.

- **Preheat oven to 325°F (160°C)**
- **12-cup muffin pan, lined with paper liners**

1½ cups	Brown Rice Flour Blend (page 187)	375 mL
1 tsp	gluten-free baking powder	5 mL
¾ tsp	baking soda	3 mL
½ tsp	salt	2 mL
¼ tsp	ground nutmeg	1 mL
½ cup	liquid honey or agave nectar	125 mL
½ cup	unsweetened light coconut milk, rice milk or hemp milk	125 mL
⅓ cup	vegetable oil	75 mL
1 tbsp	cider vinegar	15 mL
1¼ cups	mashed ripe bananas	300 mL
1	large ripe banana, peeled and cut into ¼-inch (0.5 cm) chunks	1

1. In a large bowl, whisk together flour blend, baking powder, baking soda, salt and nutmeg.
2. In a medium bowl, whisk together honey, coconut milk, oil and vinegar until blended. Stir in mashed bananas.
3. Add the honey mixture to the flour mixture and stir until just blended. Gently fold in diced banana.
4. Divide batter equally among prepared muffin cups.
5. Bake in preheated oven for 22 to 25 minutes or until tops are golden and a toothpick inserted in the center comes out clean. Let cool in pan on a wire rack for 3 minutes, then transfer to the rack to cool.

> **Snack Idea:** Enjoy ½ cup (125 mL) enriched non-dairy yogurt with one of these muffins for a delicious mid-afternoon snack. If you have an allergy to soy protein, substitute ½ cup (125 mL) calcium-enriched orange juice for the yogurt.

NUTRIENTS
PER MUFFIN

Calories 210
Fat . . . . 7 g
Carbohydrate . . . . 38 g
Fiber . . . . 1 g
Protein . . . . 2 g
Iron . . . . 0.4 mg
Calcium . . . . 19 mg

Favorite Blueberry Muffins

Makes 12 muffins

These tender-as-can-be muffins have an easy style, their sapphire, tart-sweet berries harmonizing with a vanilla-scented batter.

- **Preheat oven to 350°F (180°C)**
- **12-cup muffin pan, greased**

2 cups	Brown Rice Flour Blend (page 187)	500 mL
2-1/2 tsp	gluten-free baking powder	12 mL
1/2 tsp	baking soda	2 mL
1/2 tsp	salt	2 mL
3/4 cup	unsweetened applesauce	175 mL
1/2 cup	agave nectar or liquid honey	125 mL
1/2 cup	mashed ripe banana	125 mL
1/4 cup	vegetable oil	60 mL
1 tsp	gluten-free vanilla extract	5 mL
2 cups	blueberries	500 mL
2 tbsp	turbinado sugar (optional)	30 mL

1. In a large bowl, whisk together flour blend, baking powder, baking soda and salt.
2. In a medium bowl, whisk together applesauce, agave nectar, banana, oil and vanilla until well blended.
3. Add the applesauce mixture to the flour mixture and stir until just blended. Gently fold in blueberries.
4. Divide batter equally among prepared muffin cups. Sprinkle with turbinado sugar, if desired.
5. Bake in preheated oven for 18 to 22 minutes or until tops are golden brown and a toothpick inserted in the center comes out clean. Let cool in pan on a wire rack for 3 minutes, then transfer to the rack to cool.

Breakfast Idea: Pair one of these muffins with 1 cup (250 mL) lactose-free milk or enriched non-dairy milk.

NUTRIENTS
PER MUFFIN

Calories	210
Fat	5 g
Carbohydrate	41 g
Fiber	2 g
Protein	2 g
Iron	0.5 mg
Calcium	11 mg

Pumpkin Spice Muffins

Embrace the flavors of autumn with these moist, delicious muffins. The pumpkin lends richness and color, and is one of the healthiest ingredients you can keep on your pantry shelf.

Tips

Look for a brand of pumpkin pie spice that is free of added sulfites.

To maximize your nutrient intake, make sure to select an enriched hemp or rice milk.

- **Preheat oven to 400°F (200°C)**
- **12-cup muffin pan, greased**

1½ cups	Brown Rice Flour Blend (page 187)	375 mL
¼ cup	ground flax seeds (flaxseed meal)	60 mL
1 tbsp	gluten-free baking powder	15 mL
2½ tsp	pumpkin pie spice	12 mL
¾ tsp	salt	3 mL
1 cup	pumpkin purée (not pie filling)	250 mL
⅔ cup	agave nectar or liquid honey	150 mL
½ cup	mashed ripe banana	125 mL
½ cup	vegetable oil	125 mL
⅓ cup	hemp or rice milk	75 mL
1½ tsp	gluten-free vanilla extract	7 mL

1. In a large bowl, whisk together flour blend, flax seeds, baking powder, pumpkin pie spice and salt.
2. In a medium bowl, whisk together pumpkin, agave nectar, banana, oil, hemp milk and vanilla until well blended.
3. Add the pumpkin mixture to the flour mixture and stir until just blended.
4. Divide batter equally among prepared muffin cups.
5. Bake in preheated oven for 18 to 22 minutes or until a toothpick inserted in the center comes out clean. Let cool in pan on a wire rack for 3 minutes, then transfer to the rack to cool.

Snack Idea: Pair one of these muffins with a smoothie such as The Antioxidizer (page 331) for a great mid-morning snack.

NUTRIENTS
PER MUFFIN

Calories	240
Fat	11 g
Carbohydrate	37 g
Fiber	3 g
Protein	2 g
Iron	1.0 mg
Calcium	37 mg

Carrot Cake Muffins

Makes 12 muffins

These delectable muffins are moist, heady with spices and just plain good!

Tip

To maximize your nutrient intake, make sure to select an enriched hemp or rice milk.

- **Preheat oven to 400°F (200°C)**
- **12-cup muffin pan, greased**

1½ cups	Brown Rice Flour Blend (page 187)	375 mL
2 tsp	gluten-free baking powder	10 mL
1 tsp	ground cinnamon	5 mL
1 tsp	ground ginger	5 mL
½ tsp	baking soda	2 mL
½ tsp	salt	2 mL
¼ tsp	ground nutmeg	1 mL
1 cup	hemp or rice milk	250 mL
½ cup	agave nectar or liquid honey	125 mL
⅓ cup	coconut oil, warmed	75 mL
1 tsp	gluten-free vanilla extract	5 mL
2 cups	shredded carrots	500 mL
½ cup	unsulfured dried currants or raisins	125 mL

1. In a large bowl, whisk together flour blend, baking powder, cinnamon, ginger, baking soda, salt and nutmeg.
2. In a medium bowl, whisk together hemp milk, agave nectar, oil and vanilla until well blended.
3. Add the milk mixture to the flour mixture and stir until just blended. Gently fold in carrots and currants.
4. Divide batter equally among prepared muffin cups.
5. Bake in preheated oven for 18 to 22 minutes or until tops are golden brown and a toothpick inserted in the center comes out clean. Let cool in pan on a wire rack for 3 minutes, then transfer to the rack to cool.

Snack Idea: Pair one of these muffins with Spicy Cinnamon Lemonade (page 333).

NUTRIENTS
PER MUFFIN

Calories	200
Fat	7 g
Carbohydrate	36 g
Fiber	2 g
Protein	2 g
Iron	0.6 mg
Calcium	49 mg

Morning Glory Muffins

Makes 12 muffins		

Classic morning glory muffins become that much more glorious when made with brown rice flour, flax seeds and plenty of fruits and vegetables.

Tip

Look for a brand of pumpkin pie spice that is free of added sulfites.

- **Preheat oven to 350°F (180°C)**
- **12-cup muffin pan, greased**

1²⁄₃ cups	Brown Rice Flour Blend (page 187)	400 mL
¹⁄₃ cup	ground flax seeds (flaxseed meal)	75 mL
2¹⁄₂ tsp	pumpkin pie spice	12 mL
2 tsp	gluten-free baking powder	10 mL
¹⁄₂ tsp	baking soda	2 mL
¹⁄₄ tsp	salt	1 mL
²⁄₃ cup	mashed ripe banana	150 mL
¹⁄₂ cup	agave nectar or liquid honey	125 mL
¹⁄₂ cup	coconut oil, warmed, or vegetable oil	125 mL
1 tsp	gluten-free vanilla extract	5 mL
1	can (8 oz/227 mL) unsweetened crushed pineapple, well drained	1
1 cup	finely shredded carrots	250 mL
¹⁄₂ cup	unsulfured raisins	125 mL
¹⁄₂ cup	sunflower seeds or green pumpkin seeds (pepitas), toasted	125 mL

1. In a large bowl, whisk together flour blend, flax seeds, pumpkin pie spice, baking powder, baking soda and salt.
2. In a medium bowl, whisk together banana, agave nectar, oil and vanilla until well blended.
3. Add the banana mixture to the flour mixture and stir until just blended. Gently fold in pineapple, carrots, raisins and sunflower seeds.
4. Divide batter equally among prepared muffin cups.
5. Bake in preheated oven for 22 to 25 minutes or until a toothpick inserted in the center comes out clean. Let cool in pan on a wire rack for 5 minutes, then transfer to the rack to cool.

Snack Idea: These muffins are nutritionally dense. Pair one with a serving of fresh fruit.

NUTRIENTS
PER MUFFIN

Calories	290
Fat	13 g
Carbohydrate	42 g
Fiber	3 g
Protein	3 g
Iron	1.0 mg
Calcium	30 mg

Multigrain Quinoa Muffins

Makes 18 muffins

Indigenous to the Andes, quinoa was called "the mother grain" by the Incas, who considered the plant sacred. And while much has been made of quinoa's nutritional properties, its nutty flavor in this recipe is a revelation.

- **Blender**
- **Two 12-cup muffin pans, 18 cups greased**

½ cup	quinoa, rinsed	125 mL
⅔ cup	boiling water	150 mL
2 cups	Brown Rice Flour Blend (page 187)	500 mL
½ cup	pure, uncontaminated large-flake (old-fashioned) rolled oats	125 mL
2 tsp	baking powder	10 mL
1 tsp	baking soda	5 mL
1 tsp	ground cinnamon	5 mL
½ tsp	salt	2 mL
2 tbsp	ground flax seeds (flaxseed meal)	30 mL
1½ cups	unsweetened applesauce	375 mL
½ cup	agave nectar or liquid honey	125 mL
¼ cup	vegetable oil	60 mL
½ cup	unsulfured dried blueberries or raisins	125 mL

1. In a small bowl, combine quinoa and boiling water. Let stand for 20 minutes.
2. Preheat oven to 375°F (190°C).
3. In a large bowl, whisk together flour blend, oats, baking powder, baking soda, cinnamon and salt until blended.
4. In blender, process flax seeds, applesauce, agave nectar and oil for 1 minute or until just blended.
5. Add the applesauce mixture to the flour mixture and stir until just blended. Gently fold in quinoa and blueberries.
6. Divide batter equally among prepared muffin cups.
7. Bake for 18 to 23 minutes or until tops are golden and a toothpick inserted in the center comes out clean. Let cool in pans on a wire rack for 5 minutes, then transfer to the rack to cool.

> **Breakfast Idea:** For a complete breakfast, pair one of these muffins with 1 cup (250 mL) lactose-free milk or enriched non-dairy milk.

NUTRIENTS
PER MUFFIN

Calories	250
Fat	6 g
Carbohydrate	47 g
Fiber	3 g
Protein	3 g
Iron	1.1 mg
Calcium	19 mg

Agave Flax Muffins

Makes 12 muffins

These muffins are remarkably sweet, despite having no sugar except for a small amount of agave nectar. Sorghum flour is part of the secret: it has a natural sweetness that makes any morning muffin extra-delicious. Ground flax seeds contribute moistness and nutrients.

Tip

To maximize your nutrient intake, make sure to select an enriched hemp or rice milk.

- **Preheat oven to 350°F (180°C)**
- **12-cup muffin pan, lined with paper liners**

1 cup	sorghum flour	250 mL
1 cup	Brown Rice Flour Blend (page 187)	250 mL
1/4 cup	ground flax seeds (flaxseed meal)	60 mL
1 tbsp	gluten-free baking powder	15 mL
1/2 tsp	ground cinnamon	2 mL
1/2 tsp	salt	2 mL
1/2 tsp	xanthan gum	2 mL
1/4 tsp	ground cloves	1 mL
1/4 cup	unsweetened applesauce	60 mL
1/4 cup	vegetable oil	60 mL
1/4 cup	agave nectar	60 mL
1 1/4 cups	hemp or rice milk	300 mL

1. In a large bowl, whisk together sorghum flour, flour blend, flax seeds, baking powder, cinnamon, salt, xanthan gum and cloves.
2. In a medium bowl, whisk together applesauce, oil and agave nectar until well blended. Whisk in hemp milk until blended.
3. Add the applesauce mixture to the flour mixture and stir until just blended.
4. Divide batter equally among prepared muffin cups.
5. Bake in preheated oven for 18 to 22 minutes or until a toothpick inserted in the center comes out clean. Let cool in pan on a wire rack for 5 minutes, then transfer to the rack to cool.

> **Breakfast Idea:** Pair one of these muffins with 3/4 cup (175 mL) yogurt or enriched non-dairy yogurt and 1/2 cup (125 mL) fresh fruit.

NUTRIENTS
PER MUFFIN

Calories	180
Fat	6 g
Carbohydrate	29 g
Fiber	2 g
Protein	3 g
Iron	1.0 mg
Calcium	49 mg

Breads and Snacks

Gluten-Free, Egg-Free, Corn-Free, Dairy-Free, Soy-Free Brown Bread

I had the privilege of counseling a patient whose family suffered from combined multiple allergies that included soy, dairy and egg. In addition, one family member had celiac disease. I wish I'd had this bread recipe for them at the time.

Tips

Don't be alarmed when this one turns out shorter than some loaves.

If you are sensitive to sulfites, look for unsulfered molasses or substitute 1 tbsp (15 mL) packed brown sugar. You can also replace the cider vinegar with white vinegar.

Variation

The rice bran can be replaced by an equal amount of pure, uncontaminated oat bran or brown or white rice flour.

NUTRIENTS
PER SLICE

Calories	139
Fat	4 g
Carbohydrate	24 g
Fiber	3 g
Protein	3 g
Iron	2.0 mg
Calcium	23 mg

- 9- by 5-inch (23 by 12.5 cm) loaf pan, lightly greased

¼ cup	flax flour or ground flax seeds	60 mL
⅓ cup	warm water	75 mL
1¼ cups	brown rice flour	300 mL
¾ cup	sorghum flour	175 mL
⅓ cup	rice bran	75 mL
3 tbsp	tapioca starch	45 mL
1 tbsp	xanthan gum	15 mL
1 tbsp	bread machine or instant yeast	15 mL
1¼ tsp	salt	6 mL
1 cup	water	250 mL
2 tbsp	vegetable oil	30 mL
3 tbsp	liquid honey	45 mL
1 tbsp	light (fancy) molasses	15 mL
1 tsp	cider vinegar	5 mL

1. In a small bowl or measuring cup, combine flax flour and ⅓ cup (75 mL) warm water; set aside for 5 minutes.

2. In a large bowl or plastic bag, combine brown rice flour, sorghum flour, rice bran, tapioca starch, xanthan gum, yeast and salt. Mix well and set aside.

3. In a separate bowl, using a heavy-duty electric mixer with paddle attachment, combine 1 cup (250 mL) water, oil, honey, molasses, vinegar and flax flour mixture until well blended. With the mixer on its lowest speed, slowly add the dry ingredients until combined. Stop the machine and scrape the bottom and sides of the bowl with a rubber spatula. With the mixer on medium speed, beat for 1 minute or until smooth.

4. Spoon dough into prepared pan. Let rise, uncovered, in a warm, draft-free place for 75 to 90 minutes or until dough has risen almost to the top of the pan. Meanwhile, preheat oven to 350°F (180°C).

5. Bake for 25 minutes. Check to see if loaf is getting too dark and tent with foil if necessary. Bake for 10 to 20 minutes or until internal temperature of loaf registers 200°F (100°C) on an instant-read thermometer. Remove from the pan immediately and let cool completely on a rack.

Gluten-Free, Egg-Free, Corn-Free, Lactose-Free Brown Bread

Makes 15 slices

Here's another variation on brown bread. This one uses rice bran to up the fiber quotient — a great call, as many gluten-free breads are low in fiber.

Tips

Slice this or any bread with an electric knife for thin, even sandwich slices.

For a milder-flavored bread, substitute 2 tbsp (30 mL) packed brown sugar for the molasses.

The rice bran can be replaced by an equal amount of brown or white rice flour.

If you are sensitive to sulfites, look for unsulfered molasses or substitute 1 tbsp (15 mL) packed brown sugar. You can also replace the cider vinegar with white vinegar.

NUTRIENTS
PER SLICE

Calories	140
Fat	4 g
Carbohydrate	25 g
Fiber	3 g
Protein	3 g
Iron	1.6 mg
Calcium	4 mg

- **9- by 5-inch (23 by 12.5 cm) loaf pan, lightly greased**

1¼ cups	brown rice flour	300 mL
½ cup	sorghum flour	125 mL
½ cup	rice bran	125 mL
¼ cup	tapioca starch	60 mL
1 tbsp	powdered egg replacer (see tip, page 198)	15 mL
1 tbsp	xanthan gum	15 mL
1 tbsp	bread machine or instant yeast	15 mL
1¼ tsp	salt	6 mL
1⅓ cups	water	325 mL
2 tbsp	vegetable oil	30 mL
2 tbsp	liquid honey	30 mL
1 tbsp	light (fancy) molasses	15 mL
1 tsp	cider vinegar	5 mL

1. In a large bowl or plastic bag, combine brown rice flour, sorghum flour, rice bran, tapioca starch, egg replacer, xanthan gum, yeast and salt. Mix well and set aside.

2. In a separate bowl, using a heavy-duty electric mixer with paddle attachment, combine water, oil, honey, molasses and vinegar until well blended. With the mixer on its lowest speed, slowly add the dry ingredients until combined. Stop the machine and scrape the bottom and sides of the bowl with a rubber spatula. With the mixer on medium speed, beat for 4 minutes.

3. Spoon into prepared pan. Let rise, uncovered, in a warm, draft-free place for 60 to 75 minutes, or until dough has risen to the top of the pan. Meanwhile, preheat oven to 350°F (180°C).

4. Bake for 35 to 45 minutes or until loaf sounds hollow when tapped on the bottom. Remove from the pan immediately and let cool completely on a rack.

Lunch Idea: Use 2 slices of this bread to make hearty sandwiches or enjoy 1 slice as an accompaniment to 1 serving of any of the soups in this book.

Gluten-Free, Egg-Free, Corn-Free, Dairy-Free, Soy-Free White Dinner Rolls

Makes 5 rolls

Enjoy these rolls with any vegetable- or bean-based soups. Adding raw sunflower or pumpkin seeds to the mix (see the variation, below) boosts the iron, magnesium, calcium and protein.

Tips

Egg replacer is a white powder containing a combination of baking powder and starches. It is added with the dry ingredients so that it is well mixed in before it touches the liquids.

If you are sensitive to sulfites, replace the cider vinegar with white vinegar.

Variation

Add ¼ cup (60 mL) unsalted raw sunflower seeds or green pumpkin seeds with the dry ingredients.

NUTRIENTS PER ROLL

Calories	189
Fat	7 g
Carbohydrate	30 g
Fiber	3 g
Protein	3 g
Iron	2.0 mg
Calcium	14 mg

- **Baking sheet, lightly greased**

¾ cup	brown rice flour	175 mL
¼ cup	amaranth flour	60 mL
¼ cup	tapioca starch	60 mL
1 tbsp	powdered egg replacer (see tip, at left)	15 mL
1 tbsp	granulated sugar	15 mL
2½ tsp	xanthan gum	12 mL
1 tbsp	bread machine or instant yeast	15 mL
¾ tsp	salt	3 mL
¾ cup	water	175 mL
2 tbsp	vegetable oil	30 mL
1 tsp	cider vinegar	5 mL

1. In a bowl or plastic bag, combine brown rice flour, amaranth flour, tapioca starch, egg replacer, sugar, xanthan gum, yeast and salt. Mix well and set aside.

2. In a separate bowl, using a heavy-duty electric mixer with paddle attachment, combine water, oil and vinegar until well blended. With the mixer on its lowest speed, slowly add the dry ingredients until combined. Stop the machine and scrape the bottom and sides of the bowl with a rubber spatula. With the mixer on medium speed, beat for 1 minute or until smooth.

3. Using a ¼-cup (60 mL) scoop, drop 5 scoops of dough at least 2 inches (5 cm) apart onto prepared baking sheet. Let rise, uncovered, in a warm, draft-free place for 75 minutes. Meanwhile, preheat oven to 350°F (180°C).

4. Bake for 20 to 22 minutes or until internal temperature of rolls registers 200°F (100°C) on an instant-read thermometer. Remove from the pan immediately and let cool completely on a rack.

Lunch Idea: Spread 1 tbsp (15 mL) Santorini-Style Fava Spread (page 209) on 1 dinner roll. Enjoy it with the filling Soup à la Mom (page 223).

Focaccia

Focaccia can be cut into finger-width slices and served with a bean dip as an appetizer. It also makes a great on-the-go snack. Pea flour (or any bean flour) is a great way to boost the nutritional value of bread, especially its fiber, protein and iron content.

Tips

If you have a wheat allergy or celiac disease, ensure that the pea flour is labeled "gluten-free."

If you are sensitive to sulfites, replace the cider vinegar with white vinegar.

Reheat leftovers under the broiler to enjoy crisp focaccia.

Before serving, sprinkle with pure, cold-pressed olive oil and dried rosemary for a classic Italian taste.

NUTRIENTS
PER PIECE

Calories 126
Fat . . . . .3 g
Carbohydrate . . . . .21 g
Fiber . . . . .2 g
Protein . . . . .4 g
Iron . . . . .2.0 mg
Calcium . . . . 22 mg

- **8-inch (20 cm) square baking pan, lightly greased and lined with parchment paper**

⅓ cup	amaranth flour	75 mL
¼ cup	pea flour	60 mL
3 tbsp	potato starch	45 mL
2 tbsp	tapioca starch	30 mL
1 tsp	granulated sugar	5 mL
1 tsp	xanthan gum	5 mL
1 tbsp	bread machine or instant yeast	15 mL
½ tsp	salt	2 mL
¾ cup	water	175 mL
2 tsp	extra virgin olive oil	10 mL
1 tsp	cider vinegar	5 mL

1. In a bowl or plastic bag, combine amaranth flour, pea flour, potato starch, tapioca starch, sugar, xanthan gum, yeast and salt. Mix well and set aside.

2. In a separate bowl, using a heavy-duty electric mixer with paddle attachment, combine water, oil and vinegar until well blended. With the mixer on its lowest speed, slowly add the dry ingredients until combined. Stop the machine and scrape the bottom and sides of the bowl with a rubber spatula. With the mixer on medium speed, beat for 1 minute or until smooth.

3. Gently transfer dough to prepared pan and spread evenly to the edges, leaving the top rough and uneven. Do not smooth. Let rise, uncovered, in a warm, draft-free place for 30 minutes or until almost doubled in volume. Meanwhile, preheat oven to 400°F (200°C).

4. Bake for 30 to 35 minutes or until golden. Remove from the pan immediately. Cut into 4 pieces and serve hot.

Snack Idea: Enjoy a piece of focaccia with ¼ cup (60 mL) Spicy Black Bean Dip (page 207) or Italian White Bean Spread (page 208) and ½ cup (125 mL) baby carrots.

Lunch Idea: Serve a piece of focaccia with 1 serving of any of the soup recipes in this book.

Pizza Crust

Why not make your own pizza for a Friday-night family gathering! Top this yummy, nutritious crust with your favorite vegetables and condiments.

Tips

If you are sensitive to sulfites, replace the cider vinegar with white vinegar.

If you don't have an 8-inch (20 cm) round pizza pan, use a 12-inch (30 cm) pan. After transferring dough to the pan, top it with waxed paper and roll out to an 8½-inch (21 cm) circle. Form a ¼-inch (3 mm) ridge all the way around the edge.

- **Preheat oven to 400°F (200°C), with rack set in the bottom third**
- **8-inch (20 cm) round pizza pan, lightly greased**

¼ cup	sorghum flour	60 mL
¼ cup	quinoa flour	60 mL
1 tbsp	tapioca starch	15 mL
1 tsp	granulated sugar	5 mL
2 tsp	xanthan gum	10 mL
1 tbsp	bread machine or instant yeast	15 mL
¼ tsp	salt	1 mL
⅓ cup	water	75 mL
1 tbsp	extra virgin olive oil	15 mL
1 tsp	cider vinegar	5 mL

1. In a bowl or plastic bag, combine sorghum flour, quinoa flour, tapioca starch, sugar, xanthan gum, yeast and salt. Mix well and set aside.

2. In a separate bowl, using a heavy-duty electric mixer with paddle attachment, combine water, oil and vinegar until well blended. With the mixer on its lowest speed, slowly add the dry ingredients until combined. Stop the machine and scrape the bottom and sides of the bowl with a rubber spatula. With the mixer on medium speed, beat for 1 minute or until smooth.

3. Gently transfer dough to prepared pan. Using a moist rubber spatula, carefully spread to the edges.

4. Bake in preheated oven for 10 minutes or until bottom is golden and crust is partially baked.

5. Use right away to make pizza with your favorite toppings, or wrap airtight and store in the freezer for up to 1 month. Thaw in the refrigerator overnight before using.

> **Lunch Idea:** To make pizza, add your favorite toppings and bake until crust is brown and crisp and top is bubbly. Enjoy ½ serving of pizza with 1 serving of Health Salad (page 233) for a complete lunch.

NUTRIENTS PER SERVING

Calories	230
Fat	9 g
Carbohydrate	33 g
Fiber	7 g
Protein	7 g
Iron	3.0 mg
Calcium	19 mg

Thin Pizza Crust

Makes 1 to 2 servings

For those who are watching their caloric intake, this recipe is a lighter version of the one on page 200.

Tips

If you are sensitive to sulfites, replace the cider vinegar with white vinegar.

This recipe can easily be doubled to make 2 pizza crusts. Partially bake both, then top one to bake immediately and freeze the other for a future meal.

Warming leftover pizza for 5 to 10 minutes in the oven results in a very crisp crust.

If you don't have an 8-inch (20 cm) round pizza pan, use a 12-inch (30 cm) pan. After transferring dough to the pan, top it with waxed paper and roll out to an 8½-inch (21 cm) circle. Form a ¼-inch (3 mm) ridge all the way around the edge.

- **8-inch (20 cm) round pizza pan, lightly greased**

¼ cup	brown rice flour	60 mL
2 tbsp	potato starch	30 mL
1 tsp	granulated sugar	5 mL
½ tsp	xanthan gum	2 mL
1 tsp	bread machine or instant yeast	5 mL
¼ tsp	salt	1 mL
1 tsp	dried oregano, basil, marjoram or thyme	5 mL
¼ cup	water	60 mL
1 tbsp	vegetable oil	15 mL
1 tsp	cider vinegar	5 mL

1. In a bowl or plastic bag, combine brown rice flour, potato starch, sugar, xanthan gum, yeast, salt and oregano. Mix well and set aside.

2. In a separate bowl, using a heavy-duty electric mixer with paddle attachment, combine water, oil and vinegar until well blended. With the mixer on its lowest speed, slowly add the dry ingredients until combined. Stop the machine and scrape the bottom and sides of the bowl with a rubber spatula. With the mixer on medium speed, beat for 1 minute or until smooth.

3. Gently transfer dough to prepared pan. Using a moist rubber spatula, carefully spread to the edges.

4. Place in a cold oven and set oven temperature to 400°F (200°C). Bake for 12 to 17 minutes or until bottom is golden and crust is partially baked.

5. Use right away to make pizza with your favorite toppings, or wrap airtight and store in the freezer for up to 1 month. Thaw in the refrigerator overnight before using.

> **Lunch Idea:** To make pizza, add your favorite topping ingredients and bake until crust is brown and crisp and top is bubbly.

NUTRIENTS
PER SERVING

Calories	181
Fat	8 g
Carbohydrate	26 g
Fiber	2 g
Protein	2 g
Iron	1.0 mg
Calcium	17 mg

Oat Pizza Crust

For a healthier alternative to your store-bought gluten-free pizza crust, try this one made from pure, uncontaminated oat flour.

Tips

Oat flour provides fiber, protein and iron. In addition, oats are a natural source of the B vitamins niacin, thiamin and riboflavin, which help us metabolize food, support the nervous system and contribute to eye health.

Potato flour and potato starch are two completely different ingredients and cannot be substituted for one another.

You may need to dust your hands with potato flour if the dough is a little sticky.

If you are sensitive to sulfites, replace the cider vinegar with white vinegar.

NUTRIENTS PER SERVING

Calories	114
Fat	3 g
Carbohydrate	19 g
Fiber	3 g
Protein	3 g
Iron	1.0 mg
Calcium	15 mg

- **Preheat oven to 400°F (200°C)**
- **12-inch (30 cm) pizza pan, lightly greased**

1¼ cups	pure, uncontaminated oat flour	300 mL
¼ cup	potato flour (not potato starch)	60 mL
¼ cup	tapioca starch	60 mL
1 tsp	granulated sugar	5 mL
2 tsp	xanthan gum	10 mL
1 tbsp	bread machine or instant yeast	15 mL
¾ tsp	salt	3 mL
1¼ cups	water	300 mL
1 tbsp	extra virgin olive oil	15 mL
1 tsp	cider vinegar	5 mL

Bread Machine Method

1. In a large bowl or plastic bag, combine oat flour, potato flour, tapioca starch, sugar, xanthan gum, yeast and salt. Mix well and set aside.

2. Pour water, oil and vinegar into the bread machine baking pan. Select the Dough Cycle. Allow the liquids to mix until combined. As the machine is mixing, gradually add the dry ingredients, scraping bottom and sides of pan with a rubber spatula. Try to incorporate all the dry ingredients within 1 to 2 minutes. Stop bread machine as soon as the kneading portion of the cycle is complete. Do not let bread machine finish cycle.

Mixer Method

1. In a large bowl or plastic bag, combine oat flour, potato flour, tapioca starch, sugar, xanthan gum, yeast and salt. Mix well and set aside.

2. In a separate bowl, using a heavy-duty electric mixer with paddle attachment, combine water, oil and vinegar until well blended. With the mixer on its lowest speed, slowly add the dry ingredients until combined. Stop the machine and scrape the bottom and sides of the bowl with a rubber spatula. With the mixer on medium speed, beat for 4 minutes.

Tip

Partially baked pizza crust can be wrapped airtight and frozen for up to 4 weeks. Thaw in the refrigerator overnight before using to make pizza.

Variation

Add 2 tsp (10 mL) dried oregano to the dry ingredients. Dried oregano is an excellent source of disease-fighting antioxidants.

For Both Methods

3. Gently transfer dough to prepared pan and, using a moistened rubber spatula, spread evenly to the edges. Do not smooth top.

4. Bake in preheated oven for 12 minutes or until bottom is golden and crust is partially baked.

This recipe courtesy of Beth Armour, Cream Hill Estates.

Lunch Idea: To make pizza, add your favorite topping ingredients and bake until crust is brown and crisp and top is bubbly.

Crispy Multi-Seed Crackers

Makes about 40 crackers

These wholesome crackers are a great accompaniment to bean soups and grainy salads. They also pair well with any vegetarian dip.

Tips

If you have an allergy to sesame seeds, replace them with pumpkin or sunflower seeds.

If you are sensitive to sulfites, replace the cider vinegar with white vinegar.

Parmesan cheese is naturally lactose-free, but if you have an allergy to cow's milk protein, substitute rice- or soy-based Parmesan-style cheese alternative.

Buy ground flax seeds or grind your own in a clean coffee grinder. For a thin, crisp cracker, roll dough to an even thickness as thinly as possible. Don't worry if it breaks into pieces.

NUTRIENTS
PER 1/20 RECIPE

Calories	80
Fat	4 g
Carbohydrate	9 g
Fiber	2 g
Protein	2 g
Iron	1.0 mg
Calcium	51 mg

- **Preheat oven to 375°F (190°C)**
- **Baking sheets, ungreased**

1/2 cup	water	125 mL
2 tbsp	extra virgin olive oil	30 mL
1 tsp	cider vinegar	5 mL
1/2 cup	brown rice flour	125 mL
1/2 cup	sorghum flour	125 mL
1/4 cup	cornstarch	60 mL
1/3 cup	ground flax seeds (flaxseed meal)	75 mL
1 1/2 tsp	xanthan gum	7 mL
1/2 tsp	gluten-free baking powder	2 mL
1 tsp	salt	5 mL
1/4 cup	freshly grated Parmesan cheese or non-dairy alternative	60 mL
1/4 cup	sesame seeds	60 mL
3 tbsp	dried oregano	45 mL
2 tbsp	poppy seeds	30 mL

1. In a small bowl, combine water, olive oil and vinegar. Mix well and set aside.

2. In a food processor, pulse brown rice flour, sorghum flour, cornstarch, ground flax seeds, xanthan gum, baking powder, salt, Parmesan, sesame seeds, oregano and poppy seeds until mixed. With machine running, add liquid mixture through feed tube in a slow, steady stream. Process until dough forms a ball.

3. Divide dough into four pieces. Place each on plastic wrap and flatten into a disk; wrap well. Let dough rest in refrigerator for 10 minutes. Place one disk between two sheets of waxed or parchment paper. To prevent the paper from moving while you're rolling out the dough, place it on a lint-free towel. Using a heavy stroke with a rolling pin, roll out the dough as thinly as possible. Carefully remove the top sheet of paper. Invert the dough onto the baking sheet. Remove the remaining sheet of paper. Repeat with the remaining dough.

Tips

Pay close attention during the last few minutes of baking, as crackers can burn easily.

If crackers become soft, re-crisp in a toaster oven or conventional oven at 350°F (180°C).

Just before baking, sprinkle with 1 tsp (5 mL) coarse salt or sesame seeds.

Substitute an equal amount of hempseed flour for the ground flax seeds (flaxseed meal).

4. Bake in preheated oven for 18 to 25 minutes, or until browned and crisp. Remove to a cooling rack and cool completely. Break into pieces. Store at room temperature in an airtight container for up to 2 weeks or freeze for up to 3 months.

Snack Idea: Serve these crackers with Ratatouille Salsa (page 213).

Lunch Idea: Enjoy 4 crackers (2 servings) with 1 serving of any of the soups (pages 216–232).

Lemon Pepper Thins

Makes about 32 crackers

These crackers are zesty and slightly spicy, thanks to the cracked black pepper. They pair perfectly with a dip such as Guacamole (page 212) or Chili Dilly Eggplant (page 211).

Tips

Spread batter to an even thickness, right to the edges of the pan; this ensures that the center is cooked before the edges become too dark.

Watch these carefully during baking — even as little as 1 minute too long can cause edges to burn.

Store in an airtight container at room temperature for up to 3 weeks.

If difficult to remove from the pan, place in a 300°F (150°C) oven for 2 to 3 minutes and remove immediately.

- **Preheat oven to 300°F (150°C)**
- **15- by 10-inch (40 by 25 cm) rimmed baking sheet, lightly greased**

1/2 cup	water	125 mL
2 tbsp	grated lemon zest	30 mL
1/4 cup	freshly squeezed lemon juice	60 mL
1 tbsp	vegetable oil	15 mL
3/4 cup	amaranth flour	175 mL
1/2 tsp	baking soda	2 mL
1/2 tsp	freshly cracked black pepper	2 mL
1/4 tsp	salt	1 mL

1. In a small bowl, whisk together water, lemon zest, lemon juice and oil. Set aside.
2. In a food processor, pulse amaranth flour, baking soda, pepper and salt until combined. With the motor running, through the feed tube, gradually add water mixture in a steady stream. Process for 30 seconds or until smooth and lump-free.
3. Drop dough by heaping spoonfuls onto prepared pan. Spread evenly right to the edges with a moist rubber spatula.
4. Bake on top rack of preheated oven for 15 to 20 minutes or until golden brown. (Watch carefully, as it browns and burns quickly.) Turn off oven and let cool in the oven for 1 hour. Remove from oven and break into pieces.

Snack Idea: Enjoy 5 or 6 crackers with 1/4 cup (60 mL) Greek White Bean Spread (variation, page 208) and 1/2 cup (125 mL) cherry tomatoes.

NUTRIENTS
PER 1/16 RECIPE

Calories	30
Fat	1 g
Carbohydrate	4 g
Fiber	1 g
Protein	1 g
Iron	1.0 mg
Calcium	9 mg

Spicy Black Bean Dip

Makes about 3 cups (750 mL)

Black beans, cumin and garlic make a dynamite combination. This recipe is a perfect appetizer on a hot summer day.

Tips

There are soy- and rice-based alternatives to Monterey Jack cheese, both fortified with calcium. Choose the one that's appropriate for you.

For this quantity of beans, soak, cook and drain 1 cup (250 mL) dried black beans or drain and rinse 1 can (14 to 19 oz/398 to 540 mL) black beans.

This recipe can be partially prepared up to 2 days ahead. Complete step 1, cover and refrigerate. When you're ready to cook, continue with step 2.

Black beans are an excellent source of fiber, protein, folate and iron. The cheese provides calcium.

- **Small to medium (1½- to 3½-quart) slow cooker**
- **Food processor**

1	small red or sweet onion, coarsely chopped	1
2	cloves garlic, chopped	2
1 to 2	canned chipotle pepper(s) in adobo sauce	1 to 2
2 cups	cooked black beans (see tip, at left)	500 mL
2 tsp	ground cumin	10 mL
1 tsp	finely grated lime zest	5 mL
1 tsp	salt	5 mL
½ tsp	cracked black peppercorns	2 mL
2 cups	shredded Monterey Jack cheese or non-dairy alternative (about 8 oz/250 g)	500 mL
	Finely chopped cilantro	

1. In a food processor, combine onion, garlic and chipotle pepper. Process until finely chopped. Add beans, cumin, lime zest, salt and peppercorns and process until desired consistency is achieved.

2. Transfer to slow cooker stoneware. Stir in cheese. Cover and cook on High for 1 hour. Stir well. Cover and cook on High for 30 minutes, until mixture is hot and bubbly. Garnish with cilantro. Serve immediately or set temperature at Warm until ready to serve.

> **Appetizer Idea:** This dip pairs well with slices of refreshing cucumber or zucchini.

NUTRIENTS
PER 2 TBSP (30 ML)

Calories	60
Fat	3 g
Carbohydrates	4 g
Fiber	1 g
Protein	3 g
Iron	0.4 mg
Calcium	77 mg

Italian White Bean Spread

Makes about 2 cups (500 mL)

Growing your own herbs is easy. This recipe combines fresh parsley and basil with garlic and sun-dried tomatoes for a flavorful sandwich spread or dip.

Tips

This spread can be made up to 3 days ahead.

If you have a sulfite sensitivity, ensure that the sun-dried tomatoes have no added sulfites.

Variation

Greek White Bean Spread: Instead of fresh basil, increase chopped parsley to 2 tbsp (30 mL) and add ½ tsp (2 mL) dried oregano to the onions when cooking.

- **Food processor**

2 tbsp	olive oil	30 mL
1	small onion, finely chopped	1
2	large cloves garlic, finely chopped	2
1 tbsp	red wine vinegar	15 mL
1	can (19 oz/540 mL) white kidney beans, drained and rinsed	1
2 tbsp	finely chopped oil-packed sun-dried tomatoes	30 mL
1 tbsp	chopped fresh parsley	15 mL
1 tbsp	chopped fresh basil	15 mL
	Freshly ground black pepper	

1. In a small skillet, heat oil over medium heat. Cook onion and garlic, stirring occasionally, for 3 minutes or until softened (do not brown). Add vinegar and remove from heat.
2. In food processor, purée kidney beans and onion mixture until smooth.
3. Transfer to a bowl. Stir in sun-dried tomatoes, parsley and basil; season with pepper to taste. Cover and refrigerate.

Snack Idea: Serve ¼ cup (60 mL) of this dip (or the Greek variation) with ½ cup (125 mL) baby carrots and 5 or 6 Crispy Multi-Seed Crackers (page 204).

NUTRIENTS
PER 2 TBSP (30 ML)

Calories	35
Fat	2 g
Carbohydrates	4 g
Fiber	1 g
Protein	1 g
Iron	0.4 mg
Calcium	13 mg

Santorini-Style Fava Spread

Makes about 2 cups (500 mL)

This recipe is a great example of the Mediterranean-style diet: legumes, olive oil and dried and fresh herbs. It's great spread on sandwiches or as a dip with sliced vegetables.

Tips

Parsley is an excellent source of antioxidants, vitamin C and vitamin K — an often overlooked nutrient that's important for bone building.

If you are sensitive to sulfites, ensure that the sun-dried tomatoes have no added sulfites and replace the red wine vinegar with white vinegar.

This recipe can be partially prepared up to 2 days ahead. Complete step 1, let cool, cover and refrigerate. When you're ready to cook, heat peas on the stovetop until bubbles form around the edges. Continue with step 2.

NUTRIENTS
PER 2 TBSP (30 ML)

Calories	70
Fat	5 g
Carbohydrates	5 g
Fiber	2 g
Protein	2 g
Iron	4.4 mg
Calcium	8 mg

- **Small (1½- to 2-quart) slow cooker**
- **Food processor**

½ cup	extra virgin olive oil, divided	125 mL
½ cup	diced shallots (about 2 large)	125 mL
2 tsp	dried oregano	10 mL
1 tsp	salt	5 mL
½ tsp	cracked black peppercorns	2 mL
1 cup	yellow split peas	250 mL
4 cups	water	1 L
6	oil-packed sun-dried tomato halves, drained and coarsely chopped	6
4	cloves garlic, chopped	4
¼ cup	coarsely chopped fresh flat-leaf (Italian) parsley (see tip, at left)	60 mL
4	fresh basil leaves, hand-torn	4
3 tbsp	red wine vinegar	45 mL
	Salt and freshly ground black pepper	

1. In a skillet, heat 1 tbsp (15 mL) of the oil over medium heat. Add shallots and cook, stirring, until softened, about 3 minutes. Add oregano, salt and peppercorns and cook, stirring, for 1 minute. Add split peas and cook, stirring, until coated. Add water and bring to a boil. Boil for 2 minutes.

2. Transfer to slow cooker stoneware. Cover and cook on Low for 8 hours or on High for 4 hours, until peas have virtually disintegrated. Drain off excess water, if necessary. Transfer solids to a food processor. Add sun-dried tomatoes, garlic, parsley, basil and red wine vinegar. Pulse 7 or 8 times to chop and blend ingredients. With motor running, add the remaining olive oil in a steady stream through the feed tube. Season to taste with additional salt and pepper and drizzle with additional olive oil, if desired.

Lunch Idea: Spread 2 tbsp (30 mL) of this spread on 1 slice of bread (page 196 or 197) and enjoy with 1 serving of Lentil and Spinach Soup (page 225) or Suppertime Lentil Soup (page 226).

Spicy Hummus

This version of hummus is great for anyone with a sesame allergy, as it does not include tahini. Plus, it's an excellent source of vitamin B$_6$, folate, manganese and magnesium, and a good source of dietary fiber.

Tips

If the hummus is too thick for your taste, blend in a little water.

Hummus will keep for up to 1 week in the refrigerator.

Serve hummus in a hollowed-out red pepper for a nice presentation when entertaining.

- **Blender or food processor**

1	can (19 oz/540 mL) chickpeas, drained and rinsed (about 2 cups/500 mL)	1
2	cloves garlic	2
$\frac{1}{4}$ tsp	ground cumin	1 mL
$\frac{1}{4}$ tsp	ground coriander	1 mL
$\frac{1}{4}$ tsp	hot pepper sauce	1 mL
1 tbsp	freshly squeezed lemon juice	15 mL

1. In blender, on medium speed, blend chickpeas, garlic, cumin, coriander and hot pepper sauce for 30 seconds or until finely chopped. Add lemon juice and blend until smooth.

This recipe courtesy of Catha McMaster.

> **Snack Idea:** Serve this hummus with celery sticks and strips of Focaccia (page 199).

NUTRIENTS PER SERVING

Calories 70
Fat . . . . .1 g
Carbohydrate. . . . . .12 g
Fiber . . . . .3 g
Protein. . . . . .3 g
Iron . . . . .0.8 mg
Calcium . . . . 16 mg

Chilly Dilly Eggplant

This recipe makes a great starter to any meal. Eggplant is a nightshade vegetable, related to tomatoes and potatoes, and is a great source of cholesterol-lowering soluble fiber. When cooked, it develops a rich, complex flavor.

Tips

To sweat eggplant: Place cubed eggplant in a colander, sprinkle liberally with salt, toss well and set aside for 30 minutes to 1 hour. If time is short, blanch the pieces for a minute or two in heavily salted water. In either case, rinse thoroughly in fresh cold water and, using your hands, squeeze out the excess moisture. Pat dry with paper towels and it's ready to cook.

You'll achieve maximum results if you make this a day ahead and chill thoroughly before serving, or cook overnight, purée in the morning and chill.

NUTRIENTS
PER 2 TBSP (30 ML)

Calories	20
Fat	1 g
Carbohydrate	2 g
Fiber	1 g
Protein	1 g
Iron	0.0 mg
Calcium	0 mg

- **Small to medium (1½- to 3½-quart) slow cooker**
- **Blender or food processor**

2	eggplants, peeled, cut into 1-inch (2.5 cm) cubes and drained of excess moisture (see tip, at left)	2
2 to 3 tbsp	olive oil	30 to 45 mL
2	onions, chopped	2
4	cloves garlic, chopped	4
1 tsp	dried oregano	5 mL
1 tsp	salt	5 mL
½ tsp	freshly ground black pepper	2 mL
1 tbsp	balsamic or red wine vinegar	15 mL
½ cup	chopped fresh dill	125 mL
	Dill sprigs (optional)	
	Finely chopped black olives (optional)	

1. In a skillet, heat 2 tbsp (30 mL) oil over medium-high heat. Add eggplant, in batches, and cook, stirring and tossing, until it begins to brown, about 3 minutes per batch, adding more oil, if necessary. Transfer to slow cooker stoneware.

2. In same pan, using more oil, if necessary, cook onions over medium heat, stirring, until softened, about 3 minutes. Add garlic, oregano, salt and pepper and cook for 1 minute. Transfer to slow cooker and stir to combine thoroughly. Cover and cook on Low for 7 to 8 hours or on High for 4 hours, until vegetables are tender.

3. Transfer contents of slow cooker (in batches, if necessary) to blender. Add vinegar and dill and process until smooth, scraping down sides of bowl at halfway point. Taste for seasoning and adjust. Spoon into a small serving bowl and chill thoroughly. Garnish with sprigs of dill and chopped black olives (if using).

Snack Idea: Top 1 slice of bread (page 196 or 197) with 1 tbsp (15 mL) Santorini-Style Fava Spread (page 209) and 1 to 2 tbsp (15 to 30 mL) Chilly Dilly Eggplant.

Guacamole

Guacamole is traditionally paired with corn tortilla chips, but you can replace them with rice chips or baked lentil chips. Try making this quick, easy recipe at your next impromptu gathering.

Tip

Avocados are rich in heart-healthy fats, folate and vitamins E and K, and are a good source of fiber. But limit the serving size to $1/4$ to $1/2$ an avocado to keep calories in check.

2	Hass avocados, peeled and pitted	2
1	tomato, seeded and diced	1
$1/3$ cup	coarsely chopped fresh cilantro	75 mL
2	green onions, sliced	2
1 to 2 tbsp	minced seeded jalapeño peppers	15 to 30 mL
1 tbsp	freshly squeezed lime juice	15 mL
	Salt	
	Tortilla chips	

1. In a bowl, mash avocados with a fork. Stir in tomato, cilantro, green onions, jalapeño pepper and lime juice. Season with salt to taste.

2. Place in a serving dish and accompany with tortilla chips.

NUTRIENTS
PER SERVING

Calories 110
Fat . . . . .10 g
Carbohydrate . . . . .7 g
Fiber . . . . .5 g
Protein . . . . .2 g
Iron . . . . .0.7 mg
Calcium . . . . 12 mg

Ratatouille Salsa

Makes about 2½ cups (625 mL)

This recipe takes your favorite salsa up a notch, turning it into a versatile, satisfying snack. Serve it with corn tortilla chips, rice chips or baked lentil chips, spread it on sandwiches or use it as a pizza topping.

Tips

Some brands of salsa contain soybean oil. If you have allergy to soy, read the ingredient list carefully.

Dice vegetables into ¼-inch (3 mm) pieces.

Prepare ratatouille salsa ahead. It keeps well in an airtight container in the refrigerator for 3 days or 1 month in the freezer.

This recipe is a good source of vitamin A, and an excellent source of vitamin C and bone-building vitamin K.

- **Preheat oven to 425°F (220°C)**
- **Rimmed baking sheet, greased**

1½ cups	diced eggplant	375 mL
1½ cups	diced zucchini	375 mL
1	red bell pepper, finely chopped	1
1 tsp	dried basil	5 mL
1 tbsp	olive oil	15 mL
1½ cups	medium salsa	375 mL
¼ cup	chopped fresh parsley	60 mL
1	clove garlic, minced	1

1. Spread eggplant, zucchini and red pepper on prepared baking sheet. Sprinkle with basil; drizzle with oil. Roast in preheated oven, stirring occasionally, for about 20 minutes or until vegetables are tender and lightly colored.
2. Transfer to a bowl and stir in salsa, parsley and garlic. Cover and refrigerate.

Lunch Idea: Top a pizza crust (pages 200–202) with ½ cup (125 mL) Ratatouille Salsa and ¼ to ½ cup (60 to 125 mL) shredded part-skim mozzarella cheese or a non-dairy alternative.

NUTRIENTS
PER 2 TBSP (30 ML)

Calories 15
Fat .1 g
Carbohydrate. . . . . .3 g
Fiber . . . . .1 g
Protein. . . . . .1 g
Iron . . . . .0.5 mg
Calcium . . . . 13 mg

Pineapple Salsa

Makes about 1½ cups (375 mL)

Here's a great way to jazz up your favorite store-bought salsa. Serve with Guacamole (page 212) and Lemon Pepper Thins (page 206) or Crispy Multi-Seed Crackers (page 204).

Tips

This recipe is an excellent source of vitamin C and the antioxidant lycopene.

Store in an airtight container in the refrigerator for up to 3 days.

Variation

Peach Salsa: Substitute fresh or canned peaches for the pineapple, and mint for the cilantro.

1 cup	tomato salsa	250 mL
1 cup	diced fresh or drained canned pineapple	250 mL
¼ to ½ cup	chopped fresh cilantro	60 to 125 mL

1. In a medium bowl, combine salsa, pineapple and cilantro. Serve immediately or cover and refrigerate until ready to use.

This recipe courtesy of Eileen Campbell.

Lunch Idea: Top a pizza crust (pages 200–202) with ½ cup (125 mL) Pineapple Salsa, 3 to 4 oz (90 to 125 g) diced cooked ham and ¼ to ½ cup (60 to 125 mL) shredded part-skim mozzarella cheese or a non-dairy alternative.

NUTRIENTS
PER ¼ CUP (60 ML)

Calories	24
Fat	0 g
Carbohydrate	6 g
Fiber	1 g
Protein	1 g
Iron	0.3 mg
Calcium	16 mg

Soups and Salads

Creamy Onion Soup with Kale

Makes 6 servings

The creaminess of this healthy, rich-tasting soup is created by the potatoes, which are puréed into the soup. Kale, along with other dark leafy greens, is a good source of non-dairy calcium, and soup recipes are a great way to introduce these greens into your diet.

Tips

You can use any kind of paprika in this recipe: regular, or sweet; hot, which produces a nicely peppery version; or smoked, which adds a delicious note of smokiness to the soup. If you have regular paprika and would like a bit of heat, dissolve ¼ tsp (1 mL) cayenne pepper in the lemon juice along with the paprika.

This recipe can be partially prepared up to 2 days ahead. Complete step 1, let cool, cover and refrigerate. When you're ready to cook, continue with step 2.

NUTRIENTS
PER SERVING

Calories	130
Fat	3 g
Carbohydrate	25 g
Fiber	4 g
Protein	3 g
Iron	1.4 mg
Calcium	103 mg

- **Medium to large (3½- to 5-quart) slow cooker**
- **Immersion blender, food processor or blender**

1 tbsp	olive oil	15 mL
4	onions, thinly sliced	4
2	cloves garlic, minced	2
4	whole allspice	4
1	bay leaf	1
1 tsp	grated lemon zest	5 mL
½ tsp	cracked black peppercorns	2 mL
4 cups	ready-to-use vegetable broth	1 L
3	potatoes, peeled and diced	3
1 tsp	paprika dissolved in 2 tbsp (30 mL) freshly squeezed lemon juice (see tip, at left)	5 mL
4 cups	chopped kale	1 L

1. In a skillet, heat oil over medium heat. Add onions and cook, stirring, until softened, about 5 minutes. Add garlic, allspice, bay leaf, lemon zest and peppercorns and cook, stirring, for 1 minute. Transfer to slow cooker stoneware. Stir in broth.

2. Add potatoes and stir well. Cover and cook on Low for 8 hours or on High for 4 hours, until potatoes are tender. Discard allspice and bay leaf. Stir in paprika solution and add kale, in batches, stirring after each to submerge the leaves in the liquid. Cover and cook on High for 20 minutes, until kale is tender.

3. Purée using an immersion blender. (You can also do this in batches in a food processor or blender.) Serve immediately.

Lunch Idea: Enjoy 1 serving of this soup with a white dinner roll.

Fresh Minted Pea Soup

This refreshing, flavorful soup can be enjoyed hot or chilled — perfect for a hot summer day. Peas are a great source of vitamin C and B vitamins (including folate), and a good source of fiber, vitamin K and calcium.

Tips

Bouquet garni is a French term for a bundle of seasonings that are usually wrapped in cheesecloth and tied with kitchen string. For this recipe, try three sprigs of fresh thyme or ½ tsp (2 mL) dried thyme, 4 parsley stems and 1 bay leaf.

If you are not using an immersion blender and time permits, allow the soup to cool before puréeing. Use caution as you blend hot soup, particularly if using a blender. Fill the blender container only half-full to avoid the buildup of steam, which can cause the lid to pop off.

NUTRIENTS PER SERVING

Calories 160
Fat .6 g
Carbohydrate . . . . .24 g
Fiber . . . . .4 g
Protein . . . . .4 g
Iron . . . . .1.8 mg
Calcium . . . . 156 mg

• **Food processor, blender or immersion blender**

3 tbsp	vegetable oil	45 mL
2	leeks (white and light green parts only), thinly sliced (see tip, page 218)	2
2	shallots, finely chopped (about 3 tbsp/45 mL)	2
2	carrots, peeled and chopped	2
1 lb	frozen green peas	500 mL
3 cups	ready-to-use vegetable broth	750 mL
3 cups	enriched plain rice milk or soy milk	750 mL
1	bouquet garni (see tip, at left)	1
1 tsp	dried mint (or 1 tbsp/15 mL chopped fresh)	5 mL
¼ cup	coarsely chopped fresh Italian parsley	60 mL
2 tbsp	freshly squeezed lemon juice	30 mL
½ tsp	granulated natural cane sugar (optional)	2 mL
	Salt and freshly ground black pepper	

1. In a large pot, heat oil over medium heat for 30 seconds. Add leeks and cook, stirring, for 3 minutes or until softened. Add shallots and carrots and cook, stirring, for 3 minutes or until fragrant.

2. Stir in peas, broth, rice milk, bouquet garni and mint and bring to a boil. Reduce heat and simmer, uncovered, for 10 minutes or until peas are tender and flavor develops. Discard bouquet garni. Add parsley and let stand for 1 minute.

3. In food processor, or using an immersion blender, purée soup, in batches if necessary, until smooth or desired texture is achieved (see tip, at left). If necessary, return soup to pot and reheat until steaming.

4. Stir in lemon juice and sugar (if using). Season with salt and pepper to taste. Serve hot. If you prefer a cold soup, transfer to a bowl, cover and refrigerate for 2 to 3 hours or until thoroughly chilled.

Lunch Idea: Enjoy 1 serving of this soup with ½ of a gluten-free wrap filled with 3 oz (90 g) grilled chicken breast and 1 cup (250 mL) vegetables, such as sliced cucumber or yellow bell pepper.

Leek, Potato and Cabbage Soup

This satisfying soup is a meal in itself — a perfect choice for lunch or dinner. It's an excellent source of vitamins C and K, and a good source of B vitamins and trace minerals. To reduce the amount of fat and calories, try using turkey sausage free of gluten and/ or soy.

Tips

To clean leeks: Trim dark green tops. Cut down center almost to root end and chop. Rinse in a sink full of cold water to remove sand; scoop up leeks and place in colander to drain or use a salad spinner.

Store soup in an airtight container in the refrigerator for up to 5 days.

Make sure the sausage you choose is free of gluten and/ or soy.

2 tbsp	olive oil	30 mL
2	leeks (white and light green parts only), chopped (see tip, at left)	2
2	cloves garlic, finely chopped	2
1/4 tsp	freshly ground black pepper	1 mL
1/4 tsp	caraway seeds (optional)	1 mL
3	potatoes, such as Yukon gold, peeled and cut into 1/2-inch (1 cm) cubes	3
4 cups	finely shredded green cabbage	1 L
6 cups	ready-to-use beef broth	1.5 L
8 oz	kielbasa or other cooked smoked sausage, cut into 1/2-inch (1 cm) cubes	250 g
1/4 cup	chopped fresh parsley	60 mL

1. In a large saucepan, heat oil over medium heat. Add leeks, garlic, pepper and caraway seeds (if using); cook, stirring, for 4 minutes or until softened.

2. Stir in potatoes, cabbage and broth. Bring to a boil; reduce heat to medium-low and simmer, covered, for 20 minutes or until vegetables are tender.

3. Add sausage and parsley; cook 5 minutes more or until sausage is heated through.

NUTRIENTS PER SERVING

Calories	210
Fat	12 g
Carbohydrate	17 g
Fiber	2 g
Protein	10 g
Iron	1.4 mg
Calcium	40 mg

Vegetable Gumbo

Makes 6 to 8 servings

This vegetarian meal is prepared in the slow cooker, which means it's ready when you get home. Okra is a great source of cholesterol-lowering soluble fiber, and a good source of B vitamins (including folate), vitamin C and vitamin K.

Tips

This quantity of rice, combined with the okra, produces a dense soup, which condenses even more when refrigerated overnight. If you prefer a more soup-like consistency, add an additional cup (250 mL) of broth.

Brown rice is the most nutritious form of the grain, but you may substitute an equal quantity of white rice, if you prefer.

Okra is a great thickener for broths but be sure not to overcook it because it will become unpleasantly sticky.

NUTRIENTS PER SERVING

Calories 160
Fat .3 g
Carbohydrate . . . . .30 g
Fiber . . . . .6 g
Protein . . . . .4 g
Iron . . . . .1.9 mg
Calcium . . . . 116 mg

- **Medium to large (3½- to 5-quart) slow cooker**

1 tbsp	olive oil	15 mL
2	onions, finely chopped	2
6	stalks celery, diced	6
4	cloves garlic, minced	4
2 tsp	dried thyme, crumbled	10 mL
½ tsp	cracked black peppercorns	2 mL
1	bay leaf	1
1	can (28 oz/796 mL) diced tomatoes, with juice	1
½ cup	brown rice (see tips, at left)	125 mL
4 cups	ready-to-use vegetable broth	1 L
2 tsp	paprika, dissolved in 4 tsp (20 mL) freshly squeezed lemon juice	10 mL
	Salt (optional)	
2 cups	sliced okra (¼-inch/3 mm slices)	500 mL
1	green bell pepper, finely chopped	1

1. In a skillet, heat oil over medium heat. Add onions and celery and cook, stirring, until softened, about 5 minutes. Add garlic, thyme, peppercorns and bay leaf and cook, stirring, for 1 minute. Add tomatoes with juice and bring to a boil. Transfer to slow cooker stoneware.

2. Add brown rice and broth. Cover and cook on Low for 6 hours or on High for 3 hours, until rice is tender. Discard bay leaf. Add paprika solution and stir well. Season to taste with salt (if using). Stir in okra and green pepper. Cover and cook on High for 20 minutes, until pepper is tender.

Yellow Tomato Gazpacho with Cilantro Oil

Makes 6 servings

This chilled soup shines when tomatoes are in season. Tomatoes are high in lycopene, a cancer-fighting antioxidant, and this recipe is also an excellent source of vitamin C and a good source of vitamin A.

Tips

If yellow tomatoes are not available, red ones work just as well.

If you are sensitive to sulfites, replace the sherry vinegar with white vinegar.

• **Food processor or blender**

1	yellow bell pepper, chopped	1
½	English cucumber, peeled, seeded and chopped	½
1½ lbs	yellow tomatoes (about 5 medium), chopped	750 g
½ cup	chopped sweet onion (such as Vidalia)	125 mL
1 tsp	minced garlic	5 mL
2 tbsp	sherry vinegar	30 mL
	Salt and freshly ground black pepper	
	Cilantro Oil (see recipe, opposite)	

1. In food processor, in batches if necessary, process yellow pepper, cucumber, tomatoes, onion and garlic until almost smooth. Transfer to a bowl and stir in vinegar. Season to taste with salt and pepper. Cover and refrigerate until cold, about 3 hours. Taste and adjust seasoning with vinegar, salt and pepper, if necessary.

2. Ladle into chilled bowls and drizzle with Cilantro Oil.

Lunch Idea: Enjoy 1 serving of this soup as an appetizer, followed by 1 serving of Millet Salad with Lemony Chickpeas and Tomatoes (page 239) or Quinoa Salad (page 238).

NUTRIENTS
PER SERVING

Calories	60
Fat	0 g
Carbohydrate	11 g
Fiber	3 g
Protein	2 g
Iron	0.9 mg
Calcium	48 mg

Cilantro Oil

Cilantro provides a good source of bone-building vitamin K and many health-promoting antioxidants.

Tip

Store in an airtight container in the refrigerator for up to 3 days.

- **Blender**

2 cups	packed fresh cilantro leaves	500 mL
1/2 cup	olive oil	125 mL
1/2 cup	vegetable oil	125 mL

1. Bring a large saucepan of water to a boil. Add cilantro and blanch for 5 seconds. Drain and immediately plunge into a bowl of ice water. Drain well and squeeze out all liquid.

2. In blender, purée cilantro, olive oil and vegetable oil until smooth. Strain through several layers of cheesecloth or a paper coffee filter into a squeeze bottle, discarding solids.

NUTRIENTS
PER 1 TBSP (15 ML)

Calories 130
Fat . . . . .15 g
Carbohydrates . . . . .0 g
Fiber . . . . .0 g
Protein . . . . .0 g
Iron . . . . .0.0 mg
Calcium . . . . 0 mg

Vegetarian Harira

This vegetarian version of harira, fragrant with ginger, cinnamon, cumin and turmeric, makes a great starter to a Moroccan-themed dinner.

Tips

Tomatoes are high in vitamin C, which helps enhance the absorption of the iron found in the lentils and chickpeas.

This recipe is a good source of protein, iron and trace minerals.

3 tbsp	olive oil	45 mL
2	onions, chopped	2
2	cloves garlic, minced	2
1 tsp	ground cumin	5 mL
1/2 tsp	ground cinnamon	2 mL
1/4 tsp	ground ginger	1 mL
1/4 tsp	ground turmeric	1 mL
1	can (28 oz/796 mL) crushed tomatoes	1
8 cups	ready-to-use vegetable broth	2 L
1 cup	dried brown or green lentils, rinsed	250 mL
1 tsp	salt	5 mL
1/4 tsp	freshly ground black pepper	1 mL
2	potatoes, peeled and diced	2
1	can (14 to 19 oz/398 to 540 mL) chickpeas, drained and rinsed	1
3 tbsp	chopped fresh cilantro	45 mL
1	lemon, cut into wedges	1

1. In a large pot, heat oil over medium heat. Add onions and sauté until starting to brown, about 10 minutes. Add garlic, cumin, cinnamon, ginger and turmeric; sauté for 1 minute.

2. Add tomatoes, broth, lentils, salt and pepper; bring to a boil. Reduce heat and simmer for 25 minutes. Add potatoes and simmer for 10 minutes. Add chickpeas and simmer until potatoes and lentils are tender, about 10 minutes.

3. Ladle into heated bowls and garnish with cilantro and lemon wedges. Diners may squeeze the lemon over their soup, if they desire.

Dinner Idea: Serve this soup as a starter, followed by Lamb Tagine with Chickpeas and Apricots (page 278).

NUTRIENTS PER SERVING

Calories	220
Fat	7 g
Carbohydrate	33 g
Fiber	9 g
Protein	9 g
Iron	3.6 mg
Calcium	83 mg

Soup à la Mom

*This healthy soup is a true
delight! If you are pressed for
time, use frozen cut veggies.*

Tips

A 19-oz (540 mL) can of
chickpeas will yield about 2 cups
(500 mL) once the chickpeas are
drained and rinsed. If you have
smaller or larger cans, you can
use the volume called for or just
add the amount from your can.

The longer this soup simmers, the
better it tastes.

This soup freezes well. Let cool,
divide into individual portions and
freeze in airtight containers for up
to 1 month.

This soup is an excellent source
of fiber and vitamins A, C and K.
It is also a good source of protein,
iron, calcium and trace minerals
manganese and magnesium.

NUTRIENTS
PER SERVING

Calories	160
Fat	4 g
Carbohydrate	25 g
Fiber	7 g
Protein	8 g
Iron	2.1 mg
Calcium	56 mg

2 tbsp	grapeseed oil	30 mL
3	green onions, chopped	3
3 tbsp	chopped fresh parsley	45 mL
2	carrots, chopped	2
2	stalks celery, chopped	2
1	zucchini, chopped	1
2 cups	rinsed drained canned chickpeas (see tip, at left)	500 mL
2 cups	frozen peas	500 mL
2 cups	frozen chopped green beans	500 mL
2 cups	frozen lima or butter beans	500 mL
4 cups	ready-to-use reduced-sodium gluten-free chicken broth	1 L
1/4 cup	tomato sauce (or 1 tomato, chopped)	60 mL
1/4 tsp	salt	1 mL
1/4 tsp	freshly ground black pepper	1 mL

1. In a large pot, heat oil over medium heat. Sauté green onions and parsley for about 3 minutes or until onions are softened.

2. Stir in carrots, celery, zucchini, chickpeas, peas, green beans, lima beans, broth, 4 cups (1 L) water, tomato sauce, salt and pepper. Cover, leaving lid ajar, reduce heat to low and simmer, stirring occasionally, for 30 minutes or until vegetables are tender (or for up to 1 hour if you prefer a very soft texture).

Lunch Idea: Serve this soup with 1 serving of Focaccia (page 199).

Dinner Idea: Serve this soup as a starter, followed by Spanish Chicken and Rice (page 259).

Chard-Studded Root Vegetable and Lentil Soup

Makes 6 servings

Dark leafy greens provide great health benefits, but patients often tell me they don't know how to cook them. Here's one terrific answer.

Tips

To shred Swiss chard, remove the stems, including the thick vein that runs up the bottom of the leaf, and thoroughly wash the leaves by swishing them around in a basin full of warm water; drain well. On a cutting board, stack the leaves two or three at a time. Roll them into a cigar shape and slice as thinly as you can.

If you want to save the time of washing and cutting chard, look for frozen chopped chard.

One cup (250 mL) of Swiss chard provides almost one-third of your daily intake of calcium. It is also an excellent source of vitamins A, K and C.

NUTRIENTS PER SERVING

Calories	210
Fat	3 g
Carbohydrate	38 g
Fiber	9 g
Protein	9 g
Iron	2.9 mg
Calcium	76 mg

- Medium to large (4- to 5-quart) slow cooker

1 tbsp	olive oil	15 mL
2	onions, finely chopped	2
4	carrots, peeled and diced	4
2	stalks celery, diced	2
4	cloves garlic, minced	4
1 tsp	salt	5 mL
½ tsp	cracked black peppercorns	2 mL
1	bay leaf	1
1 cup	green or brown lentils, rinsed	250 mL
6 cups	ready-to-use vegetable broth	1.5 L
1	potato, peeled and shredded	1
¼ tsp	cayenne pepper, dissolved in 1 tbsp (15 mL) freshly squeezed lemon juice	1 mL
4 cups	packed shredded Swiss chard (see tip, at left)	1 L

1. In a skillet, heat oil over medium heat. Add onions, carrots and celery and cook, stirring, until softened, about 7 minutes. Add garlic, salt, peppercorns and bay leaf and cook, stirring, for 1 minute. Add lentils and toss until coated. Transfer to slow cooker stoneware. Stir in broth.

2. Add potato and stir well. Cover and cook on Low for 6 hours or on High for 3 hours, until lentils are tender. Add cayenne solution and stir well.

3. Add chard, in batches, stirring after each to submerge before adding the next batch. Cover and cook on High for 20 minutes, until chard is tender.

Lunch Idea: For a light meal, serve this soup with a salad of tossed greens.

Lentil and Spinach Soup

Makes 4 servings

This nutritious, tasty soup is very easy to make and is an excellent source of vitamins A, C and K, folate, protein and fiber.

Tips

A 19-oz (540 mL) can of lentils will yield about 2 cups (500 mL) once the lentils are drained and rinsed. If you have smaller or larger cans, you can use the volume called for or just add the amount from your can.

Look for bags of spinach that have been frozen in small cubes rather than in a large block. You can measure the cubes and add them to the pot without thawing them. If you can't find them, use ½ cup (125 mL) drained thawed chopped spinach.

Cooked spinach has a higher amount of bioavailable iron than raw spinach.

2 tbsp	olive oil	30 mL
2	cloves garlic, minced	2
¼ cup	chopped onion	60 mL
¼ cup	chopped celery	60 mL
½ cup	chopped carrots	125 mL
2 cups	rinsed drained canned lentils (see tip, at left)	500 mL
1 cup	frozen spinach cubes	250 mL
4 cups	ready-to-use reduced-sodium gluten-free chicken or vegetable broth	1 L
	Salt and freshly ground black pepper	

1. In a large saucepan, heat oil over medium heat. Sauté garlic, onion, celery and carrots for 3 to 4 minutes or until softened.

2. Stir in lentils, spinach and broth; bring to a boil over high heat. Cover, leaving lid ajar, reduce heat to low and simmer, stirring occasionally, for 30 minutes or until vegetables are tender (or for up to 1 hour if you prefer a very soft texture). Season to taste with salt and pepper.

Lunch Idea: Serve this soup with 1 slice of bread (page 196 or 197) topped with 1 serving of Ratatouille Salsa (page 213).

NUTRIENTS PER SERVING

Calories	220
Fat	8 g
Carbohydrate	26 g
Fiber	10 g
Protein	13 g
Iron	4.5 mg
Calcium	81 mg

Suppertime Lentil Soup

Makes 6 servings

Here's a fast, easy and healthy soup that makes a satisfying meal on its own. Lentils cook faster than beans and are equally nutritious.

Tips

To save time, chop the mushrooms, onions, carrots and celery in batches in the food processor. If you have any leftover baked ham, chop it and add to the soup along with the broth.

This soup is an excellent source of vitamin A, fiber and iron, and a good source of calcium, B vitamins (including folate), vitamin K, magnesium, manganese, phosphorus, potassium and selenium.

Variation

Lentil-Rice Soup: Use ⅔ cup (150 mL) lentils and ⅓ cup (75 mL) long-grain white or brown rice instead of 1 cup (250 mL) lentils.

8 cups	ready-to-use chicken or vegetable broth	2 L
1 cup	green lentils, rinsed and sorted	250 mL
8 oz	mushrooms, chopped	250 g
3	carrots, peeled and chopped	3
2	stalks celery, including leaves, chopped	2
1	large onion, chopped	1
2	cloves garlic, finely chopped	2
1 tsp	dried thyme or marjoram	5 mL
¼ cup	chopped fresh dill or parsley	60 mL
	Salt and freshly ground black pepper	

1. In a large Dutch oven or stockpot, combine broth, lentils, mushrooms, carrots, celery, onion, garlic and thyme.
2. Bring to a boil; reduce heat, cover and simmer 35 to 40 minutes or until lentils are tender. Stir in dill or parsley. Adjust seasoning with salt and pepper to taste.

Lunch Idea: Pair ½ serving of this soup with a sandwich or Quinoa Salad (page 238).

Dinner Idea: This is a generous serving size, so enjoy the soup on its own with 1 serving of Crispy Multi-Seed Crackers (page 204).

NUTRIENTS PER SERVING

Calories	160
Fat	1 g
Carbohydrate	31 g
Fiber	8 g
Protein	9 g
Iron	3.0 mg
Calcium	82 mg

Greek-Style Split Pea Soup

This warming soup has a tangy finish and provides a good amount of vegetarian protein. Split peas are an excellent source of fiber and folate, and a good source of iron.

Tips

Traditional wisdom suggests that yellow split peas do not need to be soaked before cooking. However, without pre-soaking they are likely to be a bit tough, possibly because most are somewhat old by the time they are purchased. The safest strategy is to give them a quick soak as per step 1.

For a smoother result, purée the cooked soup.

This recipe can be partially prepared up to 2 days ahead. Complete steps 1 and 2, let cool, cover and refrigerate. When you're ready to cook, continue with step 3.

NUTRIENTS PER SERVING

Calories	230
Fat	3 g
Carbohydrate	41 g
Fiber	17 g
Protein	11 g
Iron	1.6 mg
Calcium	61 mg

- **Medium to large (4- to 5-quart) slow cooker**

2 cups	yellow split peas (see tip, at left)	500 mL
1 tbsp	olive oil	15 mL
2	onions, finely chopped	2
4	stalks celery, diced	4
4	carrots, peeled and diced	4
4	cloves garlic, minced	4
1 tsp	dried oregano, crumbled	5 mL
½ tsp	cracked black peppercorns	2 mL
6 cups	ready-to-use vegetable broth	1.5 L
	Salt (optional)	

Persillade (Optional)

1 cup	packed fresh parsley, finely chopped	250 mL
4	cloves garlic, minced	4
4 tsp	red wine vinegar	20 mL
	Extra virgin olive oil (optional)	

1. In a large pot, combine split peas and 8 cups (2 L) cold water. Bring to a boil over medium-high heat and boil rapidly for 3 minutes. Turn off heat and set aside for 1 hour. Drain and rinse thoroughly. Set aside.

2. In a skillet, heat oil over medium heat. Add onions, celery and carrots and cook, stirring, until softened, about 7 minutes. Add garlic, oregano and peppercorns and cook, stirring, for 1 minute. Transfer to slow cooker stoneware. Add reserved split peas and broth and stir well.

3. Cover and cook on Low for 8 hours or on High for 4 hours, until peas are tender. Add salt to taste (if using).

4. *Persillade (if using):* In a bowl, combine parsley, garlic and vinegar. (You can also make this in a mini-chopper.) Set aside at room temperature for 30 minutes to allow flavors to develop.

5. To serve, ladle soup into bowls, drizzle with extra virgin olive oil (if using), and garnish with persillade (if using).

> **Lunch or Dinner Idea:** Serve this soup with 3 oz (90 g) lean cooked ham, cut into small pieces.

Cumin-Laced Chickpea Soup with Roasted Red Peppers

Makes 6 to 8 servings

This hearty soup is reminiscent of Middle Eastern cuisine. It delivers a good amount of protein, is an excellent source of fiber and vitamins A, C and B_6, and is a good source of folate, iron and trace minerals.

Tips

For a slightly creamy texture, use an immersion blender for about 30 seconds to coarsely purée the soup. Or scoop out a cup (250 mL) of the soup and purée it in a blender or food processor, then stir it back into the stoneware before serving.

Use 1 cup (250 mL) dried chickpeas, soaked, cooked and drained for this quantity. If you prefer, substitute 1 can (14 to 19 oz/398 to 540 mL) chickpeas, drained and rinsed.

NUTRIENTS PER SERVING

Calories	110
Fat	3 g
Carbohydrate	18 g
Fiber	4 g
Protein	4 g
Iron	1.2 mg
Calcium	45 mg

- **Medium to large (4- to 5-quart) slow cooker**

1 tbsp	olive oil	15 mL
2	onions, finely chopped	2
2	carrots, peeled and diced	2
2	cloves garlic, minced	2
2 tsp	ground cumin	10 mL
1 tsp	salt	5 mL
1 tsp	cracked black peppercorns	5 mL
4 cups	ready-to-use vegetable broth, divided	1 L
2 cups	drained cooked chickpeas (see tip, at left)	500 mL
2	roasted red peppers, finely chopped	2
1 to 2 tbsp	fresh squeezed lemon juice	15 to 30 mL
½ cup	finely chopped fresh parsley	125 mL
	Plain yogurt or non-dairy alternative	

1. In a skillet, heat oil over medium heat. Add onions and carrots and cook, stirring, until softened, about 7 minutes. Add garlic, cumin, salt and peppercorns and cook, stirring, for 1 minute. Add 2 cups (500 mL) of the broth and bring to a boil. Transfer to slow cooker stoneware.

2. Stir in chickpeas and the remaining broth. Cover and cook on Low for 6 hours or on High for 3 hours. Add roasted peppers, lemon juice and parsley and adjust seasoning, if necessary. Cover and cook on High for 5 minutes to meld flavors. To serve, ladle into bowls and top with a dollop of yogurt.

Dinner Idea: Serve this soup as an appetizer before Pork Tenderloin with Rhubarb Chutney (page 271).

White Bean Soup with Pancetta and Sage

Makes 6 to 8 servings

Great Northern beans are high in protein and are an excellent source of fiber and folate. One-half cup (125 mL) of cooked beans provides almost the entire recommended daily intake of folate.

Tips

Pancetta is the Italian version of bacon. If you can't find it, feel free to substitute regular bacon.

To quick-soak dried beans: In a colander, rinse beans under cold water and discard any discolored ones. In a saucepan, combine beans with enough cold water to cover them by 2 inches (5 cm). Bring to a boil over medium heat and boil for 2 minutes. Remove from heat and let soak, covered, for 1 hour.

Canned beans will also work in this recipe.

1 tbsp	olive oil	15 mL
3 oz	pancetta, minced	90 g
8	cloves garlic, chopped	8
1	large onion, chopped	1
½ cup	chopped carrot	125 mL
½ cup	chopped celery	125 mL
1½ cups	dried great Northern beans, soaked overnight or quick-soaked (see tip, at left) and drained	375 mL
1	can (14 oz/398 mL) diced tomatoes, with juice	1
8 cups	ready-to-use chicken broth	2 L
2 tbsp	chopped fresh sage	30 mL
1½ tsp	salt	7 mL
½ tsp	freshly ground black pepper	2 mL
	Extra virgin olive oil	

1. In a large pot, heat oil over medium heat. Add pancetta and sauté until golden brown and crispy, about 5 minutes. Remove with a slotted spoon to a plate lined with paper towels. Set aside.

2. Add garlic, onion, carrot and celery to the pot; sauté until softened, about 6 minutes. Add beans, tomatoes with juice, broth, sage, salt and pepper; bring to a boil. Reduce heat and simmer, stirring occasionally and thinning with hot water if necessary, until beans are tender, about 1½ hours. Taste and adjust seasoning with salt and pepper, if necessary.

3. Ladle into heated bowls, garnish with reserved pancetta and drizzle with olive oil.

Lunch Idea: For a light meal, pair 1 serving of this soup with a salad of tossed greens.

NUTRIENTS PER SERVING

Calories	150
Fat	7 g
Carbohydrate	15 g
Fiber	4 g
Protein	7 g
Iron	1.3 mg
Calcium	61 mg

Minestrone

This filling soup is satisfying to the last spoonful. Enjoy it as a light meal on its own. It delivers a good amount of vegetarian protein, is an excellent source of fiber, vitamin A, folate and vitamin C, and is a good source of iron, calcium and trace minerals.

Variations

Substitute an equal amount of shredded cabbage or cooked green beans for the spinach.

Substitute 6 slices gluten-free bacon, chopped and cooked crisp, or 1 cup (250 mL) diced cooked chicken, beef or turkey for the ham.

Sprinkle with freshly grated Parmesan cheese or a non-dairy alternative.

2 tsp	extra virgin olive oil	10 mL
2	carrots, chopped	2
1	stalk celery, chopped	1
1	clove garlic, minced	1
1	small onion, chopped	1
1	small zucchini, diced	1
1	can (28 oz/796 mL) diced tomatoes, with juice	1
1	can (14 to 19 oz/398 to 540 mL) kidney beans, drained and rinsed	1
1 cup	diced cooked gluten-free ham	250 mL
1 cup	ready-to-use gluten-free chicken or vegetable broth	250 mL
2 tbsp	tomato paste	30 mL
1 cup	packed spinach, trimmed and coarsely chopped	250 mL
1 cup	cooked small gluten-free pasta	250 mL
¼ cup	snipped fresh basil	60 mL
	Salt and freshly ground black pepper	

1. In a large saucepan, heat oil over medium-low heat. Add carrots, celery, garlic and onion; cover and cook, stirring occasionally, for about 20 minutes or until tender but not brown.

2. Add zucchini, tomatoes with juice, beans, ham, broth and tomato paste; bring to a boil over medium-high heat. Reduce heat to low and simmer for 10 minutes or until soup is hot. Stir in spinach, pasta and basil; heat until spinach is wilted. Season to taste with salt and pepper.

Lunch Idea: Enjoy 1 serving of this soup with 1 slice of bread (page 196 or 197).

NUTRIENTS
PER SERVING

Calories	130
Fat	2 g
Carbohydrate	21 g
Fiber	4 g
Protein	7 g
Iron	1.8 mg
Calcium	57 mg

Red Bean and Rice Soup

This New Orleans classic is soul food at its finest and can hold its weight as a stand-alone meal. It provides a good amount of protein, along with fiber, iron, zinc and folate.

Tips

It's important not to salt dried beans at the beginning of the cooking process. Sodium prevents the beans from becoming tender. Add salt during the last half of the cooking process (at least 30 minutes before the beans are done) so they can absorb the flavor. If you wait until the end to season with salt, the soup will only taste salty.

If you have a sulfite sensitivity, omit the sherry.

NUTRIENTS PER SERVING

Calories	230
Fat	6 g
Carbohydrate	28 g
Fiber	6 g
Protein	13 g
Iron	2.6 mg
Calcium	58 mg

3	slices bacon, cut into $\frac{1}{2}$-inch (1 cm) pieces	3
2	cloves garlic, chopped	2
1	onion, finely chopped	1
1½ cups	chopped celery	375 mL
1½ cups	chopped carrots	375 mL
1	small ham hock (about 8 oz/250 g)	1
2 cups	dried red kidney beans, soaked overnight or quick-soaked (see tip, page 229) and drained	500 mL
6 cups	ready-to-use chicken broth (approx.)	1.5 L
1	bay leaf	1
½ tsp	dried oregano	2 mL
½ tsp	dried thyme	2 mL
	Salt	
3 tbsp	dry sherry	45 mL
2 tsp	Louisiana-style hot pepper sauce (such as Tabasco)	10 mL
	Freshly ground black pepper	
2 cups	hot cooked white rice	500 mL
	Chopped green onions	

1. In a large, heavy pot, sauté bacon over medium heat until it renders its fat, about 3 minutes. Add garlic, onion, celery and carrots; sauté until softened, about 6 minutes. Add ham hock, beans, broth, bay leaf, oregano and thyme; bring to a boil. Reduce heat and simmer for 1 hour. Add 1 tsp (5 mL) salt and simmer until beans are tender, about 30 minutes. Discard bay leaf.

2. Remove ham hock from the soup and let cool slightly. Pick the meat from the bone and shred into bite-size pieces. Discard bone, fat and skin. Return meat to the soup and add sherry, hot pepper sauce and salt and pepper to taste. Thin with a little more broth, if necessary, and simmer for 5 minutes, or until hot.

3. Divide rice among heated bowls and top with soup. Garnish with green onions.

Fennel-Scented Tomato and Wild Rice Soup

Makes 8 servings

The fennel in this delightful soup adds a luscious licorice flavor, and the wild rice contributes texture. Fennel is a good source of dietary fiber, potassium, manganese, zinc and copper. It is also well known for its beneficial effects on gastrointestinal health.

Tips

To toast fennel seeds: Stir seeds in a dry skillet over medium heat until fragrant, about 3 minutes. Immediately transfer to a mortar or spice grinder and grind finely.

To prepare bulb fennel: Before removing the core, chop off the top shoots (which resemble celery) and discard. If desired, save the feathery green fronds to use as a garnish. If the outer sections of the bulb seem old and dry, peel them with a vegetable peeler before using.

NUTRIENTS PER SERVING

Calories	140
Fat	3 g
Carbohydrate	27 g
Fiber	6 g
Protein	5 g
Iron	2.9 mg
Calcium	104 mg

- **Immersion blender, food processor or blender**
- **Medium to large (3½- to 5-quart) slow cooker**

1 tbsp	vegetable oil	15 mL
2	leeks (white and light green parts only), sliced (see tip, page 218)	2
1	bulb fennel, cored and thinly sliced on the vertical (see tip, at left)	1
3	cloves garlic, sliced	3
1 tsp	fennel seeds, toasted and ground (see tip, at left)	5 mL
½ tsp	salt (optional)	2 mL
½ tsp	freshly ground black pepper	2 mL
1	can (28 oz/796 mL) crushed tomatoes	1
4 cups	ready-to-use vegetable broth, divided	1 L
¾ cup	wild rice, rinsed and drained	175 mL
	Heavy or whipping (35%) cream or non-dairy alternative (optional)	
	Finely chopped fennel fronds or flat-leaf (Italian) parsley	

1. In a large skillet, heat oil over medium heat. Add leeks and sliced fennel and cook, stirring, until softened, about 7 minutes. Add garlic, fennel seeds, salt (if using) and pepper and cook, stirring, for 1 minute. Stir in tomatoes and 2 cups (500 mL) of the broth. Remove from heat.

2. Purée using an immersion blender. (You can also do this in batches in a food processor or blender.) Transfer to slow cooker stoneware.

3. Add wild rice and the remaining broth. Cover and cook on Low for 6 hours or on High for 3 hours, until rice is tender and grains have begun to split. Ladle into bowls, drizzle with cream (if using) and garnish with fennel fronds.

Health Salad

This colorful, flavorful salad makes a great accompaniment to many meals. It actually improves after a day or two, as the vegetables become infused with the dressing.

Tips

If you are sensitive to sulfites, replace the cider vinegar with white or rice vinegar.

In many locations, green onions are known as scallions.

Variations

Substitute 1 tsp (5 mL) of a flavored oil, such as sesame or garlic-infused oil, for the olive oil.

Add ½ tsp (2 mL) hot pepper sauce or a pinch of hot pepper flakes to the dressing.

Add 1 tbsp (15 mL) chopped fresh herbs, such as basil, dill, oregano or thyme, to the cabbage mixture along with the dressing.

1	large apple (unpeeled), coarsely grated	1
1	small bulb fennel, cored and thinly sliced	1
2 tbsp	freshly squeezed lemon juice	30 mL
6 cups	thinly sliced red or green cabbage (about ½ head)	1.5 L
2	carrots, peeled and grated	2
1	red bell pepper, cut into quarters and thinly sliced crosswise	1

Dressing

3	green onions (white and green parts), finely chopped	3
½ cup	cider vinegar	125 mL
3 tbsp	coarsely chopped fresh flat-leaf (Italian) parsley	45 mL
2 tbsp	olive oil	30 mL
1 tbsp	granulated natural cane sugar or other dry sweetener	15 mL
	Salt and freshly ground black pepper	

1. In a large bowl, combine apple, fennel and lemon juice. Toss to coat. Add cabbage, carrots and red pepper and toss to combine.
2. *Dressing:* In a small bowl, whisk together green onions, vinegar, parsley, olive oil and sugar. Add to cabbage mixture, season with salt and pepper to taste and toss to coat. Cover and refrigerate for at least 2 hours or until flavors are developed, or for up to 2 days.

**NUTRIENTS
PER SERVING**

Calories 90
Fat .5 g
Carbohydrate . . . . .14 g
Fiber . . . . .3 g
Protein . . . . .1 g
Iron . . . . .0.8 mg
Calcium . . . . 33 mg

Asian Carrot Cucumber Pickle

This crisp, refreshing salad makes a superb accompaniment to Asian-themed mains such as Orange Ginger Beef (page 274). It is an excellent source of vitamin A and a good source of fiber.

Tips

This refreshing, light salad needs to be made just before you serve it. If kept for longer than a few hours, the vegetables will go limp. If you need to make it ahead, prepare the marinade and keep it separate from the vegetables. Combine just before serving.

If you prefer, you can seed the cucumbers for a cleaner look.

Variations

A little chopped red chile pepper is a nice addition for those who like heat.

If you don't have rice wine vinegar, white vinegar will work, but the flavor will be slightly different.

NUTRIENTS PER SERVING

Calories	72
Fat	1 g
Carbohydrate	16 g
Fiber	2 g
Protein	1 g
Iron	0.4 mg
Calcium	29 mg

1/2 cup	rice wine vinegar	125 mL
2 tbsp	granulated sugar	30 mL
1 tsp	olive oil	5 mL
1/2 tsp	salt	2 mL
1/4 tsp	freshly ground black pepper	1 mL
1/2	large English cucumber, halved and thinly sliced	1/2
2 cups	thinly sliced carrots	500 mL
2 tbsp	finely chopped red bell pepper	30 mL

1. In a medium bowl, whisk vinegar, sugar, oil, salt and pepper until sugar is dissolved. Add cucumber, carrots and red pepper; toss to coat. Serve right away or cover and refrigerate for up to 30 minutes.

This recipe courtesy of Eileen Campbell.

Lemon Lovers' Tabbouleh

Makes 10 side servings

Tabbouleh is a versatile grain salad that can be enjoyed on its own, as an appetizer or as a side to marinated chicken or beef. The assertive lemon flavor makes it a perfect choice for a hot summer day. The gluten-free variations of this salad (see below) are an excellent source of vitamin K and manganese, and a good source of protein, vitamins A and C, folate, iron and magnesium.

Variations

Quinoa Tabbouleh: Skip step 1. Substitute 4 cups (1 L) cooked quinoa, cooled, for the bulgur.

Millet Tabbouleh: Skip step 1. Substitute 4 cups (1 L) cooked toasted millet, cooled, for the bulgur.

1½ cups	medium or fine bulgur	375 mL
2 cups	ice water	500 mL
⅓ cup	freshly squeezed lemon juice	75 mL
1 tsp	ground cumin	5 mL
1 tsp	salt	5 mL
	Freshly ground black pepper	
⅓ cup	extra virgin olive oil	75 mL
2 cups	loosely packed fresh parsley leaves, finely chopped	500 mL
2 cups	diced seedless cucumber	500 mL
2 cups	diced seeded peeled tomatoes (see tips, at left)	500 mL
½ cup	loosely packed fresh mint leaves, finely chopped	125 mL
½ cup	chopped green onions, white part only	125 mL
	Hearts of romaine (optional)	

1. In a bowl, combine bulgur and cold water. Stir well and set aside until liquid is absorbed, about 10 minutes.

2. Meanwhile, in a small bowl, combine lemon juice, cumin, salt and pepper to taste. Whisk in olive oil. Add to bulgur and set aside until liquid is absorbed, about 15 minutes.

3. Add parsley, cucumber, tomatoes, mint and green onions and toss well. Cover and chill thoroughly. If using the lettuce, line a serving bowl with hearts of romaine and add tabbouleh or serve romaine as a dipper to scoop the salad.

> **Lunch Idea:** Combine 1 serving of this salad with 1 serving of Lemon Garlic Chicken (page 251) or Grilled Chicken Kabobs (page 261).

NUTRIENTS
PER SERVING

Calories 160
Fat .8 g
Carbohydrate . . . . .20 g
Fiber . . . . .5 g
Protein . . . . .3 g
Iron . . . . .1.8 mg
Calcium . . . . 34 mg

Quinoa Salad with Grapefruit and Avocado

The colors and textures in this salad make it perfect for a festive occasion or a lunch served al fresco.

Tip

To prevent the avocado from discoloring, don't peel or cut it until you are ready to serve the salad.

Variations

To boost the calcium content and crunch factor in this salad, garnish with a sprinkling of salted roasted pumpkin seeds.

Substitute fresh cilantro for the mint.

Substitute 2 oranges or 2 blood oranges for the grapefruit.

2 cups	water	500 mL
1 tsp	salt	5 mL
1 cup	quinoa, washed, rinsed and drained	250 mL
2 tbsp	chopped fresh mint	30 mL
2 tbsp	freshly squeezed lime juice	30 mL
2 tsp	granulated natural cane sugar or other dry sweetener	10 mL
1/2 tsp	salt	2 mL
Pinch	freshly ground black pepper	Pinch
1/3 cup	vegetable oil	75 mL
1	red grapefruit, peeled, sectioned and each section cut into thirds	1
1	avocado, peeled, pitted and cut into 3/4-inch (2 cm) cubes (see tip, at left)	1
1/3 cup	Pickled Pink Onion Relish (see recipe, opposite)	75 mL

1. In a pot, bring water and salt to a boil over high heat. Add quinoa, stirring to prevent lumps from forming, and return to a boil. Cover, reduce heat to low and simmer for 15 minutes or until tender and liquid is absorbed. Remove from heat and let stand, uncovered, for 5 minutes or until it reaches room temperature. Transfer to a serving bowl.

2. Meanwhile, in a small bowl, whisk together mint, lime juice, sugar, salt and pepper. Whisk in oil. Add grapefruit pieces, avocado and onion relish and toss lightly to coat. Spoon over quinoa, letting dressing drizzle down through the salad. Serve immediately.

> **Lunch Idea:** For a vegetarian lunch, serve this salad with Lentil and Spinach Soup (page 225).

NUTRIENTS
PER SERVING

Calories 260
Fat . . . . 17 g
Carbohydrate . . . . 24 g
Fiber . . . . 4 g
Protein . . . . 4 g
Iron . . . . 1.4 mg
Calcium . . . . 23 mg

Pickled Pink Onion Relish

This bright pink relish is a perfect condiment for many sandwiches and salads. It is also a colorful way to top off hors d'oeuvres.

Tip

The color of this relish will deepen with time. Any juice leftover once the onions have been used up can be used to make tasty salad dressings and marinades.

Variations

Add ½ tsp (2 mL) of your favorite dried herb, such as thyme, tarragon or basil, along with the vinegar.

Use ½ cup (125 mL) freshly squeezed lemon juice or another flavored vinegar instead of the rice vinegar to steep the onions. Add 2 tsp (10 mL) granulated natural cane sugar or other dry sweetener. Avoid balsamic vinegar, as the dark brown color overpowers the pink onions.

NUTRIENTS
PER 1 TBSP (15 ML)

Calories 2
Fat . . . . 0 g
Carbohydrate . . . . 0 g
Fiber . . . . 0 g
Protein . . . . 0 g
Iron . . . . 0.0 mg
Calcium . . . . 0 mg

6 cups	water	1.5 L
1 tsp	salt	5 mL
1	red onion, cut in half from stem to root, then crosswise and thinly sliced	1
½ cup	seasoned rice vinegar	125 mL

1. In a pot over high heat, bring water and salt to a boil. Add onion and return to a boil (about 45 seconds). Drain and immediately transfer to a nonreactive container. Add vinegar and toss to coat evenly.

2. Let cool to room temperature. Cover and refrigerate for 2 hours or until chilled and deep pink.

Quinoa Salad

Quinoa is a source of high-quality protein, which makes this salad easy to enjoy on its own. The peas make it even more wholesome and enjoyable.

Tip

This salad is an excellent source of vitamin C, vitamin K and manganese. It is a good source of protein, dietary fiber, folate and trace minerals.

Variation

If you're making this salad for non-vegetarians, you can substitute ready-to-use reduced-sodium gluten-free chicken or turkey broth for the vegetable broth.

1¼ cups	ready-to-use reduced-sodium gluten-free vegetable broth	300 mL
¾ cup	quinoa, rinsed	175 mL
½ cup	thawed frozen peas	125 mL
¼ cup	finely chopped orange bell pepper	60 mL
¼ cup	finely chopped yellow bell pepper	60 mL
1 tbsp	finely chopped red onion	15 mL
2 tbsp	extra virgin olive oil	30 mL
1 tbsp	chopped fresh parsley	15 mL
1 tsp	dried thyme	5 mL
1 tsp	freshly squeezed lemon juice	5 mL
	Salt and freshly ground black pepper	

1. In a saucepan, bring broth to a boil over high heat. Add quinoa, reduce heat to low, cover and simmer for 20 minutes or until quinoa is tender and liquid is almost absorbed. Remove from heat and let stand, covered, for 5 minutes or until liquid is absorbed.

2. In a large bowl, combine quinoa, peas, orange pepper, yellow pepper and red onion.

3. In a small bowl, whisk together oil, parsley, thyme and lemon juice. Drizzle over salad and toss to coat. Season to taste with salt and pepper. Serve warm or cover and refrigerate for 1 hour, until chilled, and serve cold.

> **Lunch Idea:** Combine 1 serving of this salad with 1 serving of Greek-Style Split Pea Soup (page 227).

NUTRIENTS PER SERVING

Calories 210
Fat . . . . .9 g
Carbohydrate . . . . .26 g
Fiber . . . . .4 g
Protein . . . . .6 g
Iron . . . . .2.2 mg
Calcium . . . . 34 mg

Millet Salad with Lemony Chickpeas and Tomatoes

The flavors of the Mediterranean come together perfectly in this recipe, making it a great complement to many different mains. Serve it over hearts of romaine for an appetizing presentation.

Tips

For this quantity of chickpeas, soak and cook 1 cup (250 mL) dried chickpeas. Or use 1 can (14 to 19 oz/398 to 540 mL) chickpeas, drained and rinsed.

This salad is a good source of protein, iron and trace minerals.

If field tomatoes are in season, substitute an equal quantity of seeded diced tomatoes for the cherry tomatoes.

1 cup	millet	250 mL
2 cups	water or ready-to-use vegetable broth	500 mL
2 cups	halved cherry tomatoes (see tip, at left)	500 mL
2 cups	cooked chickpeas (see tip, at left)	500 mL
8	green onions, white part only, finely chopped	8
2 cups	thinly sliced radishes	500 mL
	Hearts of romaine (optional)	

Dressing

1/4 cup	freshly squeezed lemon juice	60 mL
1/2 tsp	salt	2 mL
Pinch	cayenne pepper (optional)	Pinch
	Freshly ground black pepper	
6 tbsp	extra virgin olive oil	90 mL
1/4 cup	finely chopped parsley or dill	60 mL

1. In a saucepan over medium heat, toast millet, stirring, until it crackles and releases its aroma, about 5 minutes. Transfer to a bowl. Add water to saucepan and bring to a boil. Stir in millet and return to a boil. Reduce heat to low. Cover and simmer until water is absorbed, about 25 minutes. Remove from heat and let stand, covered, for 10 minutes. Transfer to a serving bowl and fluff with a fork. Set aside and let cool.

2. *Dressing:* Meanwhile, in a small bowl, combine lemon juice, salt, cayenne (if using) and pepper to taste, stirring until salt dissolves. Whisk in olive oil. Add parsley. Set aside.

3. Add tomatoes, chickpeas, green onions and radishes to millet and toss. Add dressing and toss well. Cover and chill. If using lettuce, line a serving bowl with hearts of romaine and add salad. Or serve salad as an appetizer and use romaine as dippers.

NUTRIENTS PER SERVING

Calories	210
Fat	10 g
Carbohydrate	24 g
Fiber	5 g
Protein	5 g
Iron	1.6 mg
Calcium	38 mg

Dinner Idea: Serve this salad as a side dish to Grilled Chicken Kabobs (page 261) or Chicken Cacciatore (page 258).

Taco Salad

Nutritious and easy to make, this recipe is perfect for a weekday dinner. It's an excellent source of protein, fiber and iron.

Tips

You can choose a hot or mild barbecue sauce; just be sure it is free of allergens, such as gluten, soy, mustard and fish. Make your own, if you prefer.

If you purchase a sirloin steak, cut it across the grain into thin strips for a tender result.

Variation

Top the salad with guacamole, salsa or shredded cheese (such as naturally lactose-free Monterey Jack) or a non-dairy alternative. Adding lactose-free cheese or an enriched non-dairy alternative will boost the calcium content.

2	Tortilla Bowls (see recipe, opposite)	2
4 cups	shredded lettuce	1 L
2	tomatoes, diced	2
1/4	orange bell pepper, finely chopped	1/4
1/4	yellow bell pepper, finely chopped	1/4
1/4 cup	gluten-free barbecue sauce	60 mL
3/4 tsp	gluten-free chili powder	3 mL
Pinch	ground hot pepper	Pinch
1 tsp	extra virgin olive oil	5 mL
6 oz	beef sirloin stir-fry strips	175 g

1. Place tortilla bowls on individual plates. Divide the lettuce evenly among the tortilla bowls. Top each with tomatoes, orange pepper and yellow pepper. Set aside.

2. In a small bowl, combine barbecue sauce, chili powder and hot pepper. Set aside.

3. In a skillet, heat oil over medium-high heat. Brown beef strips, turning occasionally, for 2 to 3 minutes or until just slightly pink in the center. Pour in the barbecue sauce mixture and heat just until steaming.

4. Top each tortilla bowl with half the beef mixture.

NUTRIENTS PER SERVING

Calories	344
Fat	8 g
Carbohydrate	45 g
Fiber	8 g
Protein	24 g
Iron	4.0 mg
Calcium	159 mg

Tortilla Bowls

Makes 2 servings

Make these neat containers to hold anything from salads to entrées. Children and adults alike will love to eat from them.

Tip

Warm the tortillas in the oven slightly before molding them into the bowl, for easier handling.

- **Preheat oven to 350°F (180°C)**
- **5½-inch (14 cm) ovenproof bowl, at least 3½ inches (9 cm) deep**

| 2 | 8-inch (20 cm) gluten-free tortillas | 2 |

1. Gently place a tortilla in the bowl, easing it in to fit the bottom and up the sides. Bake in preheated oven for 15 minutes or until crisp. Let cool in bowl for 5 minutes. Carefully remove from bowl and repeat for the remaining tortilla. Let cool completely before filling.

NUTRIENTS PER SERVING

Calories	130
Fat	3 g
Carbohydrates	24 g
Fiber	2 g
Protein	2 g
Iron	0.7 mg
Calcium	0 mg

Black Bean Salad

Black beans are an excellent source of protein, fiber and iron. Enjoy this Mexican-inspired salad over a bed of greens.

Tips

If you're using 19-oz (540 mL) cans of beans, add an additional 1 tsp (5 mL) lime juice, 1/4 tsp (1 mL) cumin and a pinch of adobo seasoning.

Adobo seasoning is a spice mixture composed of salt, garlic, black pepper, oregano and turmeric. Make sure the spice blend you choose is free of allergens, such as gluten and sulfites. If you can't find adobo seasoning, substitute a pinch each of garlic powder, ground oregano and turmeric and salt and black pepper to taste.

You can use 1¾ cups (425 mL) frozen corn kernels, thawed and drained, instead of the canned corn.

3 tbsp	olive oil, divided	45 mL
1	red onion, finely chopped (about 1½ cups/375 mL)	1
1	clove garlic, minced (about 1 tsp/5 mL)	1
2	cans (each 14 to 19 oz/398 to 540 mL) black beans, drained and rinsed (see tip, at left)	2
2½ tbsp	freshly squeezed lime juice	37 mL
2 tsp	granulated natural cane sugar, or to taste	10 mL
1 tsp	ground cumin	5 mL
½ tsp	adobo seasoning or Mexican spice blend (see tip, at left)	2 mL
¼ tsp	hot pepper sauce, or to taste	1 mL
2	cans (each 7 oz/213 mL) corn kernels, drained (see tip, at left)	2
2	large tomatoes, seeded and finely diced	2
½ cup	coarsely chopped fresh cilantro	125 mL
	Salt and freshly ground black pepper	

1. In a large skillet, heat 1 tbsp (15 mL) oil over medium heat for 30 seconds. Add onion and cook, stirring, for 3 minutes or until softened. Add garlic and cook, stirring, for 1 minute. Stir in beans and reduce heat to medium-low. Cook for 4 minutes or until beans are heated through.

2. Meanwhile, in a small bowl, whisk together lime juice, sugar, cumin, adobo seasoning, hot pepper sauce and the remaining olive oil until well blended.

3. In a serving bowl, combine bean mixture, corn, tomatoes and cilantro. Add dressing and toss until evenly coated. Season with salt and pepper to taste. Cover and refrigerate for 2 hours or until chilled. This salad can be refrigerated in an airtight container for up to 3 days.

Lunch Idea: Serve ½ serving of this salad in a Tortilla Bowl (page 241).

NUTRIENTS PER SERVING

Calories	260
Fat	8 g
Carbohydrate	38 g
Fiber	7 g
Protein	9 g
Iron	2.0 mg
Calcium	60 mg

Main Dishes

Ratatouille

This dish, loaded with tender Mediterranean vegetables, can be enjoyed hot or cold. Traditional ratatouille can be time-consuming, but this version emphasizes convenience.

Tips

This dish is a good source of cholesterol-lowering soluble fiber, along with many types of antioxidants.

If you don't like the bitter flavor of some eggplant, salting it with coarse salt, such as kosher or sea salt, and allowing it to "sweat" reduces some of the bitterness.

Use canned tomatoes with or without seasoning for this recipe.

Ratatouille will keep, covered, in the refrigerator for up to 3 days.

Variation

Add 1 cup (250 mL) quartered button mushrooms along with the peppers.

NUTRIENTS PER SERVING

Calories	120
Fat	6 g
Carbohydrate	15 g
Fiber	5 g
Protein	3 g
Iron	1.4 mg
Calcium	47 mg

1	eggplant (about 1¼ lb/625 g), unpeeled, cut into ½-inch (1 cm) cubes	1
2 tbsp	kosher or coarse sea salt	30 mL
3 tbsp	olive or vegetable oil	45 mL
1	large onion, sliced on the vertical (¼ inch/0.5 cm)	1
5	cloves garlic, minced (about 1½ tbsp/22 mL)	5
2	green bell peppers, cut into ½-inch (1 cm) squares	2
2	zucchini, quartered lengthwise and cut into ½-inch (1 cm) thick slices	2
⅓ cup	dry white wine, water or ready-to-use vegetable broth	75 mL
1	bay leaf	1
1 tsp	dried thyme	5 mL
1	can (28 oz/796 mL) diced tomatoes, with juice	1
	Salt and freshly ground black pepper	
2 tbsp	chopped fresh flat-leaf (Italian) parsley	30 mL

1. In a colander over the sink, toss eggplant with salt. Let drain for 20 minutes. Rinse and pat dry.

2. In a large pot, heat oil over medium heat for 30 seconds. Add onion and cook, stirring, for 3 minutes or until softened. Add garlic and cook, stirring, for 1 minute. Add eggplant and cook, stirring occasionally, for 5 minutes. Add peppers and cook, stirring, for 1 minute.

3. Stir in zucchini, white wine, bay leaf, thyme and tomatoes and cook until small bubbles begin to form on surface. Reduce heat to maintain a gentle simmer. Cover and cook, stirring occasionally, for 15 to 20 minutes or until eggplant is tender and mixture is thickened. Season with salt and pepper to taste. Discard bay leaf. Serve hot, let cool to room temperature or cover, chill and serve cold. Sprinkle with parsley before serving.

Dinner Idea: Combine 1 serving of Ratatouille with 1 serving of Pork Tenderloin (page 270) or Roast Pork with Red Rice and Beans (page 268).

Tagine of Squash and Chickpeas with Mushrooms

The beans and vegetables in this slow-cooking stew absorb the exotic flavor of the ginger, turmeric and cinnamon for a delightful meal. The currants and the bittersweet mixture of honey and lemon add a perfect finish.

Tips

This dish is an excellent source of protein, fiber and vitamin A, and a good source of iron, folate and trace minerals.

For this quantity of chickpeas, use 1 can (14 to 19 oz/398 to 540 mL) drained and rinsed, or cook 1 cup (250 mL) dried chickpeas.

This recipe can be partially prepared up to 2 days ahead. Complete step 1, let cool, cover and refrigerate. When you're ready to cook, continue with step 2.

NUTRIENTS
PER SERVING

Calories 200
Fat .4 g
Carbohydrate. . . . . .37 g
Fiber . . . . .7 g
Protein. . . . . .7 g
Iron . . . . .2.4 mg
Calcium . . . . 92 mg

- **Medium to large (3½- to 5-quart) slow cooker**

1 tbsp	vegetable oil	15 mL
1	onion, finely chopped	1
2	carrots, peeled and diced (about 1 cup/250 mL)	2
4	cloves garlic, minced	4
1	2-inch (5 cm) cinnamon stick	1
2 tbsp	minced gingerroot	30 mL
1 tsp	ground turmeric	5 mL
½ tsp	salt	2 mL
½ tsp	cracked black peppercorns	2 mL
1	can (28 oz/796 mL) tomatoes, with juice, coarsely chopped	1
3 cups	cubed peeled butternut squash or pumpkin (1 inch/2.5 cm cubes)	750 mL
2 cups	drained cooked chickpeas (see tip, at left)	500 mL
8 oz	cremini mushrooms, stemmed and halved	250 g
1 tbsp	liquid honey	15 mL
1 tbsp	freshly squeezed lemon juice	15 mL
¼ cup	currants (optional)	60 mL

1. In a large skillet, heat oil over medium heat. Add onion and carrots and cook, stirring, until carrots are softened, about 7 minutes. Add garlic, cinnamon stick, ginger, turmeric, salt and peppercorns and cook, stirring, for 1 minute. Add tomatoes with juice and bring to a boil. Transfer to slow cooker stoneware.

2. Stir in squash, chickpeas and mushrooms. Cover and cook on Low for 8 hours or on High for 4 hours, until vegetables are tender. Discard cinnamon stick.

3. In a small bowl, combine honey and lemon juice. Add to slow cooker and stir well. When serving, sprinkle with currants (if using).

> **Dinner Idea:** Enjoy 1 serving of this dish with 1 cup (250 mL) sautéed spinach or Swiss chard.

Curried Chickpeas

The entire family will enjoy this quick, nutritious dish, which provides a good amount of protein, fiber, iron, folate and other B vitamins. Serving it with steamed or sautéed greens boosts the calcium content.

Tips

Precooking curry powder in oil helps maximize its flavor and mitigate any potential harshness. In this recipe, it is cooked with other ingredients for convenience.

Although coconut milk adds the best flavor to this dish, it is very high in saturated fats. You can replace all or a portion of it with enriched almond milk or any other non-dairy beverage if you prefer.

2 tbsp	vegetable oil	30 mL
1	Spanish onion, thinly sliced (about 1½ cups/375 mL)	1
3	garlic cloves, minced (about 1 tbsp/15 mL)	3
1 tbsp	gluten-free curry powder	15 mL
1	can (14 oz/398 mL) coconut milk	1
1	can (14 to 19 oz/398 to 540 mL) chickpeas, drained and rinsed	1
1 lb	frozen mixed bell peppers, thawed, or fresh bell peppers, cut into 2-inch by ¼-inch (5 cm by 0.5 cm) strips	500 g
2 tbsp	tomato paste	30 mL
1 tbsp	packed brown sugar or granulated natural cane sugar	15 mL
1 tbsp	freshly squeezed lemon juice	15 mL
1 tsp	salt, or to taste	5 mL
Pinch	hot pepper flakes or dash hot pepper sauce	Pinch
2 tbsp	chopped fresh cilantro or parsley (optional)	30 mL

1. In a large skillet, heat oil over medium heat for about 30 seconds. Add onion and cook, stirring, for 3 minutes or until softened. Add garlic and curry powder and cook, stirring, for 1 minute.

2. Stir in coconut milk, chickpeas, peppers, tomato paste, brown sugar, lemon juice, salt and hot pepper flakes and bring to a boil. Reduce heat and simmer, uncovered, for 20 to 25 minutes or until sauce is thickened and vegetables are tender. Serve sprinkled with cilantro (if using).

Dinner Idea: Enjoy 1 serving of this dish with 1 cup (250 mL) steamed or sautéed kale, bok choy or collard greens and 1 cup (250 mL) cooked basmati rice for a satisfying vegetarian meal.

NUTRIENTS PER SERVING

Calories	410
Fat	27 g
Carbohydrate	37 g
Fiber	8 g
Protein	9 g
Iron	5.2 mg
Calcium	70 mg

Mixed Vegetable Coconut Curry

This rich, slow-cooked curry is sure to delight with its aromatic blend of ginger, cumin, coriander and turmeric. It can be enjoyed on its own for a light meal or with a grain salad for a more special occasion.

Tips

This recipe is an excellent source of vitamins A and C.

For the best flavor, toast the cumin and coriander seeds and grind them yourself. To toast seeds: Place in a dry skillet over medium heat and cook, stirring, until fragrant, about 3 minutes. Immediately transfer to a spice grinder or mortar and grind finely.

This recipe can be partially prepared up to 2 days ahead. Complete step 1, let cool, cover and refrigerate. When you're ready to cook, continue with step 2.

NUTRIENTS PER SERVING

Calories	160
Fat	4 g
Carbohydrate	29 g
Fiber	6 g
Protein	4 g
Iron	2.2 mg
Calcium	113 mg

- **Medium to large (4- to 5-quart) slow cooker**

1 tbsp	vegetable or coconut oil	15 mL
3 cups	cubed peeled carrots (about 4 medium, cut into 1/2-inch/1 cm cubes)	750 mL
2	onions, finely chopped	2
2	stalks celery, diced	2
4	cloves garlic, minced	4
1 tbsp	minced gingerroot	15 mL
2 tsp	ground cumin (see tip, at left)	10 mL
2 tsp	ground coriander	10 mL
1 tsp	salt	5 mL
1 tsp	cracked black peppercorns	5 mL
1/2 tsp	ground turmeric	2 mL
1	bay leaf	1
1	can (28 oz/796 mL) diced tomatoes, with juice	1
4 cups	cubed peeled winter squash (1-inch/2.5 cm cubes)	1 L
1 cup	enriched coconut milk	250 mL
1	red bell pepper, finely chopped	1
1	long red or green chile pepper, seeded and minced	1

1. In a skillet, heat oil over medium heat. Add carrots, onions and celery and cook, stirring, until softened, about 7 minutes. Add garlic, ginger, cumin, coriander, salt, peppercorns, turmeric and bay leaf and cook, stirring, for 1 minute. Add tomatoes with juice and bring to a boil. Transfer to slow cooker stoneware.

2. Stir in squash. Cover and cook on Low for 6 hours or on High for 3 hours. Add coconut milk, bell pepper and chile pepper and stir well. Cover and cook on High for 15 minutes, until peppers are tender.

Lunch Idea: Serve with Millet Salad with Lemony Chickpeas and Tomatoes (page 239).

Dinner Idea: Serve with Coconut Chicken with Quinoa (page 256) or Aloo Tikki (page 300).

Cornish Game Hens with Cranberry and Wild Rice Stuffing

Makes 4 to 6 servings

This recipe is just the thing for a festive occasion. The wild rice stuffing adds crunch and texture, and it is healthier than a traditional stuffing made with bread crumbs.

Tips

Butter is naturally lactose-free, but if you are allergic to cow's milk protein, substitute non-dairy, soy-free margarine.

When purchasing dried sage or thyme, use dried leaves and avoid the powdered variety.

This recipe makes enough stuffing for 4 to 6 Cornish game hens or a 10-lb (4.5 kg) turkey.

NUTRIENTS
PER SERVING

Calories	570
Fat	14 g
Carbohydrate	50 g
Fiber	4 g
Protein	57 g
Iron	3.5 mg
Calcium	74 mg

- **Roasting pan**

4 cups	ready-to-use gluten-free chicken broth	1 L
¾ cup	brown rice	175 mL
½ cup	wild rice, rinsed	125 mL
1 tbsp	crumbled dried sage	15 mL
1 tbsp	crumbled dried thyme	15 mL
1 tbsp	butter	15 mL
1 tbsp	vegetable oil	15 mL
1	large onion, chopped	1
1 cup	sliced cremini mushroom caps (halved, then cut into ¼-inch/0.5 cm slices)	250 mL
1 cup	diced celery	250 mL
1 cup	diced carrots	250 mL
¼ tsp	salt	1 mL
¼ tsp	freshly ground black pepper	1 mL
1 cup	dried cranberries	250 mL
2 tbsp	balsamic vinegar	30 mL
4 to 6	Cornish game hens (each about 1 to 1¼ lb/500 to 625 g)	4 to 6
	Plum Dipping Sauce (see recipe, opposite)	

1. In a large saucepan, over high heat, combine broth, brown rice, wild rice, sage and thyme and bring to a boil. Reduce heat, cover and simmer gently for 45 to 55 minutes, or until rice is tender. Remove from heat and fluff with a fork. Set aside to cool completely.

2. In a skillet, heat butter and oil over medium-high heat. Add onion, mushrooms, celery, carrots, salt and pepper and cook, stirring constantly, until tender, about 8 to 10 minutes. Stir in dried cranberries and balsamic vinegar.

3. Add vegetable mixture to rice mixture and stir gently to combine. Loosely stuff into the game hens and place them breast side up in roasting pan.

4. Preheat oven to 350°F (180°C). Roast hens, uncovered, for 45 to 60 minutes, or until meat thermometer inserted in thigh registers 180°F (82°C). Remove the stuffing immediately.

5. Serve with Plum Dipping Sauce.

Plum Dipping Sauce

This quick, easy, rich, plum-colored sauce is wonderful with Cornish Game Hens (opposite), and kids will love it with baked chicken fingers.

Tips

This sauce can be stored, covered, in the refrigerator for up to 2 weeks.

To prevent cross-contamination, set out individual bowls for dipping sauces for each person.

Serve the sauce warm or cold — it's delicious either way!

Variations

In season, 8 fresh plums can be substituted for the canned plums. For an even quicker sauce, substitute one 7.5-oz (213 mL) jar of gluten-free baby food strained plums.

To add tomato flavor, add 1 tbsp (15 mL) gluten-free ketchup to the dipping sauce.

**NUTRIENTS
PER SERVING**

Calories	35
Fat	0 g
Carbohydrate	10 g
Fiber	1 g
Protein	0 g
Iron	0.1 mg
Calcium	2 mg

- **Blender**

1	can (14 oz/398 mL) prune plums	1
⅓ cup	granulated sugar	75 mL
3 tbsp	white vinegar	45 mL

1. Drain plums, reserving 2 tbsp (30 mL) liquid. Remove pits from plums. In blender, purée plums and reserved liquid.

2. In a small saucepan, combine plum purée, sugar and vinegar. Heat over medium heat until mixture comes to a gentle boil. Remove from heat and let cool before serving.

Chicken with Root Vegetables

This hearty one-pot meal is satisfying and chock full of nutrients. Root vegetables are good sources of soluble fiber and minerals, and are typically easy to digest.

3 lb	whole chicken, skin removed	1.5 kg
	Salt and freshly ground black pepper	
8	small russet potatoes, peeled and quartered	8
4	stalks celery, peeled and coarsely chopped	4
4	carrots, peeled and coarsely chopped	4
4	parsnips, peeled and coarsely chopped	4
8 cups	ready-to-use gluten-free chicken broth	2 L
8	sprigs parsley	8
4	bay leaves	4

1. Sprinkle chicken all over (including cavity) with salt and pepper. Place in a large, heavy-bottomed pot or Dutch oven.

2. Arrange potatoes, celery, carrots and parsnips around chicken. Pour in broth, immersing chicken (add enough water to cover, if necessary). Sprinkle with parsley and bay leaves.

3. Over medium heat, simmer, uncovered and checking occasionally to ensure chicken is covered (add more water, if necessary), for 50 minutes or until drumsticks wiggle when touched, a meat thermometer inserted in the thickest part of a thigh registers 185°F (85°C) and vegetables are tender.

Dinner Idea: Serve with Quinoa Salad (page 238) for a satisfying and nutritious meal.

NUTRIENTS PER SERVING

Calories 479
Fat . . . . .7 g
Carbohydrate . . . . .49 g
Fiber . . . . .7 g
Protein . . . . .53 g
Iron . . . . 3 mg
Calcium . . . . 91 mg

Lemon Garlic Chicken

Makes 4 servings

The herbs and spices in this tangy, light dish smell wonderful when you're cooking and taste wonderful when it's time to eat.

Tips

Chicken can be marinated at room temperature for up to 30 minutes if you are short on time. Any longer, make sure it is refrigerated. Throw out the plastic bag used for marinating.

Can't find the cover that fits your casserole? Cover it with foil, dull side out. Trace around the rim with your fingers to be sure foil forms a tight seal.

Variations

Rather than baking the chicken, barbecue or grill it for 5 to 8 minutes per side.

Substitute an equal amount of oregano for the thyme. Or use 1 tbsp (15 mL) snipped fresh thyme or oregano.

NUTRIENTS PER SERVING

Calories 170
Fat .7 g
Carbohydrate . . . . .1 g
Fiber . . . . .0 g
Protein . . . . .25 g
Iron . . . . .1.0 mg
Calcium . . . . 14 mg

- **8-cup (2 L) covered casserole dish**

1	clove garlic, minced	1
2 tbsp	freshly squeezed lemon juice	30 mL
1 tbsp	extra virgin olive oil	15 mL
1 tsp	dried thyme	5 mL
1/4 tsp	salt	1 mL
Pinch	ground nutmeg	Pinch
Pinch	paprika	Pinch
Pinch	freshly ground white pepper	Pinch
4	boneless skinless chicken breasts	4

1. In a sealable plastic freezer bag set in a bowl, combine garlic, lemon juice, olive oil, thyme, salt, nutmeg, paprika and white pepper. Add chicken breasts to marinade, seal bag and refrigerate for 1 hour.

2. Preheat oven to 375°F (190°C). Place chicken breasts with marinade in the casserole dish and cover tightly. Bake for 45 minutes, or until chicken is no longer pink inside and a meat thermometer inserted in the thickest part of a breast registers 165°F (74°C).

Dinner Idea: Serve with Health Salad (page 233) and either Lemon Jasmine Rice Pilaf (page 302) or Millet Salad with Lemony Chickpeas and Tomatoes (page 239).

Southwestern-Style Chile Chicken with Wehani Rice

Makes 8 servings

Wehani rice is a type of red rice grown by the popular Lundberg Family Farms. It has a robust, chewy flavor that anchors the meal well, and it has a lower glycemic index than plain white rice.

Tips

This meal is an excellent source of niacin and selenium, a good source of vitamin A, B vitamins, phosphorus, iron and magnesium, and a source of fiber.

Bhutanese, Thai or Camargue red rice can be substituted for the Wehani rice, although the cooking times vary. If you prefer, cook the rice in a rice cooker.

For best results, toast and grind cumin seeds yourself. To toast seeds: Place in a dry skillet over medium heat and cook, stirring, until fragrant, about 3 minutes. Immediately transfer to a spice grinder or mortar and grind finely.

NUTRIENTS PER SERVING

Calories	410
Fat	18 g
Carbohydrate	28 g
Fiber	4 g
Protein	34 g
Iron	3.1 mg
Calcium	46 mg

• Blender

3 cups	ready-to-use reduced-sodium chicken broth, divided	750 mL
1 cup	Wehani rice, rinsed and drained (see tip, at left)	250 mL
4	dried ancho, mild New Mexico or guajillo chiles	4
2 cups	boiling water	500 mL
1 cup	packed coarsely chopped cilantro (stems and leaves)	250 mL
2 tbsp	red wine vinegar	30 mL
1 tbsp	extra virgin olive oil (approx.)	15 mL
3 lbs	skin-on bone-in chicken breasts, cut into serving-size pieces, rinsed and patted dry	1.5 kg
2	onions, finely chopped	2
4	cloves garlic, minced	4
1 tbsp	ground cumin (see tip, at left)	15 mL
1 tsp	dried oregano (preferably Mexican)	5 mL
1/2 tsp	cracked black peppercorns	2 mL
	Salt (optional)	
	Additional finely chopped cilantro	

1. In a saucepan with a tight-fitting lid over medium-high heat, bring 2 cups (500 mL) of the broth to a boil. Add rice and stir well. Return to a rapid boil. Reduce heat to low (see tip, at right). Cover and cook until liquid is absorbed and rice is tender, about 45 minutes.

2. Meanwhile, in a heatproof bowl, soak dried chiles in boiling water for 30 minutes, weighing down with a cup to ensure they remain submerged. Drain, discarding soaking liquid and stems. Pat dry, chop finely and transfer to blender. Add the remaining broth, cilantro and vinegar. Purée and set aside.

3. Meanwhile, in a Dutch oven, heat oil over medium-high heat for 30 seconds. Add chicken, in batches, and cook, turning once, until skin is browned and crispy, about 10 minutes per batch, adding more oil, if necessary. Transfer to a plate and set aside. Drain off all but 1 tbsp (15 mL) fat from pan. Reduce heat to medium.

Tips

Make sure the red wine vinegar you choose is free of sulfites. If you prefer, you can substitute white vinegar.

Unless you have a stove with a true simmer, after reducing the heat to low, place a heat diffuser under the pot to prevent the mixture from boiling. This device also helps to ensure the grains will cook evenly and prevents hot spots, which might cause scorching. Heat diffusers are available at kitchen supply and hardware stores and are made to work on gas or electric stoves.

4. Add onions to pan and cook, stirring, until softened, about 3 minutes. Add garlic, cumin, oregano and peppercorns and cook, stirring, for 1 minute. Stir in reserved chile mixture. Season with salt (if using). Return chicken to pan, skin side up, and spoon a little sauce over each piece. Reduce heat to low. Cover and simmer until chicken is no longer pink inside, about 30 minutes, turning the chicken over to cook in the sauce for the last 5 minutes of cooking.

5. To serve: On a deep platter, arrange rice in a ring around the edge, leaving the center hollow. Spoon chicken and sauce into the center and garnish with additional cilantro.

> **Dinner Idea:** Serve this meal with a tossed green salad or Cumin Beets (page 281).

Fruity Sautéed Chicken

Makes 4 servings

This light supper offers an interesting way to introduce fruit into your diet. It is a excellent source of protein, zinc and niacin, and is high in magnesium, vitamin C and other B vitamins.

8	boneless skinless chicken thighs	8
	Salt and freshly ground black pepper	
2 tsp	canola oil, divided	10 mL
½ cup	orange juice	125 mL
2	large cooking apples, chopped	2
1	large pear, chopped	1
½ cup	halved seedless grapes	125 mL
3	thin slices gingerroot (optional)	3
1	4-inch (10 cm) cinnamon stick (optional)	1
2 tbsp	chopped fresh parsley	30 mL

1. Sprinkle chicken with a pinch each of salt and pepper. In a Dutch oven or large pot, heat 1 tsp (5 mL) oil over medium-high heat. Add half the chicken and cook, turning once, for 3 to 4 minutes per side or until lightly browned. Transfer to a bowl and set aside. Add the remaining oil to the pot and brown the remaining chicken. Transfer to bowl.

2. Add orange juice and deglaze the pot, scraping up any brown bits. Return chicken and any accumulated juices to the pot. Stir in apples, pear, grapes, ginger (if using), cinnamon stick (if using), ½ tsp (2 mL) salt and ½ tsp (2 mL) pepper; bring to a boil. Reduce heat to medium, cover and simmer for 15 minutes or until fruit is soft. Uncover and simmer for 5 minutes or until sauce is slightly thickened and juices run clear when chicken is pierced. Discard cinnamon stick and ginger. Serve garnished with parsley.

This recipe courtesy of Christine D. Lee.

Dinner Idea: Pair 1 serving of this meal with 1 cup (250 mL) cooked millet or quinoa.

NUTRIENTS
PER SERVING

Calories 280
Fat .8 g
Carbohydrate. . . . . .30 g
Fiber . . . . .4 g
Protein. . . . . .23 g
Iron . . . . .1.7 mg
Calcium . . . . 31 mg

Peppery Chicken Quinoa

Makes 4 servings

This colorful meal is very easy to make on busy weeknights. It's an excellent source of vitamins A and C, niacin, iron and trace minerals, a good source of B vitamins, and a source of calcium.

Tips

Harissa is a North African chili paste that is often added to couscous to give it some bite. If you don't have it, pass your favorite hot pepper sauce at the table to satisfy any heat seekers in the group.

If you are sensitive to sulfites, replace the sherry vinegar with white or rice vinegar.

Variation

Instead of quinoa, serve this over couscous or brown or red rice.

3 cups	ready-to-use reduced-sodium chicken broth, divided	750 mL
1 tbsp	harissa (optional)	15 mL
1 cup	quinoa, rinsed and drained	250 mL
3 tbsp	extra virgin olive oil, divided	45 mL
½ tsp	cracked black peppercorns	2 mL
1 lb	skinless boneless chicken breasts, thinly sliced	500 g
4	cloves garlic, thinly sliced	4
3	red bell peppers, cut into thin strips	3
2 tbsp	sherry vinegar	30 mL
¼ cup	finely chopped fresh parsley	60 mL

1. In a saucepan over medium heat, bring 2 cups (500 mL) of the broth to a boil. Stir in harissa (if using). Add quinoa in a steady steam, stirring constantly, and return to a boil. Reduce heat to low. Cover and simmer until tender, about 15 minutes. Remove from heat and let stand for 5 minutes. Fluff with a fork.

2. Meanwhile, in a large skillet or wok, heat 1 tbsp (15 mL) of the olive oil over medium-high heat. Add black peppercorns and stir well. Add chicken and cook, stirring, until it turns white and almost cooks through, about 5 minutes. Transfer to a plate.

3. Add the remaining oil to pan. Add garlic and cook, stirring, just until it begins to turn golden, about 2 minutes. Add bell peppers and cook, stirring, until they begin to shimmer, about 2 minutes. Add sherry vinegar and the remaining broth and cook until mixture is reduced by half, about 8 minutes. Return chicken to pan and toss until heated through. Remove from heat.

4. To serve: Spread cooked quinoa over a deep platter and scoop out an indentation in the middle. Fill with chicken mixture and garnish with parsley.

Dinner Idea: Serve this meal with Peas and Mushrooms (page 286).

NUTRIENTS PER SERVING

Calories	420
Fat	16 g
Carbohydrate	35 g
Fiber	5 g
Protein	33 g
Iron	3.3 mg
Calcium	43 mg

Coconut Chicken with Quinoa

Makes 4 servings

This rich dish boasts mouthwatering flavors and is very nutritious. It's an excellent source of vitamin C, niacin, iron and trace minerals, and a good source of B vitamins and fiber.

Tips

If you prefer, you can substitute already ground spices for the cumin seeds and allspice and skip the toasting step. Use 1 tsp (5 mL) ground cumin and ½ tsp (2 mL) ground allspice.

The crispy chicken skin adds texture and flavor to this dish, but it also adds fat. If you want to reduce the quantity of fat, remove the skin. Most of the saturated fat comes from the chicken skin and the coconut milk.

Choose enriched coconut milk to up your calcium intake.

2 tsp	cumin seeds (see tip, at left)	10 mL
1 tsp	whole allspice	5 mL
1 tbsp	olive oil	15 mL
1½ lbs	skin-on bone-in chicken breasts, rinsed and patted dry	750 g
1	onion, finely chopped	1
1	red bell pepper, finely chopped	1
1	green bell pepper, finely chopped	1
6	cloves garlic, minced	6
½ to 1	chile pepper, seeded and minced (optional)	½ to 1
1 tsp	gluten-free curry powder	5 mL
½ tsp	salt	2 mL
½ tsp	freshly ground black pepper	2 mL
¾ cup	quinoa, rinsed and drained	175 mL
1½ cups	ready-to-use reduced-sodium chicken broth	375 mL
½ cup	enriched coconut milk	125 mL

1. In a dry large skillet over medium heat, combine cumin seeds and allspice. Toast, stirring constantly, until fragrant, about 4 minutes. Immediately transfer to a mortar or a spice grinder and grind. Set aside.

2. In same skillet, heat oil over medium heat for 30 seconds. Add chicken, in batches, skin side down, and brown well, about 4 minutes. Turn over, cover and cook for 10 minutes. Remove from pan and keep warm. Drain all but 1 tbsp (15 mL) fat from pan.

3. Add onion, bell peppers, garlic and chile pepper (if using) and cook, stirring, until vegetables are softened, about 5 minutes. Add curry powder, salt, black pepper, reserved ground spices and quinoa and cook, stirring, until quinoa is well integrated into mixture, about 1 minute. Add broth and coconut milk and bring to a boil. Lay chicken, skin side up, over mixture. Reduce heat to low. Cover and cook until chicken is no longer pink inside, about 30 minutes.

Dinner Idea: Serve this meal with 1 to 2 cups (250 to 500 mL) steamed or sautéed bok choy or collard greens.

NUTRIENTS PER SERVING

Calories	460
Fat	20 g
Carbohydrate	32 g
Fiber	5 g
Protein	37 g
Iron	5.4 mg
Calcium	102 mg

French-Style Red Rice with Chicken

Camargue red rice, which is available in North America at stores specializing in products from France, has a delicate nutty flavor. If you can't find it, other varieties of red rice work well, but you'll need to adjust the cooking time. You want the rice to be tender to the bite, but not fully cooked, when the dish is placed in the oven.

Tips

This dish is an excellent source of vitamin A, vitamin C, niacin, iron and selenium, and a good source of vitamin E and trace minerals.

If you're a heat seeker, you can use 2 chile peppers when making this recipe.

If you are sensitive to sulfites, make sure the olives have no added sulfites.

NUTRIENTS
PER SERVING

Calories	480
Fat	16 g
Carbohydrate	53 g
Fiber	6 g
Protein	31 g
Iron	4.2 mg
Calcium	59 mg

- **Preheat oven to 350°F (180°C)**
- **12-cup (3 L) baking dish**

1½ cups	Camargue or other red rice, rinsed	375 mL
3 cups	ready-to-use reduced-sodium chicken broth	750 mL
1 tbsp	olive oil	15 mL
2 lbs	skin-on bone-in chicken breasts, cut into serving-size pieces, rinsed and patted dry	1 kg
2	onions, finely chopped	2
1	green bell pepper, finely chopped	1
1	red bell pepper, finely chopped	1
1	long red or green chile pepper, seeded and minced (see tip, at left)	1
4	cloves garlic, minced	4
1 tbsp	sweet paprika	15 mL
½ tsp	salt	2 mL
¼ tsp	cracked black peppercorns	1 mL
1	can (28 oz/796 mL) no-salt-added diced tomatoes, with juice	1
½ cup	chopped pitted black olives	125 mL
2 tbsp	finely chopped fresh parsley	30 mL

1. In a heavy saucepan with a tight-fitting lid, combine rice and broth. Bring to a rapid boil over high heat. Reduce heat to low. Cover and simmer until rice is tender to the bite, about 30 minutes. Remove from heat and set aside.

2. Meanwhile, in a skillet, heat oil over medium-high heat for 30 seconds. Add chicken, in batches, and cook, turning once, until nicely browned, about 5 minutes per batch. Transfer to a plate and set aside. Drain off all but 2 tbsp (30 mL) fat from pan.

3. Reduce heat to medium. Add onions, bell peppers, chile pepper and garlic and cook, stirring, until peppers have softened, about 5 minutes. Add paprika, salt and peppercorns and cook, stirring, for 1 minute. Add tomatoes with juice and bring to a boil. Cook, stirring, until mixture amalgamates and some of the liquid evaporates, about 2 minutes. Stir in rice with liquid and boil for 1 minute. Stir in olives and parsley. Transfer to baking dish and arrange chicken over top. Cover and bake in preheated oven until rice is tender and chicken is no longer pink, about 40 minutes.

Chicken Cacciatore

Makes 4 to 6 servings

Traditionally, this dish is prepared with mushrooms. If you wish, add 1 cup (250 mL) sliced mushrooms when sautéing the vegetables.

Tip

This meal is an excellent source of vitamins A and C, protein, niacin, iron and selenium.

2 tsp	grapeseed oil	10 mL
1½ lbs	boneless skinless chicken thighs	750 g
½ cup	chopped onion	125 mL
½ cup	chopped red bell pepper	125 mL
½ cup	chopped yellow bell pepper	125 mL
1 tsp	dried thyme	5 mL
1 tsp	dried basil	5 mL
1 tsp	dried marjoram	5 mL
2 cups	ready-to-use reduced-sodium gluten-free chicken or vegetable broth	500 mL
½ cup	tomato sauce	125 mL
	Salt and freshly ground black pepper	

1. In a large saucepan, heat oil over medium-high heat. Cook chicken for 5 minutes per side or until browned on both sides.

2. Reduce heat to medium. Add onion, red pepper, yellow pepper, thyme, basil and marjoram; sauté for 3 to 4 minutes or until softened.

3. Stir in broth and tomato sauce; bring to a boil, scraping up any brown bits from pan. Reduce heat to low, cover and simmer, stirring occasionally, for about 45 minutes or until stew is thickened and juices run clear when chicken is pierced. Season to taste with salt and pepper.

> **Dinner Idea:** To increase the calcium content, serve with quinoa pasta or Teff Polenta (page 304).

NUTRIENTS
PER SERVING

Calories	190
Fat	6 g
Carbohydrate	5 g
Fiber	2 g
Protein	29 g
Iron	2.7 mg
Calcium	34 mg

Spanish Chicken and Rice

This delicious meal uses ingredients you are likely to have on hand. It is high in protein and is an excellent source of vitamins A and C, niacin, iron and selenium. Thanks to the herbs and spices, it is also a source of antioxidants.

Tip

To microwave the rice: In an 8-cup (2 L) casserole dish, combine 2 cups (500 mL) broth and 1 cup (250 mL) long-grain white rice. Microwave, covered, on High for 4 to 6 minutes or until boiling. Microwave on Medium (50%) for 10 to 14 minutes or until most of the liquid is absorbed. Let stand for 10 minutes. Makes 3 cups (750 mL) rice.

2 cups	ready-to-use chicken broth	500 mL
1 cup	long-grain white rice	250 mL
1 lb	lean ground chicken, turkey or beef	500 g
1 tbsp	vegetable oil	15 mL
2	cloves garlic, finely chopped	2
1	small onion, finely chopped	1
1	green bell pepper, finely chopped	1
1	large stalk celery, finely chopped	1
1½ tsp	gluten-free chili powder	7 mL
1 tsp	dried oregano	5 mL
1 tsp	paprika	5 mL
½ tsp	salt	2 mL
¼ tsp	freshly ground black pepper	1 mL
1	can (14 oz/398 mL) diced tomatoes, with juice	1

1. In a medium saucepan, bring broth to a boil. Add rice, reduce heat, cover and simmer for 20 minutes or until liquid is absorbed and rice is tender.

2. In a large saucepan over medium-high heat, cook chicken, breaking up with a wooden spoon, for 5 minutes or until no longer pink. Transfer to a bowl.

3. Add oil to pan. Cook garlic, onion, green pepper, celery, chili powder, oregano, paprika, salt and pepper, stirring often, for 4 minutes or until vegetables are softened.

4. Return chicken to pan, along with tomatoes and their juice; bring to a boil. Reduce heat to medium-low, cover and simmer for 10 minutes or until vegetables are tender.

5. Stir in cooked rice. Cover and let stand for 5 minutes to blend the flavors.

NUTRIENTS PER SERVING

Calories 350
Fat . . . . .13 g
Carbohydrate . . . . .34 g
Fiber . . . . .3 g
Protein . . . . .24 g
Iron . . . . .3.1 mg
Calcium . . . . 62 mg

Dinner Idea: Serve this dish with a green-leaf lettuce salad on the side.

Italian-Style Chicken and Rice

This variation on the theme of chicken and rice is just as satisfying and tasty as the Spanish version on page 259. Try serving it with Veggie Kabobs (page 288).

Tips

Pancetta is a kind of Italian bacon, made from cured pork belly. It has a unique flavor, but if you can't find it, you can substitute an equal quantity of bacon.

This dish is high in protein and B vitamins, such as niacin and B_6. It is also a great source of phosphorus and selenium.

- **Preheat oven to 350°F (180°C)**
- **10-cup (2.5 L) baking dish with cover**

1 cup	short-grain brown rice	250 mL
2½ cups	ready-to-use reduced-sodium chicken broth or water	625 mL
1 tbsp	olive oil	15 mL
2 lbs	skin-on bone-in chicken breasts, cut into serving-size pieces, rinsed and patted dry	1 kg
2 oz	chunk of pancetta (see tip, at left), finely chopped	60 g
2	onions, thinly sliced on the vertical	2
4	cloves garlic, minced	4
2	dried red cayenne peppers	2
1 tbsp	finely grated lemon zest	15 mL
1½ tsp	dried Italian seasoning	7 mL
	Coarse sea salt	
	Freshly ground black pepper	
2 tbsp	freshly squeezed lemon juice	30 mL
	Extra virgin olive oil	

1. In a heavy saucepan with a tight-fitting lid, combine rice and broth. Bring to a rapid boil over high heat. Reduce heat to low. Cover and simmer for 15 minutes. Remove from heat and set aside.

2. Meanwhile, in a large skillet, heat oil over medium-high heat for 30 seconds. Add chicken, in batches, and cook, turning once, until nicely browned, about 5 minutes per batch. Transfer to a plate and set aside. Drain off all but 1 tbsp (15 mL) fat from pan.

3. Reduce heat to medium. Add pancetta and cook, stirring, for 2 minutes. Add onions and cook, stirring, until softened, about 3 minutes. Add garlic, dried peppers, lemon zest and Italian seasoning and cook, stirring, for 1 minute. Add reserved rice with liquid and bring to a boil.

4. Transfer to baking dish. Arrange chicken over top. Cover and bake in preheated oven until chicken is no longer pink inside and rice is tender, about 45 minutes. Remove and discard cayenne peppers.

5. Sprinkle chicken with sea salt and pepper to taste. Drizzle with lemon juice and olive oil.

NUTRIENTS
PER SERVING

Calories	370
Fat	17 g
Carbohydrate	33 g
Fiber	3 g
Protein	24 g
Iron	1.3 mg
Calcium	30 mg

Grilled Chicken Kabobs

Makes 4 servings

This simple yet delicious seasoned chicken is wonderful for a summer patio lunch or dinner!

• **Four 8- or 9-inch (20 or 23 cm) metal or wooden skewers**

2 to 3	cloves garlic, minced	2 to 3
1½ tbsp	olive oil	22 mL
1 tsp	dried parsley	5 mL
½ tsp	dried oregano	2 mL
1 lb	boneless skinless chicken breasts, cut into 1½-inch (4 cm) cubes	500 g
	Salt and freshly ground black pepper	

1. In a large sealable plastic bag, combine garlic to taste, oil, parsley and oregano. Add chicken, seal and toss to coat. Refrigerate for at least 6 hours or overnight.

2. Preheat barbecue grill to medium. If using wooden skewers, soak them in water for 10 minutes.

3. Remove chicken from marinade, discarding marinade. Thread chicken onto skewers, leaving space between pieces. Grill chicken, turning often, for 7 to 10 minutes per side or until chicken is no longer pink inside. Season to taste with salt and pepper.

> **Dinner Idea:** Serve this meal with Oven-Roasted Lemon Potatoes (page 292) and a tossed salad.

NUTRIENTS
PER SERVING

Calories	180
Fat	8 g
Carbohydrate	1 g
Fiber	0 g
Protein	24 g
Iron	0.6 mg
Calcium	12 mg

Light and Easy Chicken Chili

This lighter version of a classic meal is sure to bring comfort on cold winter nights. It is an excellent source of iron, folate, vitamin A and vitamin K, and a good source of calcium and other trace minerals.

Tip

Cumin is a spice of Egyptian descent. It is available as seeds and in ground form. The seeds are sometimes toasted whole and then ground, particularly for curry dishes.

1 tbsp	canola oil	15 mL
2 cups	chopped onions	500 mL
1 cup	chopped carrots	250 mL
1 cup	chopped celery	250 mL
1 cup	chopped red bell pepper	250 mL
2	cloves garlic, minced	2
1 lb	boneless skinless chicken breasts, cut into 1-inch (2.5 cm) cubes	500 g
2 to 3 tbsp	chili powder	30 to 45 mL
2 tsp	ground cumin	10 mL
1 tsp	dried oregano	5 mL
1/2 tsp	salt	2 mL
1/4 tsp	hot pepper flakes	1 mL
1	can (19 oz/540 mL) red kidney beans, drained and rinsed	1
1	can (19 oz/540 mL) chickpeas, drained and rinsed	1
1	can (28 oz/796 mL) diced tomatoes, with juice	1
1/4 cup	chopped fresh parsley	60 mL

1. In a large pot, heat oil over medium-high heat. Sauté onions, carrots, celery and red pepper for 4 to 5 minutes or until softened. Add garlic and sauté for 30 seconds.

2. Add chicken and cook, stirring occasionally, for 7 to 8 minutes or until starting to brown. Add chili powder, cumin, oregano, salt and hot pepper flakes; sauté for 1 to 2 minutes or until fragrant.

3. Stir in kidney beans, chickpeas and tomatoes; bring to a boil, stirring. Reduce heat and simmer, stirring occasionally, for 30 minutes or until sauce is slightly thickened and chicken is no longer pink inside. Serve garnished with parsley.

This recipe courtesy of Phyllis Quarrie.

Dinner Idea: Enjoy this chili with 1 slice of bread (page 196 or 197), or on its own with a tossed green salad.

NUTRIENTS
PER SERVING

Calories	251
Fat	4 g
Carbohydrate	34 g
Fiber	9 g
Protein	21 g
Iron	3.6 mg
Calcium	99 mg

Three-Bean Chili with Turkey

Makes 8 servings		

This filling chili boasts both flavor and nutritious ingredients. Serve it on its own or alongside a tossed green salad.

Tips

This chili is an excellent source of fiber, vitamin A, B vitamins (including folate) and some trace minerals, and a good source of calcium, magnesium and copper.

After emptying the tomatoes from the can, rinse the can with the water (the amount of water specified in step 2 is one full can) before adding it to the pan, to capture all the juices that cling to the sides.

A 19-oz (540 mL) can of beans will yield about 2 cups (500 mL) once the beans are drained and rinsed. If you have smaller or larger cans, you can use the volume called for or just add the amount from your can.

1 tsp	grapeseed oil	5 mL
1 lb	lean ground turkey	500 g
1	clove garlic, minced	1
1 cup	chopped onion	250 mL
1 cup	chopped celery	250 mL
1 cup	chopped carrots	250 mL
1	can (28 oz/796 mL) crushed tomatoes (see tip, at left)	1
2 cups	rinsed drained canned romano beans	500 mL
2 cups	rinsed drained canned black beans	500 mL
2 cups	rinsed drained canned lentils	500 mL
1 tsp	dried oregano	5 mL
1 tsp	cayenne pepper	5 mL
1/2 tsp	ground cumin	2 mL
1/2 tsp	ground coriander	2 mL
1/4 tsp	salt	1 mL

1. In a large saucepan, heat oil over medium-high heat. Cook turkey, breaking it up with the back of a spoon, for about 7 minutes or until no longer pink. Add garlic, onion, celery and carrots; sauté for 3 to 4 minutes or until tender.

2. Stir in tomatoes, $3\frac{1}{4}$ cups (800 mL) water, romano beans, black beans, lentils, oregano, cayenne, cumin, coriander and salt; bring to a boil. Cover, leaving lid ajar, reduce heat to low and simmer, stirring occasionally, for $1\frac{1}{2}$ hours to blend the flavors.

NUTRIENTS PER SERVING

Calories	260
Fat	5 g
Carbohydrate	33 g
Fiber	11 g
Protein	22 g
Iron	4.0 mg
Calcium	109 mg

Turkey Sausage with Lima Bean Medley

This weeknight dinner takes very little time to prepare. It is also very tasty and highly nutritious.

Tips

Vegetables of the Brassicae family, such as broccoli, chard, kale and collard greens, are sources of non-dairy calcium.

This meal is an excellent source of vitamin C, vitamin K and iron, a good source of fiber and trace minerals, and a source of calcium.

If you are sensitive to sulfites, replace the red wine vinegar with white vinegar.

2 tbsp	grapeseed oil	30 mL
1 lb	turkey sausages (about 4), removed from casings	500 g
1 cup	sliced mushrooms	250 mL
½ cup	chopped onion	125 mL
1 cup	frozen chopped broccoli	250 mL
1 cup	frozen lima beans	250 mL
1 tbsp	chopped fresh parsley	15 mL
1 tbsp	red wine vinegar	15 mL
	Salt and freshly ground black pepper	

1. In a large skillet, heat oil over medium heat. Cook sausage, breaking it up with the back of a spoon, for 7 to 10 minutes or until no longer pink. Using a slotted spoon, transfer to a plate lined with paper towels.

2. Add mushrooms and onion to skillet; sauté for about 5 minutes or until mushrooms are browned and crisp. Add broccoli, beans, parsley and vinegar; sauté for 5 to 8 minutes or until tender. Return sausage to skillet and simmer, stirring, until heated through. Season to taste with salt and pepper.

> **Dinner Idea:** To increase the absorption of iron from this meal, pair it with Asian Carrot Cucumber Pickle (page 234) or a green-leaf lettuce salad with oil-and-vinegar dressing.

NUTRIENTS PER SERVING

Calories	280
Fat	16 g
Carbohydrate	16 g
Fiber	4 g
Protein	19 g
Iron	3.0 mg
Calcium	59 mg

Sausage-Spiked Peas 'n' Rice

Makes 6 servings

This dish has a tempting combination of flavors and textures. And if you prepare it in the slow cooker, it'll be ready when you arrive home from work.

Tips

This dish is an excellent source of B vitamins, including folate and B_2, as well as trace minerals. It is a good source of fiber.

Make sure the sausage is free of allergens, such as wheat or soy.

You can cook the split peas yourself, reserving ¼ cup (60 mL) of the cooking liquid, or you can use a can (14 to 19 oz/398 to 540 mL) yellow split peas, rinsed and drained, plus ¼ cup (60 mL) water. The canned peas will be much higher in sodium than those you cook yourself.

If you have fresh thyme on hand, substitute 2 whole sprigs for the dried. Discard before serving.

2 cups	cooked yellow split peas, with ¼ cup (60 mL) cooking liquid (see tip, at left)	500 mL
1 tbsp	olive oil	15 mL
12 oz	hot or mild Italian sausage, removed from casings	375 g
1	bulb fennel, cored and chopped	1
1	onion, finely chopped	1
4	cloves garlic, minced	4
1 tsp	dried thyme (see tip, at left)	5 mL
	Freshly ground black pepper	
1 cup	brown and wild rice mixture, rinsed and drained	250 mL
2 cups	ready-to-use reduced-sodium chicken broth	500 mL

1. In a large saucepan with a tight-fitting lid or Dutch oven, heat oil over medium heat for 30 seconds. Add sausage, fennel and onion and cook, stirring and breaking sausage up with a spoon, until meat is cooked through, about 6 minutes. Add garlic, thyme, pepper to taste and rice and cook, stirring, for 1 minute. Stir in peas with reserved liquid and broth and bring to a boil.

Stovetop Method

2. Reduce heat to low. Cover tightly and simmer until grains of wild rice begin to split, about 50 minutes. Ladle into soup plates.

Slow Cooker Method

2. Complete step 1. Transfer mixture to slow cooker stoneware. Cover and cook on Low for 8 hours or on High for 4 hours, until wild rice is tender and grains begin to split.

> **Dinner Idea:** Pair this meal with Baked Portobello Mushrooms (page 285) or 1 cup (250 mL) steamed dark leafy greens, such as spinach or bok choy.

NUTRIENTS
PER SERVING

Calories	410
Fat	16 g
Carbohydrate	48 g
Fiber	9 g
Protein	18 g
Iron	2.7 mg
Calcium	74 mg

Mushroom, Sausage and Wild Rice Stir-Fry

Makes 6 servings

Stir-frying is a quick and easy way to prepare a nutritious meal when you are pressed for time. This dish is an excellent source of vitamin C, B vitamins and trace minerals.

Tips

Butter is lactose-free, but if you have an allergy to cow's milk protein, substitute a non-dairy, soy-free alternative.

Use half long-grain brown and half wild rice or a packaged blend of brown and wild rice. Cook according to package directions.

Use hot or mild Italian sausage to suit your taste. Make sure it's free of allergens, such as wheat or soy.

3 cups	cooked brown and wild rice mixture (see tip, at left)	750 mL
1 tbsp	butter	15 mL
1 lb	mushrooms, thinly sliced	500 g
	Salt and freshly ground black pepper	
1 tbsp	freshly squeezed lemon juice	15 mL
1 tbsp	olive oil	15 mL
8 oz	Italian sausage (see tip, at left), removed from casings	250 g
1	onion, finely chopped	1
2	red bell peppers, finely chopped	2
4	cloves garlic, minced	4
1 tbsp	dried Italian seasoning	15 mL
1/2 cup	dry white wine or ready-to-use chicken broth	125 mL

1. In a large skillet, melt butter over medium-high heat. Add mushrooms and cook, stirring, until they release their liquid, about 7 minutes. Continue to cook until most of the liquid evaporates, about 2 minutes. Remove from heat. Season to taste with salt and black pepper and stir in lemon juice. Transfer to a bowl. Return skillet to medium heat.

2. Add oil to pan and heat for 30 seconds. Add sausage, onion, bell peppers and garlic. Cook, stirring and breaking sausage up with a spoon, until vegetables are very tender and sausage is no longer pink, about 7 minutes. Add Italian seasoning and cook, stirring, for 1 minute. Add wine and bring to a boil. Cook until reduced by half, about 2 minutes. Stir in rice and reserved mushrooms and cook until heated through, about 3 minutes.

Lunch Idea: For a complete meal, enjoy 1/2 serving of this dish with 1 serving of Summer Fruit Compote (page 314).

NUTRIENTS
PER SERVING

Calories 290
Fat . . . . 13 g
Carbohydrate . . . . 33 g
Fiber . . . . 4 g
Protein . . . . 11 g
Iron . . . . 1.4 mg
Calcium . . . . 57 mg

Hawaiian Pizza

This pizza is quick and easy to put together. Serve it with a tossed green salad to complete a nutritious meal.

Tips

Keep one of these pizzas wrapped airtight in the freezer for up to 1 month, for when you are invited to a pizza party. Reheat in a 400°F (200°C) oven for 12 to 15 minutes or until cheese is bubbly and crust is crisp.

Cut into bite-size appetizers or wedges for your next party.

Variations

Substitute Asiago, fontina or provolone cheese for the mozzarella. All of these cheeses are lactose-free. If you have an allergy to cow's milk protein, substitute a non-dairy alternative.

Replace the ham with 1 cup (250 mL) of cooked cubed chicken.

NUTRIENTS
PER SERVING

Calories	461
Fat	20 g
Carbohydrate	41 g
Fiber	4 g
Protein	29 g
Iron	2.0 mg
Calcium	451 mg

• **Preheat oven to 400°F (200°C)**

1	partially baked Thin Pizza Crust (page 201), at room temperature	1
½ cup	gluten-free pizza sauce	125 mL
¾ cup	cubed gluten-free cooked ham	175 mL
½ cup	drained pineapple tidbits	125 mL
⅓ cup	thinly sliced green bell pepper	75 mL
1 cup	shredded mozzarella cheese	250 mL

1. Spread sauce over crust to within $\frac{1}{4}$ inch (0.5 cm) of the edges. Sprinkle with ham, pineapple, green pepper and mozzarella.

2. Bake in preheated oven for 20 to 25 minutes or until cheese is bubbly and crust is golden. Transfer to a cutting board and cut into wedges. Serve immediately. Transfer any extra wedges to a wire rack to prevent the crust from getting soggy.

Roast Pork with Red Rice and Beans

This yummy, nutritious dish is great for a special family occasion. It is an excellent source of protein, fiber, B vitamins, iron, magnesium and manganese. Serve it on a bed of collard greens, seasoned with a bit of oil and vinegar, to boost the calcium content of the meal.

Tips

The cooking time for red rice depends upon the variety you use. These instructions work for longer-cooking varieties, such as Camargue and Wehani. Thai red rice should be added to the beans after they have cooked for 30 minutes in total. If you're using quick-cooking Bhutanese red rice, add it to the beans after they have cooked for 45 minutes in total.

You can also make this recipe using a single-loin roast of the same weight, in which case it will cook more quickly, in about 1 hour.

NUTRIENTS PER SERVING

Calories 390
Fat . . . . 7 g
Carbohydrate . . . . 45 g
Fiber . . . . 7 g
Protein . . . . 37 g
Iron . . . . 4.8 mg
Calcium . . . . 71 mg

- **Roasting pan**

1½ cups	red rice, rinsed and drained (see tip, at left)	375 mL
1½ cups	dried navy beans	375 mL
5 cups	ready-to-use reduced-sodium chicken broth, divided	1.25 L
1 tbsp	coarse salt	15 mL
1 tbsp	herbes de Provence	15 mL
6	cloves garlic, finely grated or put through a press	6
1 tsp	cracked black peppercorns	5 mL
1 tbsp	olive oil (approx.)	15 mL
3 lbs	boneless pork double-loin roast, trimmed and tied (see tip, at left)	1.5 kg
3	leeks (white and light green parts only), thinly sliced (see tip, page 218)	3
6	stalks celery, diced	6
30	fresh sage leaves, finely chopped	30
2 tsp	poultry seasoning	10 mL
1 tsp	paprika	5 mL
1 cup	dry white wine	250 mL
1 tbsp	demi-glace concentrate (optional)	15 mL
	Salt and freshly ground black pepper	

1. In a bowl, combine red rice with 2½ cups (625 mL) water. Set aside for 1 hour.

2. In a large saucepan over medium-high heat, combine beans and 4 cups (1 L) water. Bring to a boil and boil rapidly for 3 minutes. Remove from heat and let stand for 1 hour. Drain and rinse thoroughly under cold running water. Return to saucepan and add 4 cups (1 L) of the broth. Bring to a boil. Reduce heat to low and simmer, uncovered, for 15 minutes. Add red rice with soaking liquid and bring to boil. Cover and cook until rice and beans are tender, about 50 minutes.

3. In a separate bowl, combine coarse salt, herbes de Provence, garlic and peppercorns. Mix well and stir in 1 tbsp (15 mL) olive oil. Rub all over pork. Place pork in a roasting pan and set aside at room temperature for 30 minutes.

Tips

If you are sensitive to sulfites, replace the wine with chicken or vegetable broth.

Demi-glace concentrate is available in specialty stores and well-stocked supermarkets. This dish is tasty without it, but it adds luscious depth to the rice and bean mixture.

Variation

Substitute an equal quantity of dried flageolet for the navy beans. They are slightly sweeter and more buttery and are available in well-stocked supermarkets and specialty stores.

4. Meanwhile, preheat oven to 350°F (180°C). Roast pork in preheated oven until an instant-read thermometer inserted into the thickest part of the meat registers 160°F (71°C), about 1 hour and 15 minutes. Transfer to a platter, cover loosely with foil and keep warm. Drain off all but 2 tbsp (30 mL) of the fat in roasting pan (or, if necessary, add olive oil to make 2 tbsp/30 mL), and place roasting pan on stove over medium heat.

5. Add leeks, celery and sage to roasting pan and cook, stirring, until vegetables are very soft, about 10 minutes. Add poultry seasoning and paprika and stir well. Increase heat to high and add wine and remaining 1 cup (250 mL) of chicken stock. Cook, stirring, until reduced by half, about 3 minutes. Add demi-glace concentrate, if using, and any juice from the pork that has collected on the platter, and cook, stirring, until concentrate has completely dissolved. Add beans and rice with cooking liquid and cook, stirring, to meld flavors, about 5 minutes. Season to taste with salt and pepper.

6. *To serve:* Spread rice and beans on a large deep platter. Slice pork thinly and lay on top.

Dinner Idea: Serve this dish with Sweet-and-Spicy Cabbage (page 282).

Pork Tenderloin

Makes 8 servings

Here's a dish that's perfect for a special family event. The ruby red color of the cranberry sauce makes for an appetizing presentation.

Tip

This dish provides low-fat protein and is an excellent source of vitamin C.

- **Preheat oven to 450°F (230°C)**
- **Large, heavy-bottomed ovenproof skillet**

2 lbs	pork tenderloin, trimmed	1 kg
	Salt and freshly ground black pepper	
1/3 cup	olive oil, divided	75 mL
1 1/3 cups	canned whole-berry cranberry sauce	325 mL
1 cup	ready-to-use gluten-free vegetarian chicken-flavored broth	250 mL
1/4 cup	balsamic vinegar	60 mL
2 tbsp	chopped fresh rosemary	30 mL

1. Sprinkle pork all over with salt and pepper. In skillet, heat 1/4 cup (60 mL) of the oil over medium-high heat. Sear pork for 2 minutes on each side. Transfer skillet to preheated oven and bake, uncovered, for 35 minutes or until a meat thermometer inserted in the thickest part of the tenderloin registers 160°F (71°C).

2. Meanwhile, in a small saucepan, heat the remaining oil over medium-high heat. Whisk in cranberry sauce, broth, vinegar and rosemary for about 2 minutes or until cranberry sauce has melted. Reduce heat to low and keep warm.

3. Transfer pork to a cutting board. Cover with foil and let rest for 10 minutes.

4. Pour cooking juices and any scrapings from skillet into cranberry mixture and bring to a boil over medium heat. Cook, stirring occasionally, for 15 to 20 minutes or until thickened enough to generously coat a spoon. Season to taste with salt and pepper.

5. Slice pork and serve with sauce.

Dinner Idea: Pair this dish with Oven-Baked Potato Wedges (page 291).

NUTRIENTS
PER SERVING

Calories	251
Fat	7 g
Carbohydrate	20 g
Fiber	1 g
Protein	26 g
Iron	1.0 mg
Calcium	12 mg

Pork Tenderloin with Rhubarb Chutney

Rhubarb boasts many nutritional qualities and has a delicate tart taste. The delightful rhubarb chutney pairs extremely well with pork. Serve this dish with Butternut Squash with Snow Peas and Red Pepper (page 287).

Tips

This dish provides low-fat protein, is an excellent source of zinc and B vitamins, and is a good source of magnesium.

If you are sensitive to sulfites, replace the white wine vinegar with white vinegar.

Variation

Replace half the rhubarb with sliced strawberries to make strawberry rhubarb chutney.

NUTRIENTS
PER SERVING

Calories	296
Fat	3 g
Carbohydrate	41 g
Fiber	3 g
Protein	27 g
Iron	3.1 mg
Calcium	113 mg

- **Preheat oven to 375°F (190°C)**
- **Small roasting pan, greased**

Rhubarb Chutney

¾ cup	granulated sugar	175 mL
2 tbsp	minced gingerroot	30 mL
2 tbsp	minced garlic (about 6 cloves)	30 mL
2 tsp	ground cumin	10 mL
1 tsp	ground cinnamon	5 mL
1 tsp	ground cloves	5 mL
½ tsp	hot pepper flakes	2 mL
⅓ cup	white wine vinegar	75 mL
½	red onion, chopped	½
4 cups	chopped rhubarb	1 L
⅓ cup	raisins	75 mL

Pork

1 tbsp	ground cumin	15 mL
1 tsp	garlic powder	5 mL
½ tsp	freshly ground black pepper	2 mL
2	pork tenderloins (each about 12 oz/375 g), trimmed	2

1. *Chutney:* In a large saucepan, combine sugar, ginger, garlic, cumin, cinnamon, cloves, hot pepper flakes and vinegar. Bring to a simmer over medium heat, stirring occasionally, until sugar dissolves. Stir in red onion, rhubarb and raisins; bring to a boil, stirring often. Reduce heat and simmer, stirring occasionally, for about 20 minutes or until rhubarb is tender and mixture thickens and becomes syrupy.

2. *Pork:* Meanwhile, in a small bowl, combine cumin, garlic powder and pepper. Rub all over tenderloin. Place pork in prepared roasting pan. Roast in preheated oven for 20 minutes. Spread half the chutney over pork. Roast for 5 to 10 minutes or until a meat thermometer inserted in the thickest part of the tenderloin registers 155°F (68°C). Transfer to a cutting board, tent with foil and let rest for 5 to 10 minutes to allow juices to redistribute and pork to reach an internal temperature of 160°F (71°C).

3. Cut tenderloin crosswise into thin slices and serve with the remaining chutney.

This recipe courtesy of dietitian Jennifer Miller.

Stewed Pork with Greens

Dark leafy greens, such as bok choy, rapini and collard greens, are a good source of non-dairy calcium. They also pair very well with pork.

Tips

This dish provides a good amount of low-fat protein and is a good source of vitamin A, calcium, iron and other trace minerals.

A medium lemon yields about 3 tbsp (45 mL) lemon juice.

Variation

Substitute cubed stewing beef for the pork.

- **Large, heavy-bottomed pot with tight-fitting lid or Dutch oven**

1 tbsp	olive oil	15 mL
1 lb	boneless pork shoulder, cubed	500 g
1	can (14 oz/398 mL) diced tomatoes, with juice	1
3 cups	ready-to-use gluten-free vegetable broth	750 mL
2 cups	coarsely chopped trimmed green beans	500 mL
1 cup	coarsely chopped bok choy	250 mL
$\frac{1}{4}$ cup	freshly squeezed lemon juice	60 mL
	Salt	

1. In large pot, heat oil over medium-high heat. Cook pork, turning, for 10 to 15 minutes or until browned all over. Using tongs, remove pork and set aside. Drain fat from pot.

2. Return pork to pot and add tomatoes and juice, broth, green beans, bok choy, lemon juice and salt to taste. Bring to a boil over medium-high heat and cook for 2 to 3 minutes. Reduce heat to medium-low, cover and cook, stirring occasionally, for about $1\frac{1}{2}$ to 2 hours or until pork is very tender.

3. With a slotted spoon, transfer solids to a bowl, cover with foil and keep warm. Increase heat to high, bring cooking liquid to a boil and simmer until reduced to 1 cup (250 mL) or less.

4. Return solids to cooking liquid. Reduce heat to medium and cook, gently stirring, until heated through.

> **Dinner Idea:** Pair this dish with Lightened-Up Scalloped Potatoes (page 296).

NUTRIENTS PER SERVING

Calories	140
Fat	7 g
Carbohydrate	7 g
Fiber	2 g
Protein	13 g
Iron	2.0 mg
Calcium	53 mg

Beef with Cumin and Lime

Lime juice adds extra tanginess to this Mexican-inspired dish. Serve on a bed of rice or, for a nice change of pace, with vegetables in a gluten-free tortilla.

Tip

This dish is very high in zinc, vitamin B_{12} and niacin, and is a good source of magnesium and other B vitamins.

1 tsp	ground cumin	5 mL
1/4 tsp	salt	1 mL
1/4 tsp	freshly ground black pepper	1 mL
1/8 tsp	cayenne pepper	0.5 mL
1 tsp	olive oil	5 mL
2 lbs	stewing beef, cubed	1 kg
1 cup	water	250 mL
2	whole cloves	2
1 tbsp	freshly squeezed lime juice	15 mL
1/4 cup	chopped fresh cilantro	60 mL

1. In a small bowl, stir together cumin, salt, pepper and cayenne.

2. In a large nonstick skillet, heat oil over medium-high heat. Brown beef on all sides. Sprinkle cumin mixture over beef and stir in cloves, water and lime juice. Reduce heat to medium, cover and simmer, adding more water if mixture becomes dry, for 1 hour or until beef is tender.

3. Remove and discard cloves. Using a slotted spoon, transfer beef to a plate. Cover with foil and keep warm. Increase heat to high and boil cooking liquid for 5 to 10 minutes or until reduced to 1/4 cup (60 mL). Stir in cilantro. Divide beef evenly among 8 individual serving plates. Spoon sauce on top.

> **Dinner Idea:** For a comforting meal, serve this dish with Yam Fries (page 289).

NUTRIENTS
PER SERVING

Calories 171
Fat . . . . .9 g
Carbohydrate . . . . .1 g
Fiber . . . . .0 g
Protein . . . . .22 g
Iron . . . . .3.0 mg
Calcium . . . . 12 mg

Orange Ginger Beef

Makes 4 servings

Ginger, garlic and orange make a great combination in this stir-fry. Hoisin sauce contains many allergens, including sesame, soy and wheat, so omit it if you have allergies or intolerances to these ingredients.

Tips

This dish is very high in zinc, vitamin B_{12} and niacin, and is a good source of magnesium and other B vitamins.

If you are allergic to corn, replace the cornstarch with tapioca starch.

Eye of round is a lean cut of beef. Marinating it before cooking maximizes its tenderness.

Be sure not to crowd the beef while sautéing it, or it will steam instead of brown. You may need to brown it in three batches if you have a smaller skillet.

Variation

Use trimmed snow peas instead of mushrooms.

2 tbsp	minced gingerroot	30 mL
1 tbsp	minced garlic	15 mL
1 tsp	freshly ground black pepper	5 mL
2 tbsp	canola oil, divided	30 mL
1 tbsp	hoisin sauce	15 mL
1 lb	beef eye of round marinating steak, cut into 3- by $\frac{1}{2}$-inch (7.5 by 1 cm) strips	500 g
1 tbsp	cornstarch	15 mL
1 tbsp	grated orange zest	15 mL
$\frac{3}{4}$ cup	orange juice	175 mL
2 cups	quartered mushrooms	500 mL
2 tbsp	chopped fresh cilantro	30 mL

1. In a shallow bowl, combine ginger, garlic, pepper, 1 tbsp (15 mL) of the oil and hoisin sauce. Add beef and stir to coat well. Cover and refrigerate for at least 4 hours or up to 12 hours.

2. Drain marinade from beef, discarding marinade. Pat beef strips dry with paper towels. Heat a large nonstick skillet over medium heat. Add half the beef and sauté for 3 to 4 minutes or until lightly browned. Transfer to a bowl and set aside. Repeat with the remaining beef.

3. In a small bowl, whisk together cornstarch and orange juice.

4. Add the remaining oil to skillet and sauté mushrooms for 3 to 4 minutes or until lightly browned. Return beef and accumulated juices to skillet. Stir in cornstarch mixture and cook, stirring, for about 3 minutes or until sauce is thickened. Serve garnished with orange zest and cilantro.

This recipe courtesy of dietitian Jennifer Garus.

Dinner Idea: Pair each serving of this dish with 1 to 2 cups (250 to 500 mL) steamed or sautéed broccoli and 1 cup (250 mL) cooked quinoa.

NUTRIENTS PER SERVING

Calories 269
Fat . . . . 12 g
Carbohydrate. . . . . 12 g
Fiber . . . . 1 g
Protein. . . . . 28 g
Iron . . . . 2.2 mg
Calcium . . . . 24 mg

Skillet Shepherd's Pie

This no-fuss version of the traditional dish requires hardly any cleanup — perfect for busy weeknights.

Tips

This dish is very high in zinc, vitamin B_{12}, vitamin K and niacin, and is a good source of calcium, iron, magnesium and other trace minerals.

Whenever you can, try to use beef from locally raised, grass-fed cattle.

For the frozen vegetables, try a combination of small-cut carrots, corn, beans and peas.

You can leave the skins on the potatoes if you prefer. It adds more fiber to the dish and makes it look hearty and comforting.

- **Large ovenproof skillet**

1 lb	potatoes, peeled and chopped	500 g
1/4 cup	enriched gluten-free non-dairy milk or lactose-free 1% milk	60 mL
2 tbsp	non-dairy, soy-free margarine or butter	30 mL
1 cup	shredded reduced-fat Cheddar cheese or Cheddar-style rice cheese	250 mL
1 lb	extra-lean ground beef	500 g
1/2 cup	chopped onion	125 mL
1	clove garlic, minced	1
1 tbsp	chopped fresh parsley	15 mL
2 tsp	dried basil	10 mL
1 cup	frozen mixed vegetables	250 mL

1. Place potatoes in a large pot and add enough water to cover. Bring to a boil over high heat. Reduce heat to medium-low and boil for 15 to 20 minutes or until potatoes are tender.

2. Drain potatoes and return to pot. Add milk and margarine; using a potato masher, mash potatoes until smooth. Stir in cheese and set aside.

3. In ovenproof skillet, cook beef over medium-high heat, breaking it up with the back of a spoon, for 7 minutes or until no longer pink. Add onion, garlic, parsley and basil; cook, stirring, for 3 to 4 minutes or until tender. Add mixed vegetables and cook, stirring, for 5 minutes. Meanwhile, preheat broiler.

4. Spread mashed potatoes on top of beef mixture. Broil for 5 to 10 minutes or until potatoes are golden.

> **Dinner Idea:** Pair this dish with a tossed green salad.

NUTRIENTS PER SERVING

Calories 370
Fat . . . . .13 g
Carbohydrate . . . . .31 g
Fiber . . . . .3 g
Protein . . . . .33 g
Iron . . . . .3.2 mg
Calcium . . . . 178 mg

Spaghetti Sauce

Spaghetti is a mainstay in many households. Here's a sauce recipe than can be frozen and used as the base for a quick, nutritious dinner when you are rushed.

Tip

This recipe is very high in vitamin B_{12} and high in iron, niacin and zinc.

12 oz	lean ground beef	375 g
1	small onion, chopped	1
1	clove garlic, minced	1
1	can (19 oz/540 mL) stewed tomatoes, with juice, chopped	1
1	can (5½ oz/156 mL) tomato paste	1
¼ cup	chopped green bell pepper	60 mL
1 tbsp	dried basil	15 mL
½ tsp	crushed fennel seeds	2 mL
Pinch	freshly ground black pepper	Pinch

1. In a large skillet, over medium heat, brown ground beef, breaking up chunks. Add onion, garlic, tomatoes, tomato paste, green pepper, basil, fennel seeds and pepper; bring to a boil. Reduce heat and simmer, stirring occasionally, for 20 to 30 minutes or until vegetables are tender and flavor is well developed.

This recipe courtesy of dietitian Judy Jenkins.

Dinner Idea: Ladle each serving of sauce over 1 cup (250 mL) cooked quinoa pasta or rice bran pasta. Serve Health Salad (page 233) on the side.

NUTRIENTS
PER ½ CUP (125 ML)

Calories	114
Fat	5 g
Carbohydrate	8 g
Fiber	2 g
Protein	8 g
Iron	2.1 mg
Calcium	37 mg

Stuffed Cabbage Rolls

Cabbage rolls are a common meal in the Balkans and parts of Eastern Europe. Large batches are usually cooked at once, and leftovers are frozen to be enjoyed at a later time.

Tips

This dish provides a good amount of protein, is an excellent source of vitamin C, niacin, vitamin B_{12}, iron and trace minerals, and is a good source of calcium.

Traditionally, cabbage rolls are served with a dollop of sour cream. If you have an allergy to cow's milk protein, use a non-dairy alternative.

Cooked cabbage rolls can be frozen for up to 2 months.

If inner cabbage leaves are not softened, blanch cabbage again in boiling water to soften leaves.

NUTRIENTS
PER SERVING

Calories	260
Fat	6 g
Carbohydrate	32 g
Fiber	6 g
Protein	19 g
Iron	3.4 mg
Calcium	121 mg

- **Preheat oven to 350°F (180°C)**
- **Food processor**
- **12-cup (3 L) casserole dish**

1	head green cabbage, cored (about 3 lbs/1.5 kg)	1
1 tbsp	vegetable oil	15 mL
1	large onion, finely chopped	1
2	large cloves garlic, finely chopped	2
1 tsp	paprika	5 mL
1½ cups	cooked rice	375 mL
1 lb	lean ground beef	500 g
	Salt and freshly ground black pepper	
1	can (28 oz/796 mL) plum tomatoes, including juice	1
2 tsp	packed brown sugar	10 mL

1. In a large pot of boiling salted water, cook cabbage for 5 to 6 minutes or until leaves are softened. Drain, rinse under cold water, carefully separating 12 leaves. Using a knife, trim coarse veins from cabbage leaves.

2. In a large saucepan, heat oil over medium heat; cook onion, garlic and paprika, stirring, for 5 minutes or until softened. In a bowl, combine half the onion mixture, rice, beef, ½ tsp (2 mL) salt and ½ tsp (2 mL) pepper; mix well.

3. In food processor, purée tomatoes including juice. Add with brown sugar to the remaining onion mixture in saucepan; bring to a boil. Cover and reduce heat; simmer for 15 minutes, stirring occasionally. Season with salt and pepper to taste.

4. Spoon ¼ cup (60 mL) rice mixture onto each cabbage leaf just above stem. Fold ends and sides over filling; roll up. Spoon 1 cup (250 mL) tomato sauce in bottom of casserole dish. Layer with half the cabbage rolls; pour 1 cup (250 mL) tomato sauce over. Top with the remaining cabbage rolls and pour the remaining sauce over. Cover and bake in preheated oven for 1 to 1¼ hours or until rolls are tender.

Dinner Idea: Enjoy this dish with a slice of bread (page 196 or 197) on the side.

Lamb Tagine with Chickpeas and Apricots

This Moroccan-style stew is accented with rich spices. Serve over millet or brown rice couscous.

Tips

This dish is an excellent source of vitamin A, niacin, vitamin B_{12}, iron, zinc and other trace minerals.

Buy a 3-lb (1.5 kg) leg of lamb or shoulder roast to get $1\frac{1}{2}$ lbs (750 g) boneless lamb.

To cook this in a slow cooker, follow step 1 and transfer lamb to slow cooker. Follow step 2, then stir in tomatoes and broth; bring to a boil. Transfer to slow cooker. Cover and cook on Low for 6 hours or on High for 3 hours, until almost tender. Add chickpeas, apricots and honey. Cover and cook on Low for 1 hour or on High for 30 minutes.

If you are sensitive to sulfites, make sure the dried apricots or figs have no added sulfites.

NUTRIENTS
PER SERVING

Calories	390
Fat	13 g
Carbohydrate	40 g
Fiber	6 g
Protein	29 g
Iron	4.0 mg
Calcium	73 mg

2 tbsp	olive oil (approx.)	30 mL
$1\frac{1}{2}$ lbs	lean boneless lamb, cut into 1-inch (2.5 cm) cubes	750 g
5	carrots, peeled and thickly sliced	5
1	large onion, chopped	1
3	cloves garlic, finely chopped	3
1 tsp	ground ginger	5 mL
1 tsp	ground cumin	5 mL
1 tsp	ground cinnamon	5 mL
1 tsp	ground turmeric	5 mL
$\frac{1}{2}$ tsp	salt	2 mL
$\frac{1}{2}$ tsp	freshly ground black pepper	2 mL
1	can (14 oz/398 mL) diced tomatoes, with juice	1
1 cup	ready-to-use chicken broth (approx.)	250 mL
1	can (19 oz/540 mL) chickpeas, rinsed and drained	1
$\frac{1}{2}$ cup	dried apricots or figs, roughly chopped	125 mL
$\frac{1}{4}$ cup	liquid honey	60 mL

1. In a Dutch oven, heat 1 tbsp (15 mL) oil over medium-high heat. Brown lamb, in batches, adding more oil as needed. Transfer to a plate as meat browns.

2. Reduce heat to medium. Add carrots, onion, garlic, ginger, cumin, cinnamon, turmeric, salt and pepper to pan; cook, stirring, for about 5 minutes or until onion is softened.

3. Add tomatoes, broth and lamb, along with any accumulated juices; bring to a boil. Reduce heat to medium-low, cover and simmer for $1\frac{1}{2}$ hours or until lamb is just tender.

4. Add chickpeas, apricots and honey. Add more broth, if necessary. Cover and simmer for 30 minutes or until lamb is very tender.

> **Dinner Idea:** Pair this dish with Exotic Spiced Roasties (page 294) or ladle each serving over 1 cup (250 mL) cooked millet or brown rice couscous.

Side Dishes

Stuffed Artichokes

Makes 4 servings

This delicious side dish is the perfect accompaniment for grilled poultry. It's an excellent source of fiber, vitamin C, folate and vitamin K, a good source of iron, magnesium and manganese, and a source of calcium.

Tips

Not only are artichokes a great source of iron and fiber, but they're also a great deal of fun to eat. Peel off one petal, place it between your teeth and pull, leaving the tender part in your mouth and discarding the unwanted leaf. When you reach the center, discard the choke and enjoy the tender base.

The cooking time depends on the size of the artichoke. When choosing your artichokes, make sure they are all the same size, so they'll all be done at the same time.

8	small artichokes (about 1 lb/500 g)	8
	Lemon wedges	
1/2 cup	gluten-free cracker crumbs	125 mL
2 to 3	cloves garlic, minced	2 to 3
2 tsp	dried parsley	10 mL
	Salt and freshly ground black pepper	
2 tbsp	olive oil	30 mL

1. Cut the stems off the artichokes, creating a flat base. Trim off the tough outer leaves. Cut about 1/2 inch (1 cm) off the tops, then use scissors to snip off the sharp leaf tips. Push open the leaves and rinse. Rub all cut surfaces with lemon.

2. In a small bowl, combine cracker crumbs, garlic to taste and parsley. Season with salt and pepper to taste. Stir in oil to make a paste.

3. Stuff artichokes with cracker mixture and place upright in a large pot. Add enough water to come halfway up artichokes. Cover and bring to a boil over high heat. Reduce heat to low and simmer for 45 minutes or until tender.

> **Lunch Idea:** Enjoy 2 stuffed artichokes with 1 serving of Millet Salad with Lemony Chickpeas and Tomatoes (page 239).
>
> **Dinner Idea:** Pair this dish with Mushroom, Sausage and Wild Rice Stir-Fry (page 266).

NUTRIENTS
PER SERVING

Calories 180
Fat . . . . .9 g
Carbohydrate . . . . .22 g
Fiber . . . . .8 g
Protein . . . . .5 g
Iron . . . . .2.0 mg
Calcium . . . . 74 mg

Cumin Beets

Makes 4 to 6 servings

Beets are closely related to quinoa, Swiss chard and spinach. Their ruby red color is an indication of very high antioxidant content. They are also delicious and enhance the visual appeal of any meal.

Tips

This dish is an excellent source of folate, magnesium and manganese.

Peeling the beets before they are cooked ensures that all the delicious cooking juices end up on your plate.

If you prefer a spicy dish, add hot pepper sauce, to taste, after the beets have finished cooking.

This recipe can be partially prepared up to 2 days ahead. Complete step 1, let cool, cover and refrigerate. When you're ready to cook, continue with step 2.

Small (about 2-quart) slow cooker

1 tbsp	vegetable oil	15 mL
1	onion, finely chopped	1
3	cloves garlic, minced	3
1 tsp	ground cumin	5 mL
1 tsp	salt	5 mL
½ tsp	freshly ground black pepper	2 mL
2	tomatoes, peeled and coarsely chopped	2
1 cup	water	250 mL
1 lb	beets, peeled and used whole, if small, or sliced thinly	500 g
	Hot pepper sauce (optional)	

1. In a skillet, heat oil over medium heat. Add onion and cook, stirring, until softened, about 3 minutes. Stir in garlic, cumin, salt and pepper and cook, stirring, for 1 minute. Add tomatoes and water and bring to a boil.

2. Place beets in slow cooker stoneware and pour tomato mixture over them. Cover and cook on Low for 8 hours or on High for 4 hours, until beets are tender. If desired, pass hot pepper sauce at the table.

> **Dinner Idea:** Serve this dish with Roast Pork with Red Rice and Beans (page 268).

NUTRIENTS PER SERVING

Calories	70
Fat	3 g
Carbohydrate	11 g
Fiber	3 g
Protein	2 g
Iron	1.0 mg
Calcium	27 mg

Sweet-and-Spicy Cabbage

Makes 4 servings

A new twist on a classic Oktoberfest mainstay, this side dish goes well with pork chops and roasts.

Tip

This dish is an excellent source of vitamin C and a good source of folate and calcium.

1	large pear or apple	1
2 tbsp	vegetable oil	30 mL
½	red onion, cut into thin wedges	½
½ tsp	hot pepper flakes, or to taste	2 mL
½	small savoy cabbage, finely shredded	½
2 tbsp	rice vinegar	30 mL
1 tbsp	liquid honey	15 mL
	Salt	

1. Cut pear into quarters and core (not necessary to peel). Thinly slice, then cut slices in half.
2. In a large nonstick skillet, heat oil over medium-high heat. When almost smoking, add pear, onion and hot pepper flakes; stir-fry for 1 minute. Add cabbage and stir-fry for 1 minute more or until wilted.
3. Stir in rice vinegar and honey; cook, stirring, for 30 seconds. Season with salt to taste; serve immediately.

> **Dinner Idea:** Serve this dish alongside Pork Tenderloin (page 270) or Stewed Pork with Greens (page 272).

NUTRIENTS
PER SERVING

Calories 130
Fat .7 g
Carbohydrate . . . . .17 g
Fiber . . . . .4 g
Protein . . . . .2 g
Iron . . . . .0.4 mg
Calcium . . . . 33 mg

Ginger Carrots

Here's a delicious way to enjoy carrots that will add a splash of color and a burst of flavor to any meal. A serving of these carrots provides an excellent source of vitamin A and a good source of fiber.

Tip

Use the side of a spoon to scrape the skin off gingerroot before chopping or grating. Gingerroot keeps well in the freezer for up to 3 months and can be grated from frozen.

4 cups	chopped carrots	1 L
½ cup	ready-to-use vegetable or chicken broth	125 mL
2 tsp	minced gingerroot	10 mL
1 tsp	minced garlic	5 mL
1 tsp	packed brown sugar	5 mL
¼ tsp	freshly squeezed lemon juice	1 mL

1. In a large saucepan, combine carrots, broth, ginger, garlic, brown sugar and lemon juice. Bring to a boil, then reduce heat, cover and simmer for about 20 minutes or until carrots are tender-crisp and liquid is absorbed.

This recipe courtesy of dietitian Roberta Lowcay.

Dinner Idea: Pair this dish with Fruity Sautéed Chicken (page 254).

NUTRIENTS PER SERVING

Calories 34
Fat .0 g
Carbohydrate. . . . . .8 g
Fiber . . . . .2 g
Protein. . . . . .1 g
Iron . . . . .0.3 mg
Calcium . . . . 25 mg

Fennel and Sun-Dried Tomatoes

Sautéed fennel has a mild licorice flavor. This side dish is an excellent source of fiber, vitamin C, manganese and potassium, and a good source of calcium, iron and other trace minerals.

Tips

If you have a sulfite sensitivity, look for sun-dried tomatoes with no added sulfites.

Fennel is well known for its ability to calm symptoms of irritable bowel syndrome.

1 tbsp	grapeseed oil	15 mL
1	fennel bulb, trimmed and cut into 1/4-inch (0.5 cm) thick slices	1
1/4 cup	sliced drained oil-packed sun-dried tomatoes	60 mL
1 tbsp	chopped fresh parsley	15 mL
	Salt and freshly ground black pepper	

1. In a skillet, heat oil over medium heat. Sauté fennel for 5 to 7 minutes or until tender and golden brown. Add sun-dried tomatoes and parsley; sauté for 1 minute. Season to taste with salt and pepper.

Dinner Idea: Serve this dish with Spanish Chicken and Rice (page 259) or Italian-Style Chicken and Rice (page 260).

NUTRIENTS PER SERVING

Calories	160
Fat	9 g
Carbohydrate	20 g
Fiber	8 g
Protein	4 g
Iron	2.0 mg
Calcium	119 mg

Baked Portobello Mushrooms

Makes 4 servings

Portobello mushrooms are extremely filling and satisfying. If you are not sensitive to sulfites, add a splash of red wine in the last 5 minutes of baking to spike the flavor quotient.

Tips

When removing the mushroom stem, carefully cut it out with a paring knife to leave the cap intact.

Portobello mushrooms are a good source of fiber, B vitamins (such as niacin, riboflavin and pantothenic acid), and the trace minerals copper and selenium. They also provide vitamin D_2 — a precursor of vitamin D_3, which helps the body absorb calcium.

- **13- by 9-inch (33 by 23 cm) glass baking dish, greased**

4	portobello mushrooms, cleaned and stems removed (see tip, at left)	4

Marinade

$1/4$ cup	olive oil	60 mL
2 tbsp	balsamic vinegar	30 mL
	Salt and freshly ground black pepper	

1. *Marinade:* In a small bowl, whisk together olive oil, balsamic vinegar and salt and pepper to taste.
2. Place mushrooms in prepared baking dish, gill side up, and pour marinade over top, making sure each mushroom cap is completely covered. Cover dish and refrigerate for 1 to 2 hours to allow mushrooms to absorb some of the marinade.
3. Preheat oven to 350°F (180°C). Drain off excess marinade. Bake mushrooms in preheated oven for 35 minutes or until soft.

Dinner Idea: Serve a whole baked mushroom on a bun or soft roll. If you have an allergy to wheat, celiac disease or gluten sensitivity, use a Gluten-Free, Egg-Free, Corn-Free, Dairy-Free, Soy-Free White Dinner Roll (page 198). If desired, top the mushroom with caramelized onions. (To caramelize onions, melt 2 tbsp/30 mL non-dairy margarine in a skillet over medium heat. Add 1 large onion, thinly sliced. Sprinkle with 1 tsp/5 mL granulated natural cane sugar and cook, stirring often, for 20 minutes or until onion is soft and lightly browned.)

NUTRIENTS
PER SERVING

Calories	150
Fat	14 g
Carbohydrate	5 g
Fiber	1 g
Protein	2 g
Iron	0.3 mg
Calcium	5 mg

Peas and Mushrooms

The combination of peas and mushrooms, popular in Italian dishes, works very well with sausages or pork.

Tip

This dish is an excellent source of fiber, vitamin A, vitamin K and selenium, and a good source of folate and other B vitamins, along with the trace minerals phosphorus, copper and manganese.

2 tbsp	olive or grapeseed oil	30 mL
8 oz	mushrooms, sliced	250 g
½ cup	chopped onion	125 mL
2 cups	frozen peas	500 mL
	Salt and freshly ground black pepper	

1. In a skillet, heat oil over medium-high heat. Sauté mushrooms and onion for 5 to 7 minutes or until browned. Add peas and sauté for 5 to 7 minutes or until heated through. Season to taste with salt and pepper.

Dinner Idea: Pair this side dish with Pork Tenderloin (page 270).

NUTRIENTS
PER SERVING

Calories	150
Fat	7 g
Carbohydrate	16 g
Fiber	5 g
Protein	6 g
Iron	1.5 mg
Calcium	32 mg

Butternut Squash with Snow Peas and Red Pepper

This easy stir-fry can be made in a flash. To save time, take advantage of pre-cut butternut squash from your grocery store's produce department.

Tips

To prepare the squash for this recipe: Peel squash using a vegetable peeler or paring knife. Cut into lengthwise quarters and seed. Cut into thin 1½- by ¼-inch (4 by 0.5 cm) pieces.

This dish is an excellent source of vitamin A, vitamin C and fiber, and a good source of B vitamins, including folate.

1 tbsp	vegetable oil	15 mL
5 cups	prepared butternut squash (see tip, at left)	1.25 L
4 oz	snow peas, ends trimmed	125 g
1	red bell pepper, cut into thin strips	1
1 tbsp	packed brown sugar	15 mL
1½ tsp	grated gingerroot	7 mL
	Salt and freshly ground black pepper	

1. In a large nonstick skillet, heat oil over medium-high heat. Cook squash, stirring, for 3 to 4 minutes or until almost tender.
2. Add snow peas, red pepper, brown sugar and ginger. Cook, stirring often, for 2 minutes or until vegetables are tender-crisp. Season with salt and pepper to taste.

> **Dinner Idea:** Serve this dish alongside Sausage-Spiked Peas 'n' Rice (page 265) or Italian-Style Chicken and Rice (page 260).

NUTRIENTS
PER SERVING

Calories	140
Fat	4 g
Carbohydrate	28 g
Fiber	5 g
Protein	3 g
Iron	2.0 mg
Calcium	101 mg

Veggie Kabobs

This dish is so colorful, so easy to make and so satisfying.

Tips

This dish is an excellent source of vitamin A, vitamin C, B vitamins and fiber, and a source of antioxidants.

Zucchini, which comes in green and yellow (or golden) versions, is a type of summer squash. These kabobs are prettiest when both colors are used, but you can use all of one or the other if you prefer.

The longer the marinating time, the deeper the flavors.

Any leftover veggies from these kabobs make a perfect beginning for tasty pasta dishes or salads.

Variation

Vary the flavor by replacing the oregano with the same quantity of thyme, basil or rosemary.

NUTRIENTS PER SERVING

Calories	90
Fat	7 g
Carbohydrate	7 g
Fiber	2 g
Protein	2 g
Iron	0.6 mg
Calcium	24 mg

- **Preheat grill or broiler**
- **16 bamboo or metal skewers**

$\frac{1}{3}$ cup	freshly squeezed lemon juice	75 mL
$\frac{1}{4}$ cup	olive oil	60 mL
1	clove garlic, minced (about 1 tsp/5 mL)	1
2 tsp	dried oregano (or 2 tbsp/30 mL finely chopped fresh)	10 mL
	Salt and freshly ground black pepper	
2	bell peppers (any color), cut into 1-inch (2.5 cm) strips	2
2	small zucchini, cut into 1-inch (2.5 cm) thick slices	2
2 cups	grape tomatoes or cherry tomatoes (about 16)	500 mL
2 cups	whole button mushrooms (about 16)	500 mL
1	large onion, cut into 8 wedges and halved crosswise, separated into single layers	1
1	yellow summer squash (such as golden zucchini), cut into 1-inch (2.5 cm) cubes	1

1. In a large bowl or sealable plastic bag, combine lemon juice, olive oil, garlic, oregano and salt and pepper to taste. Add peppers, zucchini, tomatoes, mushrooms, onion and squash and stir to evenly coat. Marinate at room temperature for 15 to 20 minutes or in the refrigerator for up to 12 hours.

2. Thread vegetables onto skewers, alternating to form an attractive pattern and leaving a bit of space between the pieces to allow air to circulate.

3. Grill or broil, turning and basting often with the remaining marinade, for 8 to 10 minutes or until vegetables are browned on all sides and tender. While cooking, rotate location of the skewers on the grill or broiler to ensure even cooking.

Dinner Idea: Serve this dish alongside any roast or barbecued poultry, pork or beef.

Yam Fries

Sweet yams are perfectly enhanced by cumin and coriander to make a delicious, nutritious alternative to french fries. Serve yam fries alongside any roast poultry dish.

Tips

Yams and sweet potatoes are entirely different vegetables, with different colors, flavors and textures. The skin of yams ranges from brown to black, while the flesh can be off-white, pale yellow, purple or red.

This dish is an excellent source of vitamin A and a good source of fiber, vitamin B_6, potassium and the trace mineral manganese.

- **Preheat oven to 425°F (220°C)**
- **Two rimmed baking sheets, lined with foil**

4	large yams, peeled	4
4 tsp	olive oil	20 mL
2 tsp	ground cumin	10 mL
2 tsp	ground coriander	10 mL
	Coarse salt and freshly ground black pepper	

1. Slice yams lengthwise into $\frac{1}{2}$-inch (1 cm) thick slices. Cut slices into sticks and, as you work, immediately transfer to prepared baking sheets, drizzle with oil and roll sticks to coat all over (to prevent yams from turning black). Arrange coated sticks in single layer on sheets.

2. In a small bowl, combine cumin, coriander and salt and pepper to taste. Sprinkle over yams.

3. Bake in preheated oven, gently stirring and turning after 15 minutes, for 25 to 30 minutes or until crisp on the outside. Serve immediately.

NUTRIENTS PER SERVING

Calories 160
Fat .5 g
Carbohydrate . . . . .27 g
Fiber . . . . .4 g
Protein . . . . .2 g
Iron . . . . .1.2 mg
Calcium . . . . 49 mg

Sage Potato Crisps

The rustic look and creamy texture of fingerling potatoes pair well with the slight velvety and peppery flavor of sage, resulting in a pretty side dish.

Tips

Sea salt has a much cleaner, crisper taste and a greater mineral content than refined table salt.

This dish is an excellent source of vitamin C and a good source of fiber, vitamin B_6, potassium and the trace mineral manganese.

- **Preheat oven to 375°F (190°C)**
- **Baking dish, large enough to accommodate 12 fingerling potato halves**

12	fingerling potatoes (about 1 lb/500 g), scrubbed	12
1 tsp	salt	5 mL
24	fresh sage leaves	24
1/3 cup	olive or canola oil	75 mL
	Salt and freshly ground black pepper	

1. Place potatoes in a large saucepan and add boiling water to barely cover. Add salt, cover loosely and bring to a boil over high heat. Reduce heat and cook for 8 to 10 minutes or until potatoes still offer some resistance when pierced with a small knife. Drain well. Set aside until cool enough to handle. Slice in half lengthwise, then press a sage leaf onto cut side of each half.

2. In baking dish, arrange potatoes cut side up and drizzle with oil. Bake in preheated oven for 15 minutes or until cooked through and golden brown. Using tongs, transfer to a plate lined with paper towels. Season to taste with salt and freshly ground pepper. Serve immediately.

> **Dinner Idea:** Pair these crisps with Grilled Chicken Kabobs (page 261) or Lemon Garlic Chicken (page 251).

NUTRIENTS PER SERVING

Calories	250
Fat	14 g
Carbohydrate	27 g
Fiber	2 g
Protein	3 g
Iron	1.0 mg
Calcium	29 mg

Oven-Baked Potato Wedges

Makes 6 servings

These potato wedges are a healthier alternative to french fries. The rosemary and thyme add wonderful flavor and fragrance.

Tips

This dish is high in vitamin C, vitamin A and fiber.

Leaving the peel on shortens the preparation time and adds fiber to your meal; just be sure to scrub well with a brush under running water first. Russet potatoes are the best baking potatoes.

Variations

Different seasonings can dramatically change this potato dish. For spicy flavor, use salt and 2 tbsp (30 mL) chili powder.

If available, add a third potato color with blue (or purple) potatoes.

- **Preheat oven to 450°F (230°C)**
- **Baking sheet, lightly greased**

2 tbsp	vegetable oil	30 mL
1/2 tsp	salt	2 mL
1 tsp	dried rosemary	5 mL
1/2 tsp	dried thyme	2 mL
2	russet potatoes (unpeeled), cut into 1/2-inch (1 cm) wedges	2
1	sweet potato (unpeeled), cut into 1/2-inch (1 cm) wedges	1

1. In a large bowl, combine oil, salt, rosemary and thyme. Add potatoes and toss to coat. Transfer to prepared baking sheet.
2. Bake in preheated oven, turning wedges occasionally, for 15 to 20 minutes or until browned and tender.

This recipe courtesy of dietitian Wendy Benson.

> **Dinner Idea:** Pair these potato wedges with any roasted pork or grilled beef.

NUTRIENTS PER SERVING

Calories 124
Fat .5 g
Carbohydrate. . . . . .19 g
Fiber . . . . .2 g
Protein. . . . . .2 g
Iron . . . . .1.7 mg
Calcium . . . . 26 mg

Oven-Roasted Lemon Potatoes

Makes 6 servings

The Greek-style combination of oregano, tangy lemon and black pepper is very refreshing and makes these potatoes a great accompaniment to chicken kabobs.

Tip

This dish is an excellent source of vitamin C.

- **Preheat oven to 400°F (200°C)**
- **Large shallow roasting pan**

1½ lbs	potatoes, peeled and cut into chunks	750 g
3 tbsp	olive oil	45 mL
	Juice of 1 lemon	
½ tsp	dried oregano	2 mL
¼ tsp	freshly ground black pepper	1 mL
	Salt	
1½ cups	ready-to-use chicken broth (approx.)	375 mL

1. Place potatoes in a single layer in roasting pan. Add olive oil, lemon juice, oregano, pepper and salt to taste; toss to coat. Pour in just enough broth to half-cover potatoes.

2. Bake in preheated oven for about 1 hour or until potatoes are tender, golden-brown and crispy on the outside.

This recipe courtesy of dietitian Patti Thomson.

Dinner Idea: Pair this dish with Grilled Chicken Kabobs (page 261) or Lemon Garlic Chicken (page 251).

NUTRIENTS
PER SERVING

Calories 131
Fat . . . . .6 g
Carbohydrate . . . . .18 g
Fiber . . . . .1 g
Protein . . . . .2 g
Iron . . . . .0.5 mg
Calcium . . . . 13 mg

Oven-Roasted Potatoes and Parsnips with Curry

Makes 6 servings

Root vegetables are known for their soluble fiber and digestibility. They are very helpful for those with symptoms of irritable bowel syndrome.

Tips

This dish is an excellent source of vitamin C, folate, vitamin B$_6$, fiber, potassium and manganese.

Cut potatoes and parsnips into evenly sized pieces, not too small.

Stirring the vegetables as they cook encourages browning and slight caramelizing on as many sides as possible. Don't crowd the roasting pan, or the vegetables will steam together rather than roast.

Variation

Substitute turnips, rutabaga, beets, celeriac, carrots or sweet potatoes for the parsnips.

- **Preheat oven to 400°F (200°C)**
- **Roasting pan large enough to accommodate vegetables in a single layer**

5	large floury or all-purpose potatoes, scrubbed and cut into chunks (see tip, at left)	5
6	shallots, peeled	6
5	large parsnips, peeled and cut into chunks	5
1	head garlic, separated into cloves and peeled	1
1/3 cup	olive oil	75 mL
2 tbsp	gluten-free curry powder	30 mL
	Salt and freshly ground black pepper	

1. In a large bowl, toss potatoes, shallots, parsnips, garlic, oil and curry powder to coat. Season to taste with salt and freshly ground pepper.

2. In a large roasting pan, arrange vegetables in a single layer. Roast in preheated oven, stirring occasionally, for 45 to 60 minutes or until cooked through and potatoes and parsnips are crusty and golden brown. (If they are browning too quickly and have not yet cooked through, cover with foil.) Serve immediately.

Dinner Idea: Serve this dish alongside roasted or grilled pork or beef.

NUTRIENTS PER SERVING

Calories 340
Fat . . . . .10 g
Carbohydrate . . . . .59 g
Fiber . . . . .10 g
Protein . . . . .6 g
Iron . . . . .3.0 mg
Calcium . . . . 91 mg

Exotic Spiced Roasties

This Indian-inspired potato dish will have you coming back for more. The spice mixture is a great pantry staple that you'll find uses for in many other dishes.

Tips

This dish is an excellent source of vitamin C and potassium, and a good source of fiber. Leaving the skin on the potatoes increases the fiber content.

The spice combo in this recipe lends an Indian flavor to food. It can be used as a dry rub on boneless chicken or pork chops before grilling or searing.

Sea salt has a much cleaner, crisper taste and a greater mineral content than refined table salt.

- Preheat oven to 400°F (200°C)
- Rimmed baking sheet, lightly brushed with olive oil
- Glass jar with tight-fitting lid

Spice Mixture

1 tbsp	ground cardamom	15 mL
1 tbsp	cayenne pepper	15 mL
1 tbsp	ground coriander	15 mL
1 tbsp	ground cumin	15 mL
1 tbsp	paprika	15 mL
1 tsp	ground cinnamon	5 mL
1 tsp	ground cloves	5 mL
1 tsp	freshly ground black pepper	5 mL
1 tsp	ground nutmeg	5 mL
1 tsp	ground turmeric	5 mL
1 tsp	salt	5 mL
1 tsp	granulated sugar	5 mL

Potatoes

2 lbs	small waxy new potatoes, lightly scrubbed and thoroughly dried	1 kg
¼ cup	olive oil	60 mL

1. *Spice Mixture:* In a small bowl, combine cardamom, cayenne, coriander, cumin, paprika, cinnamon, cloves, pepper, nutmeg, turmeric, salt and sugar. Mix well. Transfer to a glass jar with a tight-fitting lid and store in a cool, dark place for up to 2 weeks. (Makes about ½ cup/125 mL.)

2. *Potatoes:* Using a fork, prick each potato a few times and transfer to a large bowl. Add oil and 1 to 2 tbsp (15 to 30 mL) of the spice mixture. Toss to coat.

3. Arrange in a single layer on prepared baking sheet. Roast in preheated oven, turning once or twice, for 45 minutes to 1 hour or until tender. Serve immediately.

Dinner Idea: Pair this side dish with Lamb Tagine with Chickpeas and Apricots (page 278).

NUTRIENTS
PER SERVING

Calories	190
Fat	10 g
Carbohydrate	25 g
Fiber	4 g
Protein	3 g
Iron	1.4 mg
Calcium	23 mg

New Potatoes with Asparagus and Prosciutto

Makes 4 to 6 servings

I love the taste of tender new potatoes and fresh, crunchy asparagus in the spring. This dish will also work as a refreshing light lunch.

Tips

To prepare the asparagus, use a vegetable peeler to lightly peel the spears, starting halfway down from the tip, to reveal the pale green. Trim off 2 inches (5 cm) from the base of each. Using kitchen string, tie the spears into a few bundles.

It's important to cover the pot only loosely when cooking the asparagus. If it's tightly covered, the asparagus will lose its bright green color.

Butter is lactose-free, but if you have an allergy to cow's milk protein, substitute non-dairy, soy-free margarine.

NUTRIENTS PER SERVING

Calories	370
Fat	19 g
Carbohydrate	35 g
Fiber	7 g
Protein	17 g
Iron	2.3 mg
Calcium	52 mg

- Deep pot (large enough to accommodate potatoes and upright asparagus)
- Large oval serving platter, warmed

2 lbs	fresh asparagus (see tips, at left)	1 kg
2 lbs	waxy new potatoes, scrubbed, halved if large	1 kg
4 oz	butter, melted	125 g
3 tbsp	freshly squeezed lemon juice	45 mL
2 tbsp	chopped fresh chives	30 mL
	Salt and freshly ground black pepper	
8 oz	thinly sliced prosciutto	250 g

1. Place potatoes in a large, deep pot and add boiling water to barely cover. Add 1 tsp (5 mL) salt and bring to a boil. Add asparagus bundles, setting upright around sides of pot. Cover loosely, reduce heat and cook for 10 to 12 minutes or just until asparagus is tender. Using tongs, remove asparagus from pot, drain well, and wrap loosely in a clean tea towel. Continue cooking potatoes until tender. Drain well. Return potatoes to pot over very low heat and shake the pot to dry them thoroughly. Cool slightly.

2. In a bowl, whisk together butter, lemon juice and chives. Season to taste with salt and pepper. Pour about half of the mixture over potatoes, carefully turning to coat.

3. Transfer potatoes to center of prepared serving platter. Arrange asparagus in bundles around potatoes, parallel to long edges of platter. Drizzle with the remaining butter mixture. Loosely drape prosciutto slices over asparagus, folding them so they don't cover asparagus completely. Serve immediately.

Lunch Idea: Serve this dish with a small salad of arugula dressed with 2 tbsp (30 mL) lemon juice, 1 tbsp (15 mL) extra virgin olive oil, salt and pepper.

Lightened-Up Scalloped Potatoes

If you want to enjoy scalloped potatoes without the creaminess of the traditional dish, here's a recipe to try.

Tip

This recipe is high in vitamins C and B$_6$.

- **Preheat oven to 450°F (230°C)**
- **11- by 7-inch (28 by 18 cm) casserole dish, lightly greased**

2 lbs	potatoes, peeled and sliced	1 kg
1	clove garlic, chopped	1
1	onion, thinly sliced	1
1 tbsp	chopped fresh rosemary	15 mL
1½ cups	ready-to-use beef broth	375 mL

1. In prepared casserole dish, layer potatoes, garlic and onion. Sprinkle with rosemary. Pour in broth.
2. Cover and bake in preheated oven for 25 minutes. Uncover and bake for 5 minutes or until potatoes are soft and tops are browned.

This recipe courtesy of dietitian Helen Haresign.

> **Dinner Idea:** Serve this dish alongside Stewed Pork with Greens (page 272).

NUTRIENTS PER SERVING

Calories	107
Fat	0 g
Carbohydrate	24 g
Fiber	2 g
Protein	3 g
Iron	0.5 mg
Calcium	17 mg

French Potato Galette

Makes 2 servings

In French, the word "galette" has many different meanings. Here, it describes a dish of ultra-thin slices of potato arranged in circular pattern and fried on both sides, ultimately resembling a giant potato chip.

Tips

You have to make these galettes one at a time, so if you plan on making a few, keep them warm in a low oven.

Sea salt has a much cleaner, crisper taste and a greater mineral content than refined table salt.

Butter is lactose-free, but if you have an allergy to cow's milk protein, replace it with non-dairy, soy-free margarine.

Potatoes are an excellent source of vitamin C.

- Mandoline or food processor fitted with the slicing blade
- Small or medium nonstick skillet or well-seasoned cast-iron pan

1	large floury potato, peeled	1
1 tbsp	butter, melted	15 mL
1 tbsp	extra virgin olive oil	15 mL
	Salt and freshly ground black pepper	

1. Using a mandoline or food processor fitted with slicing blade, slice potatoes very thinly, about $1/8$ inch (3 mm) thick. In a large bowl, combine butter and oil. Add potatoes. Season to taste with salt and freshly ground pepper. Using your hands, toss until potatoes are well coated.

2. In a skillet, working from the center and covering the bottom of the pan, arrange about 12 of the largest potato slices in a spiral, slightly overlapping edges and using smaller slices here and there between the larger ones. Using a metal spatula, gently but firmly press down on galette.

3. Cook over medium-high heat, without disturbing potatoes, for 10 to 12 minutes, until galette is crisping slightly around the edges. Using metal spatula, gently lift and loosen edges of potato cake, then shake pan to free bottom (potato slices should adhere in one mass). Flip galette and cook for 6 minutes, until it is golden brown on the underside.

4. Flip once or twice more for a total of 2 minutes or until potato is cooked through, golden brown and very crisp. Season to taste with salt and freshly ground pepper. Serve immediately.

Dinner Idea: This side dish makes an ideal partner for grilled sirloin.

NUTRIENTS PER SERVING

Calories	180
Fat	13 g
Carbohydrate	17 g
Fiber	2 g
Protein	1 g
Iron	0.3 mg
Calcium	7 mg

Crisp Potato Pakoras with Mint-Cilantro Chutney

These crispy fritters make a wonderful side dish or a terrific appetizer for an outdoor summer barbecue.

Tips

This dish is an excellent source of iron, fiber and vitamin C, and a good source of B vitamins.

Chickpea flour is used extensively in Sicilian cuisine, so look for it in Italian food shops. You may also find it in East Indian markets, labeled "besan." If you have an allergy to wheat, or celiac disease, make sure the flour is labeled "gluten-free." Some chickpea flours have been found to be contaminated with wheat.

Start by making the chutney, to allow the flavors to develop fully.

NUTRIENTS
PER SERVING

Calories	210
Fat	2 g
Carbohydrate	42 g
Fiber	5 g
Protein	8 g
Iron	1.6 mg
Calcium	22 mg

- Food processor or blender
- Large heavy pot, Dutch oven or deep fryer
- Candy/deep-frying thermometer (if not using a deep fryer)

Mint-Cilantro Chutney

2 cups	fresh mint leaves	500 mL
1 cup	fresh cilantro leaves, with some stems	250 mL
1/2 cup	unsweetened dried coconut	125 mL
1/4 cup	water	60 mL
2 tbsp	freshly squeezed lime juice	30 mL
1 tsp	packed brown sugar	5 mL
1 tsp	salt	5 mL
1/2 tsp	hot pepper flakes	2 mL
2 tsp	vegetable oil	10 mL

Pakora Batter

1 cup	chickpea flour (see tip, at left)	250 mL
2 tbsp	rice flour	30 mL
1 tbsp	freshly squeezed lime juice	15 mL
1/2 tsp	chili powder	2 mL
1/2 tsp	salt	2 mL
1/2 tsp	ground turmeric	2 mL
1/2 cup	water	125 mL
1/8 tsp	baking soda	0.5 mL

Potatoes

	Vegetable oil	
3	large floury potatoes, peeled and sliced 1/8 inch (3 mm) thick	3

1. *Mint-Cilantro Chutney:* In food processor, pulse mint, cilantro, coconut, water, lime juice, brown sugar, salt and hot pepper flakes until smooth and blended.

2. In a small saucepan, heat oil over medium heat. Add chutney mixture (be wary of spitting oil) and stir-fry until fragrant, about 10 minutes. Scrape into a small bowl and set aside to cool. Cover with plastic wrap and refrigerate until ready to serve, about an hour ahead of time.

Tips

If you slice the potatoes ahead of time, cover them with cold water until you're ready to cook, but make sure to dry thoroughly before dipping in the batter and frying.

Be sure to get the oil hot enough to ensure that the interior of the potato is cooked and the exterior is crunchy-crisp.

3. *Pakora Batter:* In a bowl, sift together chickpea and rice flours. Add lime juice, chili powder, salt and turmeric, then gradually whisk in water until mixture is consistency of heavy cream. Cover and let stand for 10 minutes. Just before you're ready to cook, add baking soda, whisking for about a minute to fully incorporate into batter.

4. *Potatoes:* Preheat oven to 140°F (60°C). Add 4 to 6 inches (10 to 15 cm) oil to a large, heavy pot. It should come a little over halfway up the sides of the pot; do not overfill, making sure to leave at least 3 inches (7.5 cm) of space at top of pot. Place over medium-high heat until thermometer registers 360°F (185°C). (If you are using a deep fryer, follow the manufacturer's instructions.)

5. Working with six slices at a time, pat potatoes dry and dip each in batter until well coated, letting excess drip back into bowl. Carefully slip into hot oil. Fry, turning once or twice, until golden on both sides, about 5 minutes. Once cooked, transfer to a baking sheet lined with paper towels and keep warm in the oven. Serve with Mint-Cilantro Chutney.

> **Lunch Idea:** Serve pakoras with Vegetarian Harira (page 222) or Suppertime Lentil Soup (page 226).

Aloo Tikki

Makes about 14 patties

These crunchy potato patties make the perfect side dish for an Indian-themed dinner. Or serve them with Spicy Hummus (page 210) as an appetizer.

Tips

This dish is an excellent source of vitamin C and vitamin K, and a good source of vitamin B₆.

This is a great use for leftover mashed potatoes, or you can plan to make them with freshly made potatoes. If you are using leftover mash that was prepared with lots of butter and cream, add a little flour to the mixture, enough to form a soft dough. One pound (500 g), or 2 large potatoes, makes about 2½ to 3 cups (625 to 750 mL) mashed potatoes.

Sea salt has a much cleaner, crisper taste and a greater mineral content than refined table salt.

4	large floury potatoes, peeled	4
2 tsp	salt, divided	10 mL
2	onions, finely chopped	2
3	cloves garlic, finely chopped	3
2 tsp	chopped gingerroot	10 mL
1 cup	chopped fresh cilantro (leaves and some stem)	250 mL
1 tsp	freshly ground black pepper	5 mL
½ tsp	ground cinnamon	2 mL
¼ cup	vegetable oil	60 mL

1. Place potatoes in a large saucepan and add cold water to barely cover. Add 1 tsp (5 mL) salt, cover loosely and bring to a boil over high heat. Reduce heat and cook for 20 minutes or until potatoes are tender. Drain well. Using a large fork, mash potatoes roughly.

2. In a large bowl, combine potatoes, onions, garlic, ginger, cilantro, remaining 1 tsp (5 mL) salt, freshly ground pepper and cinnamon. Mix well. Divide into balls the size of ping-pong balls, then flatten into disks.

3. In a skillet, heat oil over medium-high heat. Add patties, in batches, and fry until golden brown and crisp, about 2 minutes per side.

> **Dinner Idea:** Serve this dish as a starter to Mixed Vegetable Coconut Curry (page 247).

NUTRIENTS
PER PATTY

Calories 80
Fat .4 g
Carbohydrate. . . . . 11 g
Fiber . . . . .2 g
Protein. . . . . .1 g
Iron . . . . .0.3 mg
Calcium . . . . 16 mg

Minted Lentils with Vegetables

Lentils are a personal favorite because they cook so quickly and are so easily infused with the flavors of spices and herbs, such as the mint and cumin in this recipe.

Tips

This dish is an excellent source of fiber and B vitamins, including folate, and a good source of calcium.

If you prefer vegetables in smaller, more uniform pieces, dice rather than chop.

Depending on the sodium content of the broth, you may need to add a little salt.

1 tbsp	vegetable oil	15 mL
2	cloves garlic, minced	2
2	stalks celery, chopped	2
1	carrot, diced	1
1	onion, chopped	1
1	red bell pepper, chopped	1
1 tsp	ground cumin	5 mL
1 cup	dried green lentils, rinsed	250 mL
2 cups	ready-to-use gluten-free chicken broth	500 mL
1/4 cup	snipped fresh mint	60 mL

1. In a saucepan, heat oil over medium heat. Sauté garlic, celery, carrot, onion, red pepper and cumin for 5 minutes or until onion is softened.
2. Stir in lentils and broth; bring to a boil. Reduce heat and simmer gently for 30 to 40 minutes or until lentils are tender. Drain, if necessary. Stir in mint.

Dinner Idea: Add leftover diced cooked chicken, gluten-free ham or beef to turn this into a quick and easy entrée.

NUTRIENTS PER SERVING

Calories 237
Fat .4 g
Carbohydrate. . . . . .39 g
Fiber . . . . .10 g
Protein. . . . . .13 g
Iron . . . . .4.0 mg
Calcium. . . . . 101 mg

Lemon Jasmine Rice Pilaf

Makes 4 servings

This tasty side dish, high in vitamins A and C, makes the perfect accompaniment to any number of entrées.

Tips

A pilaf involves frying the rice (or any other grain) in seasonings and herbs to enhance the flavor before cooking liquid is added.

Two to 3 medium leeks yield 4 cups (1 L) sliced.

Variations

Substitute Vidalia onions for the leeks and gluten-free vegetable stock powder for the chicken stock powder.

Substitute brown, basmati or wild rice, or a combination, for the jasmine rice. Adjust the cooking time based on the package instructions.

1 tbsp	extra virgin olive oil	15 mL
4 cups	sliced leeks (white and light green parts only)	1 L
1 cup	diced carrots	250 mL
1 tsp	dried oregano	5 mL
1 cup	jasmine rice	250 mL
2 cups	water	500 mL
1 tbsp	gluten-free chicken stock powder	15 mL
2 tbsp	grated lemon zest	30 mL
2 tbsp	freshly squeezed lemon juice	30 mL
	Salt and freshly ground white pepper	

1. In a heavy saucepan, heat oil over medium-high heat. Cook leeks, carrots and oregano, stirring occasionally, for 5 to 8 minutes, or until softened. Add rice and cook for 1 minute, stirring constantly.

Stove-Top Method

2. Add water and stock powder and bring to a boil. Reduce heat to low, cover and simmer for 15 minutes, or until rice is tender. Remove saucepan from heat and let stand, covered, for 3 to 5 minutes. Stir in lemon zest and lemon juice and season to taste with salt and pepper. Fluff with a fork.

Microwave Method

2. Transfer rice mixture to an 8- to 12-cup (2 to 3 L) microwave-safe casserole dish. Add water and stock powder. Cover and cook on High for 5 minutes, or until boiling. Cook, covered, on Medium (50%) for 15 minutes until liquid is absorbed and rice is tender. Let stand, covered, for 3 to 5 minutes. Stir in lemon zest and lemon juice and season to taste with salt and pepper. Fluff with a fork.

Lunch Idea: Serve this dish with Minted Lentils with Vegetables (page 301).

NUTRIENTS PER SERVING

Calories	260
Fat	4 g
Carbohydrate	53 g
Fiber	4 g
Protein	5 g
Iron	2.5 mg
Calcium	95 mg

Mushroom Leek Pilaf

Makes 4 to 6 servings

The robust flavors of mushrooms and wild rice make this dish a good partner for beef dishes.

Tips

This dish is an excellent source of fiber, vitamin A and B vitamins (including folate), and a good source of iron and trace minerals.

For the mushrooms, try a mixture of cremini, shiitake, portobello and oyster.

Dice carrots, rather than leaving them in larger pieces, so they cook in the same time as the leek and mushrooms.

To toast quinoa: Spread quinoa seeds in a single layer in a large skillet and toast over medium heat for 3 to 4 minutes or until quinoa is golden. Quinoa will darken upon cooling.

1 tbsp	vegetable oil	15 mL
2	cloves garlic, minced	2
1	leek (white and light green parts only), chopped	1
2 cups	sliced assorted mushrooms (see tip, at left)	500 mL
1 cup	diced carrots	250 mL
3 tbsp	snipped fresh rosemary	45 mL
1/2 cup	wild rice	125 mL
1 1/2 cups	ready-to-use gluten-free chicken broth	375 mL
1/4 cup	quinoa, rinsed and toasted (see tip, at left)	60 mL
	Salt and freshly ground black pepper	

1. In a large saucepan, heat oil over medium-low heat. Sauté garlic, leek, mushrooms, carrots and rosemary for 6 to 8 minutes or until tender.

2. Add wild rice and broth; increase heat to medium-high and bring to a boil. Reduce heat to low, cover and simmer gently for 40 minutes.

3. Add quinoa, cover and simmer for 15 minutes or until quinoa is transparent and the tiny, spiral-like germ is separated, and rice is tender. Remove from heat and let stand for 5 to 10 minutes or until liquid is absorbed. Season to taste with salt and pepper.

This recipe courtesy of CanolaInfo.

Dinner Idea: Pair this dish with Chicken Cacciatore (page 258).

NUTRIENTS PER SERVING

Calories	130
Fat	3 g
Carbohydrate	22 g
Fiber	3 g
Protein	4 g
Iron	2.0 mg
Calcium	38 mg

Teff Polenta

Teff is a nutritional powerhouse — a good source of iron, calcium, protein and trace minerals. When it's turned into a hearty, delicious polenta, the dish is also an excellent source of vitamins A, C and K.

Tip

At the end of step 1, there may be some extra liquid from the tomatoes, but as long as the teff is not crunchy, the polenta is done.

- **10-inch (25 cm) skillet**
- **9-inch (23 cm) pie plate**

2 tbsp	extra virgin olive oil	30 mL
8	cloves garlic, thickly sliced	8
1 cup	coarsely chopped onion	250 mL
1 cup	chopped green bell pepper	250 mL
⅔ cup	teff grain	150 mL
2 cups	boiling water	500 mL
½ tsp	sea salt	2 mL
2 cups	chopped plum (Roma) tomatoes	500 mL
1 cup	chopped fresh basil	250 mL

1. In skillet, heat oil over medium heat. Sauté garlic and onion for 5 minutes or until tender. Add green pepper and sauté for 2 minutes or until bright green. Stir in teff. Gradually stir in boiling water and salt; simmer, stirring, for 2 minutes. Stir in tomatoes and basil; reduce heat to low, cover and simmer, stirring occasionally, for 10 to 15 minutes or until water is absorbed.

2. Transfer polenta to pie plate and let cool for 30 minutes before slicing and serving.

This recipe courtesy of Leslie Cerier (from Going Wild in the Kitchen, *Square One Publishers, 2005).*

> **Dinner Idea:** For a complete vegan meal, pair this dish with Curried Chickpeas (page 246) or Ratatouille (page 244).

NUTRIENTS PER SERVING

Calories	220
Fat	8 g
Carbohydrate	32 g
Fiber	6 g
Protein	6 g
Iron	2.7 mg
Calcium	102 mg

Desserts

Cake of Goodness

*This cake is really easy to
mix up and bake. My friend
Theresa's sons like it so
much, they dubbed it Cake
of Goodness.*

Tips

Choose your favorite enriched
gluten-free non-dairy milk, such
as soy, rice, almond or potato-
based milk, or, if you tolerate
lactose, use regular 1% milk.

Non-dairy, soy-free margarine,
such as Earth Balance vegan
buttery flavor sticks, has almost
half as much saturated fat as
regular butter and no cholesterol.
Where butter is called for in a
baking recipe, non-dairy, soy-free
margarine can be a heart-healthy,
delicious alternative.

- **Preheat oven to 350°F (180°C)**
- **8-inch (20 cm) round metal cake pan, greased, bottom
  lined with parchment paper**

1 cup	white rice flour	250 mL
¾ cup	granulated raw cane sugar	175 mL
½ cup	sorghum flour	125 mL
¼ tsp	salt	1 mL
¼ cup	cold non-dairy, soy-free margarine or butter, cut into pieces	60 mL
2 tsp	baking powder	10 mL
1 tsp	ground cinnamon	5 mL
1 cup	enriched non-dairy milk or lactose-free 1% milk	250 mL
½ tsp	vanilla extract	2 mL
½ tsp	freshly squeezed lemon juice	2 mL

1. In a large bowl, combine rice flour, sugar, sorghum
   flour and salt. Using a pastry blender or two knives,
   cut in margarine until mixture resembles coarse
   crumbs. Reserve ½ cup (125 mL) for topping.
2. To the remaining flour mixture, add baking powder,
   cinnamon, milk, vanilla and lemon juice; stir until
   just combined. Pour into prepared cake pan and
   sprinkle evenly with the reserved flour mixture.
3. Bake in preheated oven for 30 minutes or until a
   tester inserted in the center comes out clean. Let cool
   completely in pan on a wire rack.

NUTRIENTS
PER SERVING

Calories 180
Fat . . . . .5 g
Carbohydrate . . . . .30 g
Fiber . . . . .1 g
Protein . . . . .2 g
Iron . . . . .0.5 mg
Calcium . . . . 47 mg

Summer Fruit Crisp

Fruit crisp is a delicious way to enjoy seasonal fruits. Make several crisps while the fruits are at their peak of freshness and freeze some to enjoy at other times of the year.

Tips

Butter is lactose-free, but if you have an allergy to cow's milk protein, substitute non-dairy, soy-free margarine.

To store, let cool completely, wrap airtight and freeze for up to 3 months.

Variations

Recipe can be divided in half and baked in a lightly greased 9- by 5-inch (23 by 12.5 cm) glass loaf pan.

Substitute sorghum flour for the amaranth flour in both the base and the topping.

- **Preheat oven to 350°F (180°C)**
- **8-cup (2 L) shallow casserole dish, lightly greased**

Base

4	large peaches, cut into wedges	4
5	plums, cut into wedges	5
1 cup	blueberries	250 mL
3 tbsp	amaranth flour	45 mL
2 tbsp	packed brown sugar	30 mL

Topping

1½ cups	pure, uncontaminated quick-cooking rolled oats	375 mL
⅓ cup	amaranth flour	75 mL
¼ cup	packed brown sugar	60 mL
½ tsp	ground mace	2 mL
¼ cup	butter, melted	60 mL

1. *Base:* In prepared casserole dish, gently combine peaches, plums, blueberries, amaranth flour and brown sugar. Set aside.

2. *Topping:* In a bowl, combine oats, amaranth flour, brown sugar and mace. Drizzle with butter and mix just until crumbly. Sprinkle over the fruit. Do not pack.

3. Bake in preheated oven for 20 to 25 minutes or until fruit is bubbly around the edges and fork-tender, and topping is browned. Serve warm.

NUTRIENTS PER SERVING

Calories	238
Fat	7 g
Carbohydrate	40 g
Fiber	4 g
Protein	5 g
Iron	4.0 mg
Calcium	37 mg

Wholesome Rice Pudding

The ultimate comfort food, this rice pudding is the perfect finish to a special family dinner.

Tips

The pudding doesn't necessarily need to be stirred while it is cooking, but an occasional stir will help distribute the starch and aid thickening.

If you prefer a slightly thicker result, after removing the pudding from the slow cooker, chill and stir several times before serving.

- **Small (maximum 3½-quart) slow cooker**
- **Lightly greased slow cooker stoneware**

¾ cup	short-grain brown rice	175 mL
½ cup	raw cane sugar, such as Demerara or other evaporated cane juice sugar	125 mL
1 tsp	ground cinnamon	5 mL
4 cups	whole milk or enriched rice milk	1 L

1. In prepared slow cooker stoneware, combine rice, sugar and cinnamon. Stir well. Add milk and stir again. Cover and cook on High for 4 hours, until rice is tender and pudding is creamy. Stir well and transfer to a serving bowl. Let cool slightly and stir again or cover and refrigerate until ready to serve.

NUTRIENTS
PER SERVING

Calories 170
Fat . . . . .2 g
Carbohydrate. . . . . .39 g
Fiber . . . . .1 g
Protein. . . . . .1 g
Iron . . . . .0.2 mg
Calcium . . . . 205 mg

Rice Pudding with Raisins

This dessert is a classic — enjoy it with a sprinkle of cinnamon and cardamom.

Tips

If you are sensitive to sulfites, make sure the raisins have no added sulfites.

If you prefer your pudding with a thicker consistency, serve it cold. As the pudding cools, it firms up.

Variation

Add ¼ tsp (1 mL) ground cardamom along with the cinnamon.

4 cups	enriched vanilla-flavored rice milk or soy milk	1 L
1 cup	short-grain rice	250 mL
⅓ cup	granulated natural cane sugar or other dry sweetener	75 mL
½ tsp	ground cinnamon	2 mL
¼ tsp	salt	1 mL
¾ cup	dark raisins	175 mL
2 tbsp	orange juice or dark rum	30 mL
	Additional ground cinnamon (optional)	

1. In a large heavy pot, combine rice milk, rice, sugar, cinnamon and salt. Bring to a boil over medium heat, stirring constantly, until sugar is dissolved. Reduce heat to low and simmer, stirring occasionally, for 20 minutes or until rice is tender and mixture is creamy. Taste a spoonful to ensure the rice is thoroughly cooked. If not, continue cooking for a few more minutes.

2. In a small pot, over medium-high heat, combine raisins with orange juice. Cook, stirring, for 1 minute or until raisins are plump and orange juice is absorbed. Add to cooked pudding and mix thoroughly. Serve hot, or chill for at least 2 hours and serve cold, sprinkled with additional cinnamon, if desired.

NUTRIENTS PER SERVING

Calories 280
Fat .2 g
Carbohydrate. . . . . .66 g
Fiber . . . . .2 g
Protein. . . . . .3 g
Iron . . . . .1.8 mg
Calcium . . . . 213 mg

Black Sticky Rice Pudding

This Thai-style dessert is delicious even without the fruit. Savor it only occasionally, as it is quite high in saturated fats.

Tip

Thai black sticky rice is available in Asian markets. Do not use Chinese black rice, which is not sticky. To cook this quantity of black sticky rice, use about ¾ cup (175 mL) raw rice and 1½ cups (375 mL) water. Soak the rice for at least 4 hours or overnight, then bring the rice and soaking liquid to a rapid boil in a heavy pot with a tight-fitting lid. Reduce heat to low and simmer until rice is tender, 30 to 45 minutes.

1	can (14 oz/400 mL) coconut milk	1
½ cup	packed Demerara or other raw cane sugar	125 mL
½ tsp	salt	2 mL
2 cups	cooked Thai black sticky rice (see tip, at left)	500 mL
1 cup	sliced strawberries or kiwifruit or chopped peaches or mango	250 mL
¼ cup	toasted shredded sweetened coconut	60 mL
	Finely chopped mint (optional)	

1. In a saucepan, combine coconut milk, sugar and salt. Bring to a boil over medium heat and cook, stirring, until sugar dissolves. Stir in rice and cook, stirring, until thickened, about 10 minutes. Transfer to a serving bowl and chill, if desired.
2. When you're ready to serve, top with fruit and garnish with coconut and mint (if using).

NUTRIENTS
PER SERVING

Calories 280
Fat . . . . .17 g
Carbohydrate . . . . .33 g
Fiber . . . . .2 g
Protein . . . . .3 g
Iron . . . . .2.5 mg
Calcium . . . . 18 mg

Coconut Panna Cotta with Mango Ginger Sauce

Makes 6 servings

Coconut, mango, ginger and silken tofu combine to make a decadent finish to a festive meal.

Tips

If you are allergic to soy, replace the tofu with 1½ cups (375 mL) plain coconut yogurt (also known as cultured coconut milk) and increase the amount of agar powder to 2 tsp (10 mL) or substitute 2 tbsp (30 mL) agar flakes.

Arrange prepared ramekins on a tray before filling for easy transport to the refrigerator once filled.

The texture of this panna cotta can be controlled by the amount of agar powder you use. Less will produce a softer panna cotta; more will give you a firmer dessert.

NUTRIENTS PER SERVING

Calories 140
Fat .3 g
Carbohydrate. . . . . .27 g
Fiber . . . . .1 g
Protein. . . . . .3 g
Iron . . . . .0.8 mg
Calcium . . . . 73 mg

- **Food processor or blender**
- **Six ½-cup (125 mL) ramekins, lightly oiled with coconut oil**

Coconut Panna Cotta

1⅔ cups	enriched coconut milk	400 mL
6 tbsp	natural cane sugar	90 mL
½ tsp	agar powder	2 mL
1 tsp	vanilla extract	5 mL
1	package (12.3 oz/340 g) firm or extra-firm silken tofu	1

Mango Ginger Sauce

1	mango, chopped	1
2 tbsp	agave nectar	30 mL
	Grated zest of 1 lime	
2 tbsp	freshly squeezed lime juice	30 mL
1 tsp	grated gingerroot	5 mL

1. *Coconut Panna Cotta:* In a saucepan, whisk together coconut milk, sugar, agar powder and vanilla. Bring to a simmer over medium heat and cook, stirring constantly, until mixture thickens, 3 to 4 minutes. Remove from heat and let cool for 15 minutes.

2. In food processor, combine tofu and coconut milk mixture and blend until smooth. Spoon mixture into prepared ramekins, cover with plastic wrap and refrigerate until firmly set, at least 2 hours or overnight.

3. *Mango Ginger Sauce:* In clean food processor, combine mango, agave, lime zest, lime juice and ginger and process until smooth. Transfer to a bowl, cover and refrigerate until ready to serve.

4. To serve, place bottom of ramekins in hot water for a few seconds. Run a knife around the inside edge. Invert a serving plate on top of ramekin and while holding both the plate and the ramekin quickly invert. Gently shake the ramekin to loosen the panna cotta onto the plate. Top panna cotta with a spoonful of sauce and serve immediately.

Poached Pears with Cranberry Sauce

Makes 4 servings

When pears get too ripe overnight, use them to create this delicious dessert.

Tips

For the orange liqueur, choose from Grand Marnier, Triple Sec or Cointreau.

If you are sensitive to sulfites, use apple juice instead of apple cider. Make sure the liqueur you choose is free of added sulfites, or substitute an equal amount of thawed frozen orange juice concentrate.

Choose firm pears that hold up well in cooking, such as Bosc or Bartlett.

Place pears in a paper bag at room temperature to ripen. To test pears for ripeness, press lightly at the stem end. It should give slightly.

2 cups	unsweetened apple cider or apple juice	500 mL
1/2 cup	dried cranberries	125 mL
1/4 cup	packed brown sugar	60 mL
2 tsp	grated orange zest	10 mL
1 tsp	ground cardamom	5 mL
4	pears, peeled and halved lengthwise	4
2 tbsp	orange liqueur	30 mL

1. In a saucepan, combine apple cider, cranberries, brown sugar, orange zest and cardamom. Bring to a boil over medium-high heat. Reduce heat to low and simmer for 15 minutes. Add pears and simmer for 5 minutes or until tender. Remove from heat and stir in liqueur. Serve warm or chilled.

**NUTRIENTS
PER SERVING**

Calories 220
Fat . . . . 1 g
Carbohydrate . . . . 54 g
Fiber . . . . 4 g
Protein . . . . 1 g
Iron . . . . 0.6 mg
Calcium . . . . 32 mg

Caramelized Bananas with Rum Sauce

Makes 4 servings

This quick dessert is made from ingredients you may already have on hand.

Tips

If you are allergic to soy, make sure the non-dairy margarine you choose is also free of soy.

To toast coconut: Preheat oven to 325°F (160°C). Spread a thick layer of shredded coconut on a baking sheet and bake, stirring often, until golden, 8 to 10 minutes. Coconut burns quickly, so don't walk away from the oven.

Variation

Use only 2 bananas and add 2 small, peeled, halved peaches to skillet or substitute fresh pineapple spears for bananas.

- **Long-handled igniter**

3	bananas	3
1 tsp	freshly squeezed lime juice	5 mL
3 tbsp	non-dairy margarine	45 mL
6 tbsp	packed brown sugar	90 mL
1/3 cup	spiced, amber or dark rum	75 mL
1/4 tsp	freshly grated nutmeg	1 mL
2 tbsp	toasted sweetened shredded coconut (optional)	30 mL

1. Peel bananas and slice in half lengthwise, then cut each half crosswise into 4 pieces. Place in a bowl and sprinkle with lime juice. Set aside.

2. Place a large heavy-bottomed skillet over medium heat and let pan get hot. Add margarine and let it melt. Add bananas, cut side down, and cook until browned, 3 to 5 minutes. Sprinkle brown sugar over bananas and cook, shaking pan frequently, until sugar melts. Turn bananas over and cook, until caramelized, about 3 minutes.

3. Remove pan from heat and add rum. Carefully ignite with long-handled igniter. Allow flames to burn off naturally.

4. Plate each serving with 3 banana sections, a few dribbles of sauce, nutmeg and toasted coconut (if using). Serve immediately.

NUTRIENTS
PER SERVING

Calories	310
Fat	10 g
Carbohydrate	41 g
Fiber	3 g
Protein	1 g
Iron	0.5 mg
Calcium	22 mg

Summer Fruit Compote

With its blend of fresh summer fruits, vanilla and lime juice, this is no ordinary light dessert.

Tips

To get extra duty from vanilla beans, lightly rinse and air-dry them, then add the split pieces to a jar of sugar to make vanilla sugar. The split bean can stay indefinitely in the sugar jar, as you use and replenish your supply.

Add the firmest fruit, such as apples, peaches and pears, to the hot syrup first, then continue in order of the fruit's texture, ending with the most fragile fruits, such as raspberries or pieces of melon. Mix carefully so that the tender fruit doesn't break or bruise.

Variation

Use lemons or oranges instead of limes.

3½ cups	water	875 mL
1 cup	granulated natural cane sugar or other dry sweetener	250 mL
1	vanilla bean, split lengthwise (or 2 tsp/10 mL vanilla extract)	1
4	2- by ½-inch (5 by 1 cm) strips lime zest	4
2 cups	diced peeled pitted peaches, nectarines or apricots	500 mL
1 cup	diced pitted plums (about 2)	250 mL
1 cup	fresh cherries, pitted and halved	250 mL
2 cups	fresh berries (see tip, at left)	500 mL
2 cups	cantaloupe or honeydew melon balls (1-inch/2.5 cm balls)	500 mL
⅓ cup	freshly squeezed lime juice (about 3 limes)	75 mL

1. In a large pot, bring water and sugar to a boil over high heat, stirring until sugar is dissolved. Add vanilla bean and lime zest. Remove from heat, cover and let stand for 6 to 8 minutes or until fragrant.

2. Add peaches, plums, cherries, berries, then melon to syrup and stir to combine. Add lime juice and mix well. Let stand at room temperature for at least 3 hours to develop full flavor. Transfer to an airtight container and refrigerate for up to 3 days. Remove vanilla bean and lime zest before serving.

NUTRIENTS PER SERVING

Calories 110
Fat .0 g
Carbohydrate . . . . .29 g
Fiber . . . . .2 g
Protein . . . . .1 g
Iron . . . . .0.3 mg
Calcium . . . . 11 mg

Balsamic Strawberry Sauce

This well-known Italian sauce is traditionally served with a dash of freshly ground black pepper on top. Serve it warm or cold over your favorite frozen dessert.

Variation

The sauce can also be prepared without cooking. An hour before serving, place sliced berries in a bowl and add sugar. Just before serving, add the balsamic vinegar.

4 cups	sliced hulled strawberries	1 L
3 tbsp	granulated sugar	45 mL
¼ cup	balsamic vinegar	60 mL

1. In a medium saucepan, over medium heat, cook strawberries and sugar for 2 minutes or until sugar melts and starts to form a sauce. Add balsamic vinegar; cook for 2 minutes. Remove from heat.

2. Serve warm, or cover and refrigerate to serve cold.

This recipe courtesy of Eileen Campbell.

NUTRIENTS
PER SERVING

Calories	53
Fat	0 g
Carbohydrate	13 g
Fiber	2 g
Protein	1 g
Iron	0.3 mg
Calcium	13 mg

Chilled Minted Melon Soup

Makes 4 servings

Surprise guests with this ingenious melon dessert on a hot summer day.

Tip

The soup can be prepared through step 2 up to 1 day ahead.

- **Food processor or blender**

1	large honeydew melon, cut into 1-inch (2.5 cm) pieces	1
1/2 cup	loosely packed fresh mint leaves, chopped	125 mL
1/4 cup	granulated sugar	60 mL
3 tbsp	freshly squeezed lime juice	45 mL
Pinch	salt	Pinch
4	fresh mint sprigs (optional)	4

1. In a large bowl, combine melon, chopped mint, sugar, lime juice and salt. Let stand for 15 minutes.

2. In food processor, purée soup until smooth. Transfer to a large bowl, cover and refrigerate until chilled, about 3 hours.

3. Ladle into chilled bowls and garnish with mint sprigs (if using).

NUTRIENTS PER SERVING

Calories 100
Fat .0 g
Carbohydrate . . . . .26 g
Fiber . . . . .2 g
Protein . . . . .1 g
Iron . . . . .0.5 mg
Calcium . . . . 15 mg

Banana Soup with Raspberry and Mint Relish

When you grow tired of banana bread, here's another creative way to use over-ripe bananas. If the ingredients are already chilled, this soup takes very little time to prepare.

Tip

The soup can be prepared up to 2 hours ahead; cover and refrigerate until ready to serve.

Variation

For a smoothie-like rendition of this summer cooler, add 1 cup (250 mL) yogurt or non-dairy yogurt alternative and reduce the apple juice by half.

• **Food processor or blender**

4	chilled very ripe bananas, halved	4
2 cups	chilled unsweetened apple juice	500 mL
1/2 cup	chilled freshly squeezed orange juice	125 mL
2 tbsp	freshly squeezed lemon juice (approx.)	30 mL
Pinch	salt	Pinch
2 tbsp	liquid honey (optional)	30 mL
1	very ripe banana, diced	1
1 cup	raspberries	250 mL
2 tbsp	chopped fresh mint	30 mL

1. In food processor, purée halved bananas and apple juice until smooth. Transfer to a large bowl and stir in orange juice, lemon juice and salt. Taste and add honey or more lemon juice if necessary.

2. In a small bowl, combine diced banana, raspberries and mint.

3. Ladle soup into chilled bowls and top with raspberry and mint relish.

NUTRIENTS
PER SERVING

Calories 170
Fat .1 g
Carbohydrate. . . . . .42 g
Fiber . . . . .4 g
Protein. . . . . .2 g
Iron . . . . .0.6 mg
Calcium . . . . 20 mg

Lemon-Lime Sorbet

Makes 12 servings

This very citrusy sorbet is a great-tasting, low-fat alternative to ice cream.

- **Ice cream maker**

4 cups	lime-flavored club soda, divided	1 L
1 cup	granulated sugar	250 mL
1 cup	key lime preserves (without peel)	250 mL
	Juice of 2 lemons	
	Juice of 2 limes	

1. In a medium saucepan over low heat, stir together 1 cup (250 mL) of the club soda, sugar and preserves until sugar has dissolved and preserves have melted. Stir in lemon juice, lime juice and remaining soda. Pour into an airtight container and seal. Refrigerate for 2 to 3 hours or until thoroughly chilled.

2. Transfer to ice cream maker and process according to the manufacturer's instructions until mixture is the consistency of firm slush. Return to airtight container, seal and freeze for 1 hour or until mixture resembles sorbet.

NUTRIENTS
PER SERVING

Calories	96
Fat	0 g
Carbohydrate	25 g
Fiber	0 g
Protein	0 g
Iron	0 mg
Calcium	9 mg

Pomegranate, Ginger and Clove Granita

Granita makes a great palate cleanser between courses or a refreshing dessert. This one is sweet, tart and spicy all at the same time — a delight!

Tip

If desired, scrape the mixture with a fork every hour for 3 to 5 hours while it's freezing; this will promote the formation of ice crystals.

13- by 9-inch (33 by 23 cm) metal baking pan

½ cup	granulated sugar	125 mL
1 tbsp	grated gingerroot	15 mL
1 tsp	ground cloves	5 mL
4 cups	unsweetened pomegranate juice	1 L
¼ cup	pomegranate seeds	60 mL
8	fresh mint sprigs	8

1. In a large saucepan, combine sugar, ginger, cloves and pomegranate juice. Bring to a boil over high heat, stirring to dissolve sugar. Reduce heat to medium-low and simmer for 5 minutes to allow flavors to infuse juice. Strain, if desired.
2. Pour juice into baking pan. Freeze for at least 6 hours, until solid, or overnight.
3. Scrape the mixture with a fork to create a shaved ice texture. Portion into serving bowls and top with pomegranate seeds and a sprig of mint.

This recipe courtesy of dietitian Mary Sue Waisman.

NUTRIENTS
PER SERVING

Calories 121
Fat .0 g
Carbohydrate. . . . . .30 g
Fiber . . . . .0 g
Protein. . . . . .0 g
Iron . . . . .0.1 mg
Calcium . . . . 16 mg

Tropical Ice in Fruit Cups

Makes 4 servings

So simple, yet so delicious, this icy dessert will cool you down and transport you to the tropics all at once!

Tip

If baby pineapples are not available, substitute 1 large pineapple and serve tropical ice in bowls.

- **Food processor**
- **Shallow pan**

2	baby pineapples (see tip, at left)	2
¼ cup	natural cane sugar	60 mL
½ cup	water	125 mL

1. Slice pineapples in half vertically, scoop out flesh and set aside, taking care to leave pineapple shells intact. Place pineapple shells onto a baking sheet and freeze until firm.

2. In a small saucepan, combine sugar and water and bring just to a boil over medium heat, stirring to dissolve sugar. Set aside and let cool. Cover and refrigerate until chilled, about 4 hours.

3. In food processor, combine reserved pineapple fruit and ¼ cup (60 mL) cooled simple syrup and process to a smooth purée. Taste and add more simple syrup, if necessary. Pour mixture into shallow pan, cover with plastic wrap and place in freezer. Freeze until partially frozen, scraping ice crystals from sides and stirring them into mixture, about 1 hour. Return to freezer until mixture is mostly frozen but not solid, stirring occasionally to break up any large frozen pieces. Before mixture is completely frozen and while it is still granular, scoop into frozen pineapple halves and freeze to desired consistency. Remove from the freezer a few minutes before serving.

NUTRIENTS
PER SERVING

Calories	130
Fat	0 g
Carbohydrate	33 g
Fiber	2 g
Protein	1 g
Iron	1.3 mg
Calcium	25 mg

Banana Chocolate Chip Frozen Pops

Makes 6 ice pops

Here's an easy yet decadent-tasting dessert. Enjoy!

Tips

If you have an allergy to soy, cow's milk protein and/or nuts, there are a number of brands of vegan chocolate chips on the market that are free of these allergens.

The chocolate chips sink to the bottom, which, when unmolded, becomes the top. How clever.

- **Blender**
- **Six ¼-cup (60 mL) frozen pop molds**

2	bananas, cut into large pieces	2
½ cup	enriched coconut milk	125 mL
3 tbsp	agave nectar	45 mL
3 tbsp	vegan mini chocolate chips	45 mL

1. In blender, combine bananas, coconut milk and agave and purée until smooth. Divide among molds. Sprinkle 1½ tsp (7 mL) chocolate chips on top of banana mixture in each mold. Seal molds and freeze until solid, for at least 8 hours or for up to 2 weeks.

2. To serve, run mold under warm water for a few seconds then unmold pops. Serve immediately.

NUTRIENTS
PER ICE POP

Calories 80
Fat . . . . .2 g
Carbohydrate . . . . .18 g
Fiber . . . . .1 g
Protein . . . . .1 g
Iron . . . . .0.5 mg
Calcium . . . . 10 mg

Peaches and Cream Frozen Pops

Makes 6 ice pops

Ice pops are the perfect treat on a hot summer day.

NUTRIENTS
PER ICE POP

Calories	30
Fat	0 g
Carbohydrate	8 g
Fiber	0 g
Protein	0 g
Iron	0.0 mg
Calcium	2 mg

- **Blender**
- **Six ¼-cup (60 mL) frozen pop molds**

1 cup	frozen sliced peaches	250 mL
¾ cup	enriched vanilla-flavored almond milk, rice milk or coconut milk, divided	175 mL
3 tbsp	packed brown sugar	45 mL

1. In blender, combine peaches, ½ cup (125 mL) of the almond milk and brown sugar and purée until smooth. Add the remaining almond milk and process to blend. Divide among molds. Seal molds and freeze until solid, for at least 8 hours or for up to 2 weeks.
2. To serve, run mold under warm water for a few seconds then unmold pops. Serve immediately.

Frozen Tropical Vacation Pops

Makes 12 ice pops

Homemade ice pops are very easy to make.

Tip

There is no need to use a blender; in fact, it's better to make this by hand, as chunks of banana add to the texture.

NUTRIENTS
PER ICE POP

Calories	49
Fat	1 g
Carbohydrate	10 g
Fiber	0 g
Protein	1 g
Iron	0.1 mg
Calcium	32 mg

- **12 frozen pop molds or paper cups with sticks**

2	ripe bananas, mashed	2
1 cup	low-fat coconut-flavored yogurt	250 mL
1 cup	unsweetened orange juice	250 mL

1. In a bowl, combine bananas, yogurt and juice until well blended.
2. Pour banana mixture into molds and insert sticks. Freeze for at least 4 hours, until solid, or for up to 5 days.

Variation

Vary the juice and yogurt to your liking, but always use the banana for the best texture.

This recipe courtesy of Kelly Hajnik.

Beverages

Banana Blueberry Smoothie

Makes 2 servings

Bananas and blueberries are a classic combination for a satisfying smoothie, perfect as a snack or a morning pick-me-up.

NUTRIENTS
PER SERVING

Calories	230
Fat	1 g
Carbohydrate	59 g
Fiber	5 g
Protein	3 g
Iron	0.8 mg
Calcium	29 mg

- **Blender or food processor**

1½ cups	freshly squeezed orange juice	375 mL
2	bananas, cut into 1-inch (2.5 cm) pieces and frozen	2
1 cup	fresh blueberries, frozen	250 mL

1. In blender, purée orange juice, bananas and blueberries until smooth. Serve immediately.

Variation

Substitute 1 cup (250 mL) chopped fresh mango, frozen, for the blueberries.

Blue Sunset Smoothie

Makes about 1½ cups (375 mL)

Kombucha is an excellent way to consume a healthy type of active bacterial cultures.

NUTRIENTS
PER ½ CUP (125 ML)

Calories	80
Fat	3 g
Carbohydrate	11 g
Fiber	1 g
Protein	3 g
Iron	0.9 mg
Calcium	7 mg

- **Blender**

1 cup	kombucha (see tip, below)	250 mL
1	small banana	1
¼ cup	blueberries	60 mL
2 tbsp	raw shelled hemp seeds	30 mL

1. In blender, combine kombucha, banana, blueberries and hemp seeds. Blend on high speed until smooth. Serve immediately.

Tip

Kombucha is a fermented tea that aids in digestion and provides your gut with beneficial bacteria. It is available in the refrigerated section of natural foods stores and well-stocked supermarkets. If you don't have kombucha, substitute 1 cup (250 mL) filtered water and 1 tsp (5 mL) white vinegar.

Strawberry Kiwi Smoothie

Makes about 2 cups (500 mL)

Here's a delicious treat with a vitamin C punch!

NUTRIENTS
PER ½ CUP (125 ML)

Calories 90
Fat .1 g
Carbohydrate. . . . . .22 g
Fiber . . . . .3 g
Protein. . . . . .1 g
Iron . . . . .0.4 mg
Calcium. . . . . 25 mg

- **Blender**

1 cup	freshly squeezed orange juice	250 mL
2	kiwifruit, peel removed	2
1	banana	1
8 to 10	strawberries	8 to 10
1 tsp	agave nectar	5 mL
1 tsp	vanilla extract (or ¼ tsp/1 mL vanilla seeds)	5 mL

1. In blender, combine orange juice, kiwis, banana, strawberries, agave nectar and vanilla. Blend on high speed until smooth. Serve immediately.

Variation

Substitute 2 tbsp (30 mL) Date Paste (page 327) for the agave nectar.

Thank You Berry Much Smoothie

Makes about 2 cups (500 mL)

Loaded with antioxidants, this berry smoothie makes the perfect breakfast accompaniment.

NUTRIENTS
PER ½ CUP (125 ML)

Calories 70
Fat .0 g
Carbohydrate. . . . . .16 g
Fiber . . . . .2 g
Protein. . . . . .1 g
Iron . . . . .0.4 mg
Calcium. . . . . 15 mg

- **Blender**

1 cup	freshly squeezed orange juice	250 mL
6	strawberries	6
10	blueberries	10
4	blackberries	4
4	raspberries	4
1	banana	1
1	chopped pitted date	1

1. In blender, combine orange juice, strawberries, blueberries, blackberries, raspberries, banana and date. Blend on high speed until smooth. Serve immediately.

Variation

Try using gooseberries or brambleberries or even cranberries as a substitute for one of the berries. If using a less sweet fruit, add 1 to 2 tbsp (15 to 30 mL) agave nectar or ¼ cup (60 mL) Date Paste (page 327).

Lemon Meringue Smoothie

Makes about 1½ cups (375 mL)

The sweet dates and agave nectar complement the tartness of the lemon juice in this smoothie, an excellent source of low-glycemic sugars and vitamin C.

Variation

Substitute the juice of Meyer lemons for regular lemons — they are slightly sweeter.

• **Blender**

1 cup	enriched hemp milk	250 mL
¼ cup	freshly squeezed lemon juice	60 mL
1	banana	1
2 tbsp	Date Paste (see recipe, opposite)	30 mL
2 tsp	vanilla extract (or ½ tsp/2 mL vanilla seeds)	10 mL
1 tsp	agave nectar	5 mL

1. In blender, combine hemp milk, lemon juice, banana, date paste, vanilla and agave nectar. Blend on high speed until smooth.

NUTRIENTS
PER ½ CUP (125 ML)

Calories	100
Fat	1 g
Carbohydrate	20 g
Fiber	1 g
Protein	2 g
Iron	1.0 mg
Calcium	157 mg

Date Paste

This versatile recipe is a rich whole-food sweetener that makes a perfect alternative to refined sugar. It can be used as a replacement for agave nectar in many recipes and is a great finish for many desserts.

Tip

If you are sensitive to sulfites, make sure the dates are free of added sulfites.

Variation

For a sweeter paste, substitute the water with freshly squeezed orange juice, or use half of each.

- **Food processor**

10	chopped pitted dates	10
2 cups	water	500 mL
1 cup	filtered water	250 mL

1. Place dates in a bowl and add 2 cups (500 mL) water. Cover and set aside for 20 minutes. Drain, discarding soaking water.
2. In food processor, process soaked dates and filtered water until smooth. Use immediately or transfer to an airtight container and refrigerate for up to 1 week.

**NUTRIENTS
PER 2 TBSP (30 ML)**

Calories	25
Fat	0 g
Carbohydrate	7 g
Fiber	1 g
Protein	0 g
Iron	0.0 mg
Calcium	4 mg

Coconut Cardamom Smoothie

Makes about 1½ cups (375 mL)

Serve this smoothie at the end of an Indian-inspired meal, for a nutritionally dense treat.

Tip

Coconut butter is a blend of coconut oil and coconut meat that is high in healthy fats and adds creaminess to smoothies and sauces. It is available in the nut butter section of natural foods stores or well-stocked supermarkets. Don't confuse it with coconut oil.

To grind cardamom seeds: Split open the pod, extract the seeds and use a spice grinder or mortar and pestle to grind them into a fine powder. You can also use the back of a small sauté pan, applying pressure on a surface such as a cutting board.

If you are sensitive to sulfites, make sure the date is free of added sulfites.

NUTRIENTS
PER ½ CUP (125 ML)

Calories	120
Fat	5 g
Carbohydrate	20 g
Fiber	2 g
Protein	1 g
Iron	0.7 mg
Calcium	40 mg

- **Blender**

1 cup	enriched coconut milk	250 mL
1	banana	1
1	chopped pitted date	1
2 tbsp	coconut butter (see tip, at left)	30 mL
1 tbsp	agave nectar	15 mL
1 tsp	ground cardamom (see tip, at left)	5 mL
Pinch	fine sea salt	Pinch

1. In blender, combine coconut milk, banana, date, coconut butter, agave nectar, cardamom and salt. Blend on high speed until smooth. Serve immediately.

Avocado Vanilla Smoothie

Makes 1½ cups (375 mL)

Enjoy this smoothie as a filling mid-afternoon snack, and it will surely tide you over until dinner!

Tips

To remove the pit from an avocado: Use a paring knife to remove the nib at the top. Insert the blade of the knife where the nib was and turn the avocado from top to bottom to cut it in half lengthwise. Twist the two halves apart. Stick the knife into the pit and with one motion turn it 90 degrees. As you twist the knife, pull out the pit.

If you are sensitive to sulfites, make sure the date is free of added sulfites.

- **Blender**

1 cup	enriched hemp milk	250 mL
½	small avocado, pitted and peeled	½
2	chopped pitted dates	2
2 tsp	agave nectar	10 mL
2 tsp	vanilla extract (or ½ tsp/2 mL vanilla seeds)	10 mL

1. In blender, combine hemp milk, avocado, dates, agave nectar and vanilla. Blend on high speed until smooth. Serve immediately.

NUTRIENTS
PER ½ CUP (125 ML)

Calories 130
Fat .6 g
Carbohydrate. . . . . .17 g
Fiber . . . . .3 g
Protein. . . . . .2 g
Iron . . . . .1.1 mg
Calcium . . . . 160 mg

Eat Your Greens Smoothie

*This smoothie is an excellent
source of bone-building
nutrients.*

NUTRIENTS
PER ½ CUP (125 ML)

Calories. 110
Fat . . . . .2 g
Carbohydrate. . . . . .23 g
Fiber . . . . .2 g
Protein. . . . . .3 g
Iron . . . . .1.6 mg
Calcium. . . . . 183 mg

• **Blender**

1 cup	enriched hemp milk	250 mL
½ cup	chopped peeled mango	125 mL
½ cup	chopped trimmed kale	125 mL
¼ cup	chopped romaine lettuce	60 mL
¼ cup	chopped fresh parsley or cilantro	60 mL
1	banana	1
1	chopped pitted date	1

1. In blender, combine hemp milk, mango, kale, lettuce, parsley, banana and date. Blend on high speed until smooth.

Variations

Substitute chopped papaya or pear for the mango.

Replace the lettuce with arugula, spinach or mustard greens.

Bodybuilder Smoothie

Tip

If you are sensitive to sulfites, make sure the coconut water is free of added sulfites.

NUTRIENTS
PER ½ CUP (125 ML)

Calories. 110
Fat . . . . .5 g
Carbohydrate. . . . . .15 g
Fiber . . . . .2 g
Protein. . . . . .4 g
Iron . . . . .1.5 mg
Calcium. . . . . 26 mg

• **Blender**

1 cup	coconut water	250 mL
¼ cup	freshly squeezed orange juice	60 mL
¼ cup	blueberries	60 mL
¼ cup	chopped pineapple	60 mL
¼ cup	raw shelled hemp seeds	60 mL
1	banana	1

1. In blender, combine coconut water, orange juice, blueberries, pineapple, hemp seeds and banana. Blend on high speed until smooth. Serve immediately.

The Kitchen Sink

Tip

If you are sensitive to sulfites, make sure the coconut water is free of added sulfites.

NUTRIENTS PER ½ CUP (125 ML)	
Calories	35
Fat	1 g
Carbohydrate	6 g
Fiber	1 g
Protein	1 g
Iron	0.5 mg
Calcium	21 mg

- **Blender**

1 cup	coconut water	250 mL
½ cup	packed baby spinach	125 mL
¼ cup	chopped baby bok choy	60 mL
¼ cup	chopped pineapple	60 mL
¼ cup	chopped orange segments	60 mL
3	strawberries	3
5	blueberries	5
1 tbsp	raw shelled hemp seeds	15 mL

1. In blender, combine coconut water, spinach, bok choy, pineapple, orange, strawberries, blueberries and hemp seeds. Blend on high speed until smooth. Serve immediately.

Variations

Substitute an equal quantity of kale for the bok choy and/or arugula for the spinach.

In season, add half a peach, chopped, to this smoothie.

The Antioxidizer

**Makes 1½ cups
(375 mL)**

The antioxidant ingredients in this smoothie will help strengthen your immune system.

NUTRIENTS PER ½ CUP (125 ML)	
Calories	130
Fat	3 g
Carbohydrate	23 g
Fiber	3 g
Protein	4 g
Iron	1.4 mg
Calcium	166 mg

- **Blender**

1 cup	enriched hemp milk	250 mL
¼ cup	chopped trimmed kale	60 mL
8	blueberries	8
1	banana	1
2	chopped pitted dates	2
1 tbsp	raw cacao powder (see tip, page 335)	15 mL
2 tsp	raw shelled hemp seeds	10 mL

1. In blender, combine hemp milk, kale, blueberries, banana, dates, cacao powder and hemp seeds. Blend on high speed until smooth. Serve immediately.

Variation

Substitute chopped arugula, spinach or chard for the kale.

Juice in a Blender

*This refreshing drink is
perfect for those hot summer
days, when you need to stay
hydrated.*

NUTRIENTS PER ½ CUP (125 ML)	
Calories	40
Fat	0 g
Carbohydrate	10 g
Fiber	1 g
Protein	0 g
Iron	0.2 mg
Calcium	8 mg

- **Blender**

½ cup	freshly squeezed orange juice	125 mL
2	ice cubes	2
½ cup	chopped apple	125 mL
½ cup	seedless grapes (yellow, green or red)	125 mL
¼ cup	chopped pineapple	60 mL

1. In blender, combine orange juice and ice. Blend on medium speed until ice is chopped. Add apple, grapes and pineapple. Blend on high speed until smooth. Serve immediately.

Variations

Substitute other freshly squeezed juices, such as mango, pomegranate or blueberry, for the orange.

Substitute cantaloupe, honeydew or another soft melon for the pineapple.

Iron-Builder Juice

NUTRIENTS PER ½ CUP (125 ML)	
Calories	50
Fat	0 g
Carbohydrate	11 g
Fiber	0 g
Protein	1 g
Iron	0.4 mg
Calcium	13 mg

- **Juicer**

3	large red beets, sliced, divided	3
4	carrots, sliced, divided	4
½	bunch Swiss chard or beet greens, divided	½
1	small apple, sliced, divided	1

1. In juicer, process one-quarter of the beets, 1 carrot, one-quarter of the chard and one-quarter of the apple. Repeat until all the vegetables have been juiced. Whisk well and serve immediately.

Variation

Substitute 1 head of romaine lettuce or 1 bunch spinach or arugula for the chard.

Spicy Cinnamon Lemonade

Makes 4 cups (1 L)

Not your usual recipe, this lemonade will throw your palate into overdrive as it delights in the sweetness, tartness and spiciness.

NUTRIENTS
PER ½ CUP (125 ML)

Calories 110
Fat .0 g
Carbohydrate . . . . .29 g
Fiber . . . . .1 g
Protein . . . . .0 g
Iron . . . . .0.1 mg
Calcium . . . . 11 mg

- **Blender**

2 cups	freshly squeezed lemon juice (about 8 lemons)	500 mL
1 cup	filtered water	250 mL
¾ cup	agave nectar	175 mL
3	large ice cubes	3
1 tbsp	ground cinnamon	15 mL
½ tsp	cayenne pepper	2 mL

1. In blender, combine lemon juice, water, agave nectar, ice cubes, cinnamon and cayenne pepper. Blend on high speed until ice is chopped. Serve immediately.

Blueberry Lemon Elixir

Makes 1 cup (250 mL)

This juice is sweet and slightly spicy — a perfect thirst-quencher!

NUTRIENTS
PER ½ CUP (125 ML)

Calories 120
Fat .0 g
Carbohydrate . . . . .32 g
Fiber . . . . .0 g
Protein . . . . .0 g
Iron . . . . .0.1 mg
Calcium . . . . 4 mg

- **Blender**

½ cup	filtered water	125 mL
½ cup	blueberries	125 mL
¼ cup	freshly squeezed lemon juice	60 mL
3 tbsp	agave nectar	45 mL
2 tsp	chopped gingerroot	10 mL

1. In blender, combine water, blueberries, lemon juice, agave nectar and ginger. Blend on high speed until smooth.

Just Peachy Blueberry Picnic

Makes 2 cups (500 mL)

Enjoy this revitalizing smoothie in early summer, when peaches are in season.

NUTRIENTS
PER ½ CUP (125 ML)

Calories 45
Fat . . . . 1 g
Carbohydrate . . . . 9 g
Fiber . . . . 1 g
Protein . . . . 1 g
Iron . . . . 0.5 mg
Calcium . . . . 61 mg

- **Blender**

½ cup	enriched hemp milk	125 mL
1	large peach, peeled	1
½ cup	blueberries	125 mL
1 tbsp	chopped gingerroot	15 mL
1 tsp	freshly squeezed lemon juice	5 mL

1. In blender, combine hemp milk, peach, blueberries, ginger and lemon juice. Blend on high speed until smooth. Serve immediately.

Variations

Substitute an equal quantity of blackberries or brambleberries for the blueberries.

Substitute a nectarine for the peach.

Choco-Hemp-aholic

Makes 2 cups (500 mL)

This chocolatey smoothie is the perfect solution when that midday craving for something sweet hits.

NUTRIENTS
PER ½ CUP (125 ML)

Calories 110
Fat . . . . 5 g
Carbohydrate . . . . 14 g
Fiber . . . . 3 g
Protein . . . . 5 g
Iron . . . . 1.0 mg
Calcium . . . . 8 mg

- **Blender**

1 cup	filtered water	250 mL
1	banana	1
2	pitted dates	2
3 tbsp	raw shelled hemp seeds	45 mL
2 tbsp	raw cacao powder (see tip, page 335)	30 mL

1. In blender, combine water, banana, dates, hemp seeds and cacao powder. Blend on high speed until smooth.

Chocolate Cherry Delight

Makes
2 cups (500 mL)

Cacao and cherries blend nicely to make a satisfying smoothie. Enjoy it when cherries are in season.

NUTRIENTS
PER ½ CUP (125 ML)

Calories 160
Fat .5 g
Carbohydrate . . . . .24 g
Fiber . . . . .4 g
Protein . . . . .6 g
Iron . . . . .1.4 mg
Calcium . . . . 122 mg

• **Blender**

1 cup	enriched help milk	250 mL
½ cup	pitted cherries	125 mL
1	banana	1
3 tbsp	raw cacao powder (see tip, below)	45 mL
2 tbsp	raw shelled hemp seeds	30 mL
1 tbsp	agave nectar	15 mL

1. In blender, combine hemp milk, cherries, banana, cacao powder, hemp seeds and agave nectar. Blend on high speed until smooth.

Tip

Cacao powder is lactose- and dairy-free. Make sure to purchase a brand that is free of peanuts and tree nuts.

Pineapple Piña Colada

Makes 1½ cups
(375 mL)

Enjoy this rich, creamy drink as a mocktail al fresco!

NUTRIENTS
PER ½ CUP (125 ML)

Calories 130
Fat .7 g
Carbohydrate . . . . .18 g
Fiber . . . . .2 g
Protein . . . . .2 g
Iron . . . . .0.8 mg
Calcium . . . . 42 mg

• **Blender**

1 cup	enriched coconut milk	250 mL
½ cup	chopped pineapple	125 mL
3 tbsp	coconut butter (see tip, page 328)	45 mL
1	banana	1
1	chopped pitted Medjool date	1

1. In blender, combine coconut milk, pineapple, coconut butter, banana and date. Blend on high speed until smooth.

Variation

For added protein, add 2 tbsp (30 mL) raw shelled hemp seeds.

Grapefruit, Spirulina and Blackberry Frozen Martini

Makes 1½ cups (375 mL)

This versatile drink may be enjoyed for breakfast, as a snack or as a mocktail at a dinner party.

Tips

If your blender won't chop ice, put the ice cubes in a plastic bag, place on a cutting board and smash with a rolling pin until crushed. Add along with the other ingredients.

Spirulina is a blue-green alga that has many healthful properties. It has trace amounts of vitamins and minerals and is a source of phytonutrients with antioxidant properties. Spirulina can be found in the natural foods section of well-stocked grocery stores.

• Blender

½ cup	freshly squeezed grapefruit juice	125 mL
3	large ice cubes, divided (see tip, at left)	3
½ cup	frozen blackberries	125 mL
1 tsp	raw shelled hemp seeds	5 mL
1 tsp	spirulina powder (see tip, at left)	5 mL

1. In blender, combine grapefruit juice and 2 of the ice cubes. Blend on medium speed for 10 seconds. Add the remaining ice and blend on medium speed for 10 seconds. Add the frozen blackberries, hemp seeds and spirulina powder and blend on medium speed until the ice and berries are still chunky and the texture is slushy. Serve immediately.

NUTRIENTS
PER ½ CUP (125 ML)

Calories	35
Fat	1 g
Carbohydrate	7 g
Fiber	1 g
Protein	2 g
Iron	0.9 mg
Calcium	13 mg

Contributing Authors

Alexandra Anca with
Theresa Santandrea-Cull
*Complete Gluten-Free Diet &
Nutrition Guide*
Recipes from this book are found on
pages 183–185, 223, 225, 238, 258,
261, 263–64, 275, 280, 284, 286, 304
and 306.

Johanna Burkhard
500 Best Comfort Food Recipes
Recipes from this book are found on
pages 208, 212–13, 218, 226, 259,
277–78, 282 and 287.

Dietitians of Canada
Simply Great Food
Recipes from this book are found on
pages 182, 210, 214, 234, 276, 283,
291–92, 296 and 315.

Maxine Effenson Chuck & Beth Gurney
125 Best Vegan Recipes
Recipes from this book are found on
pages 217, 233, 236–37, 242, 244, 246,
285, 288, 309 and 314.

Judith Finlayson
The Complete Whole Grains Cookbook
Recipes from this book are found on
pages 179–81, 235, 239, 252–53, 255–57,
260, 265–66, 268–69 and 310.

Judith Finlayson
The Vegetarian Slow Cooker
Recipes from this book are found on
pages 207, 209, 211, 216, 219, 224,
227–28, 232, 245, 247, 281 and 308.

Douglas McNish
Eat Raw, Eat Well
Recipes from this book are found on
pages 324 (top) and 325–36.

Dr. Maitreyi Raman, Angela Sirounis
& Jennifer Shrubsole
The Complete IBS Health & Diet Guide
Recipes from this book are found on
pages 178, 250, 270, 272, 273, 289 and 318.

Deb Roussou
350 Best Vegan Recipes
Recipes from this book are found on
pages 311, 313, 320–321 and 322 (top).

Camilla Saulsbury
Recipes by this author, developed for this
book, are found on pages 186–94.

Kathleen Sloan-McIntosh
300 Best Potato Recipes
Recipes from this book are found on
pages 290, 293–95 and 297–300.

Carla Snyder & Meredith Deeds
300 Sensational Soups
Recipes from this book are found on
pages 220–22, 229, 231 and 316–17.

Mary Sue Waisman
Dietitians of Canada Cook!
Recipes from this book are found on pages
254, 262, 271, 274, 319 and 322 (bottom).

Donna Washburn & Heather Butt
250 Gluten-Free Favorites
Recipes from this book are found on
pages 176, 202–3, 206, 230, 240–41,
301, 303, 307, 312 and 324 (top).

Donna Washburn & Heather Butt
The Best Gluten-Free Family Cookbook
Recipes from this book are found on
pages 197, 204–5, 248–49, 251 and 302.

Donna Washburn & Heather Butt
The Gluten-Free Baking Book
Recipes from this book are found on
pages 196, 198–201 and 267.

Resources

Allergy Associations

American Latex Allergy Association (ALAA): www.latexallergyresources.org

Allergy/Asthma Information Association: www.aaia.ca

Anaphylaxis Canada: www.anaphylaxis.ca; www.safe4kids.ca; www.whyriskit.ca

Association Québécoise des allergies alimentaires: www.aqaa.qc.ca

Asthma and Allergy Foundation of America: www.aafa.org

Asthma Society of Canada: www.asthma.ca

Calgary Allergy Network : www.calgaryallergy.ca

The Food Allergy and Anaphylaxis Network: www.foodallergy.org

Food Allergy and Anaphylaxis Alliance: www.foodallergyalliance.org

Global Initiative for Asthma (GINA): www.ginaasthma.org

Kids with Food Allergies Foundation (online support group):
    www.community.kidswithfoodallergies.org

Managing Anaphylaxis

Canadian MedicAlert Foundation: www.medicalert.ca

EpiPen: www.epipen.com or www.epipen.ca

Twinject: www.twinject.ca

Professional Associations

American Academy of Asthma, Allergy and Clinical Immunology: www.aaaai.org

American College of Allergy, Asthma and Immunology: www.acaai.org

Allergy, Asthma and Immunology Society of Ontario: www.allergyasthma.on.ca

Canadian Society for Allergy and Clinical Immunology: www.csaci.ca

European Academy of Allergy and Clinical Immunology: www.eaaci.net

World Allergy Organization: www.worldallergy.org

Nutrition and Health Information

Canadian Food Inspection Agency: www.inspection.gc.ca

The Children's Asthma Education Centre: www.asthma-education.com

Eat Right Ontario: www.eatrightontario.ca

Health Canada: www.hc-sc.gc.ca/fn-an/securit/allerg/index-eng.php

Healthlink BC: www.healthlinkbc.ca

Sick Kids Hospital: www.aboutkidshealth.ca/En/HealthAZ/ConditionsandDiseases/
    AllergyandImmuneSystemDisorders/Pages/Food-Allergies-Home.aspx

Specialty Food Shop: www.SpecialtyFoodShop.com

Print Publications

Allergic Living Magazine: http://allergicliving.com

Living Without Magazine: www.livingwithout.com

Dietetic Associations

American Dietetic Association: www.eatright.org

British Dietetic Association: www.bda.uk.com

Dietitians of Canada: www.dietitians.ca

Celiac Disease

American Celiac Disease Alliance: www.americanceliac.org

Canadian Celiac Association: www.celiac.ca

Celiac Disease Foundation: www.celiac.org

Fondation québécoise de la maladie coeliaque: www.fqmc.org

Gluten Intolerance Group: www.gluten.net

Other Resources

Allergy Safe Communities (English and French versions):
    www.allergysafecommunities.ca; www.securite-allergie.ca

Canadian School Boards Association: http://cdnsba.org

Selected References

Chapters 1–4

Anaphylaxis Canada. *Anaphylaxis 101: The Basics*. Available at: www.anaphylaxis.ca/en/anaphylaxis101/the_basics.html. Accessed March 2012.

Bernstein IL, Li JT, Bernstein DI, et al. Allergy diagnostic testing: An updated practice parameter, Part 1. *Ann Allergy Asthma Immunol*, 2008 Mar;100(3 Suppl 3): S15–66.

Boyce JA, Assa'ad A, Burks AW, et al. Guidelines for the diagnosis and management of food allergy in the United States: Summary of the NIAID-sponsored expert panel report. *J Allergy Clin Immunol*, 2010 Dec;126(6):1105–18.

Brown SJ, Asai Y, Cordell HJ, et al. Loss-of-function variants in the filaggrin gene are a significant factor for peanut allergy. *J Allergy Clin Immunol*, 2011 Mar;127(3):661–67.

Carr S, Watson W. Eosinophilic esophagitis. *Allergy Asthma Clin Immunol*, 2011 Nov 10;7 Suppl 1:S8.

Chandra RK. Food hypersensitivity and allergic diseases. *Eur J Clin Nutr*, 2002 Aug;56 Suppl 3:S54–56.

Compalati E, Penagos M, Henley K, Canonica GW. Allergy prevalence survey by the World Allergy Organization. *Allergy Clin Immunol Int: J World Allergy Org*, 2007 May;19(3):82–90

Health Canada. Food Allergies and Intolerances. Available at: www.healthycanadians.gc.ca/init/kids-enfants/food-aliment/safety-salubrite/allergies-intolerances/index-eng.php. Accessed December 10, 2011.

Johansson SG, Bieber T, Dahl R, et al. Revised nomenclature for allergy for global use: Report of the Nomenclature Review Committee of the World Allergy Organization, October 2003. *J Allergy Clin Immunol*, 2004 May:113(5): 832–36.

Joneja JV, Bielory L. *Understanding Allergy, Sensitivity and Immunity: A Comprehensive Guide*. New Brunswick, NJ: Rutgers University Press, 1990.

Kelly CP, Schneider, LC. *Food Allergy, Intolerance, and Sensitivities*. Cambridge, MA: Harvard Health Publications, 2011.

Kim H, Fischer D. Anaphylaxis. *Allergy Asthma Clin Immunol*, 2011 Nov 10, 7 Suppl 1:S6.

Kim H, Mazza J. Asthma. *Allergy Asthma Clin Immunol*, 2011 Nov 10;7 Suppl 1:S2.

Lock RJ, Unsworth DJ. Food allergy: which tests are worth doing and which are not? *Ann Clin Biochem*, 2011 July;48(Pt 4):300–309.

McCann D, Barrett A, Cooper A, et al. Food additives and hyperactive behaviour in 3-year-old and 8/9-year-old children in the community: A randomised, double-blinded, placebo-controlled trial. *Lancet*, 2007 Nov 3; 370(9598):1560–67.

Metcalfe DD, Sampson HA, Simon RA. *Food Allergy: Adverse Reaction to Foods and Food Additives*, 4th ed. Malden, MA.: Blackwell Publishing, 2008.

Mofidi S, Bock SA. *A Health Professional's Guide to Food Challenges*. Fairfax, VA: Food Allergy and Anaphylaxis Network, 2004.

Moneret-Vautrin DA, Morisset M. Adult food allergy. *Curr Allergy Asthma Rep*, 2005 Jan;5(1):80–85.

National Institutes of Health. Defined diets and childhood hyperactivity. *Natl Inst Health Consens Dev Conf Summ*, 1982;4(3):6.

Nowak-Wegrzyn A, Assa'ad AH, Bahna SL, et al. Work Group report: Oral food challenge testing. *J Allergy Clin Immunol*, 2009 Jun; 123(6 Suppl): S365–83.

Ohman L, Simrén M. Pathogenesis of IBS: role of inflammation, immunity and neuroimmune interactions. *Nat Rev Gastroenterol Hepatol*, 2010 Mar;7(3):163–73.

Pawankar R, Canonica GW, Holgate ST, Lockey RF, eds. *WAO White Book on Allergy 2011–2012: Executive Summary*. Available at: www.worldallergy.org/publications/wao_white_book.pdf. Accessed January 8, 2012.

Philpott H, Gibson P, Thien F. Irritable bowel syndrome: An inflammatory disease involving mast cells. *Asia Pac Allergy*, 2011 Apr;1(1):36–42.

Rona RJ, Keil T, Summers C, et al. The prevalence of food allergy: a meta-analysis. *J Allergy Clin Immunol*, 2007 Sep;120(3):638–46.

Sampson HA. Update on food allergy, *J Allergy Clin Immunol*, 2004 May;113(5):805–19.

Sharief S, Jariwala S, Kumar J, et al. Vitamin D levels and food and environmental allergies in the United States: Results from the National Health and Nutrition Examination Survey 2005–2006. *J Allergy Clin Immunol*, 2011 May;127(5):1195–1202.

Sicherer SH. Food allergy: When and how to perform oral food challenges. *Pediatr Allergy Immunol*, 1999 Nov;10(4):226–34.

Sicherer S. Manifestations of food allergy: Evaluation and management. *Am Fam Physician*, 1999 Jan 15;59(2):415–24.

Simons FE, Ardusso LR, Bilò MB, et al. 2012 Update: World Allergy Organization Guidelines for the assessment and management of anaphylaxis. *Curr Opin Allergy Clin Immunol*, 2012 Aug;12(4):389–99.

Skypala I, Venter C, eds. *Food Hypersensitivity: Diagnosing and Managing Food Allergies and Intolerance*. Ames, IA: Wiley-Blackwell Publishing, 2009.

UCLA Food and Drug Allergy Care Centre. *About Allergies: Why Are Allergies Increasing?* Available at: http://fooddrugallergy.ucla.edu. Accessed January 12, 2012.

Vandenplas Y, Koletzko S, Isolauri E, et al. Guidelines for the diagnosis and management of cow's milk protein allergy in infants. *Arch Dis Child*, 2007 Oct;92(10):902–8.

von Mutius E. 99th Dahlem conference on infection, inflammation and chronic inflammatory disorders: Farm lifestyles and the hygiene hypothesis. *Clin Exp Immunol*, 2010 Apr;160(1):130–35.

Wang J, Sampson HA. Food allergy: Opportunities and challenges in the clinical practice of allergy and immunology. *Allergy Frontiers: Therapy and Prevention*, Vol. 5. Pawanker R, Holgate ST, Rosenwasser LJ, eds. Springer, 2010: 335–46.

Warrington R, Watson W, Kim HL, Antonetti FR. An introduction to immunology and immunopathology. *Allergy Asthma Clin Immunol*, 2011 Nov 10;7 Suppl 1:S1.

Waserman S, Watson W. Food allergy. *Allergy Asthma Clin Immunol*, 2011 Nov 10;7 Suppl 1:S7.

Chapters 5–7

Allergy/Asthma Information Association. Brochures: *Peanut and Nut Allergies: The Facts* (revised 2007); *Egg Allergy: The Facts* (revised 2008); *Milk Allergy: The Facts*.

Bollinger ME, Dahlquist LM, Mudd K, et al. The impact of food allergy on the daily activities of children and their families. *Ann Allergy Asthma Immunol*, 2006 Mar;96(3):415–21.

Calgary Allergy Network. Articles: *Facts on Food Hypersensitivity to Egg*; *Facts on Food Hypersensitivity to Corn*. Available at: www.calgaryallergy.ca. Accessed March–April 2012.

Canadian Food Inspection Agency. Food Allergies Fact Sheets: Egg Allergy; Milk Allergy; Peanut Allergy; Seafood Allergy; Sesame Allergy; Soy Allergy; Sulphite Sensitivity; Tree Nuts Allergy; Wheat Allergy. Available at: www.inspection.gc.ca. Accessed February–March 2012.

The Food Allergy & Anaphylaxis Network. Food Allergens: Milk; Egg; Peanuts; Tree Nuts; Wheat; Soy; Fish; Shellfish; Other. Available at www.foodallergy.org/section/common-food-allergens1. Accessed February–March 2012.

Hamilton Health Sciences, McMaster Children's Hospital. Brochures: *Egg-Free Diet*; *Milk and Dairy Free Diet*; *Soy-Free Diet*. Available at: www.hamiltonhealthsciences.ca. Accessed March 12, 2012.

Health Canada. Food Allergen Labelling. Available at: www.hc-sc.gc.ca/fn-an/label-etiquet/allergen/index-eng.php. Accessed February–March 2012.

Health Canada. Food Allergies. Information for Consumers: Peanuts; Eggs; Milk; Tree Nuts; Wheat; Soy; Sesame Seeds; Seafood (Fish, Crustaceans and Shellfish); Sulphites; Mustard: A Priority Food Allergen in Canada — A Systematic Review. Available at www.hc-sc.gc.ca/fn-an/securit/allerg/fa-aa/index-eng.php. Accessed February–March 2012.

Kim, JS, Sicherer, SH. Living with food allergy: Allergen avoidance. *Pediatr Clin N Am*, 2011 Apr;58(2):459–70.

Knibb RC, Armstrong A, Booth DA, et al. Psychological characteristics of people with perceived food intolerance in a community sample. *J Psychosom Res*, 1999 Dec;47(6):545–54.

Lopata AL, Lehrer SB. New insights into seafood allergy. *Curr Opin Allergy Clin Immunol*, 2009 June;9(3):270–77.

National Food Institute, Technical University of Denmark. Food Allergy Information. The EU Labelling Directive. Available at: www.foodallergens.info/Legal/Labelling/Labelling.html. Accessed February–March 2012.

Perry TT, Conover-Walker MK, Pomés A, et al. Distribution of peanut allergen in the environment. *J Allergy Clin Immunol*, 2004 May;113(5):973–76.

Sicherer SH, Noone SA, Muñoz-Furlong A. The impact of childhood food allergy on quality of life. *Ann Allergy Asthma Immunol*, 2001 Dec;87(6):461–64.

Sick Kids Hospital. Articles: *Egg Allergies and Nutrition*; *Soy Allergy*; *Sulphite Sensitivity*. Available at www.aboutkidshealth.ca. Accessed March–April 2012.

Skypala I, Venter C, eds. *Food Hypersensitivity: Diagnosing and Managing Food Allergies and Intolerance*. Ames, IA: Wiley-Blackwell Publishing, 2009.

United States Department of Agriculture National Agricultural Library. Allergies and Food Sensitivities. Available at: fnic.nal.usda.gov/diet-and-disease/allergies-and-food-sensitivities. Accessed February–March 2012.

U.S. Food and Drug Administration Food Safety. Food Allergens. Available at: www.fda.gov/Food/FoodSafety/FoodAllergens/default.htm. Accessed February–March 2012.

Venter C, Skypala I, Dean T. Maize allergy: What we have learned so far. *Clin Exp Allergy*, 2008 Dec;38(12):1844–46.

Vereda A, Sirvent S, Villalba M, et al. Improvement of mustard (*Sinapis alba*) allergy diagnosis and management by linking clinical features and component-resolved approaches. *J Allergy Clin Immunol*, 2011 May;127(5):1304–7.

Williams AN, Woessner KM. Monosodium glutamate "allergy": Menace or myth? *Clin Exp Allergy*, 2009 May;39(5):640–46.

Library and Archives Canada Cataloguing in Publication

Anca, Alexandra
     The total food allergy health and diet guide : includes 150 recipes for managing food allergies and intolerances by eliminating common allergens and gluten / Alexandra Anca with Gordon L. Sussman.

Includes index.
ISBN 978-0-7788-0420-8

1. Food allergy—Popular works. 2. Food allergy—Diet therapy. 3. Food allergy—Diet therapy—Recipes. 4. Cookbooks. I. Sussman, Gordon II. Title.

RC596.A53 2012   616.97'5   C2012-902824-X

Index